The Take-Out Diet

(Researching the researchers)

Science shows us how diets fail. Science and Business Practices can show us how diets work.

Dr Hugh Butler, PhD

"Half of what we know is wrong, the purpose of science is to determine which half."

Arthur Kornbeg – Nobel Laureate 1959

ISBN 9780994173300

First published in Australia Dec 2014

Acknowledgments

For Judy, Eve, Amanda, Graham and Monica. John for starting me on my journey, and for correcting the grammar and comprehension. For Kathy for encouraging me to write a book, and for all my friends and family who have had to endure my enthusiasm for information.

For all those scientists who contribute to the knowledge and understanding of our health. Biochemists, statisticians, endocrinologists, geneticists, medical researchers, sociologists, behavioural scientists, writers and commentators who take the data and try to make sense of it.

I have not done the science on nutrition or health. They have. They research, write papers and some experts have researched for 40 years or more. They may compile their specialist knowledge and our society can now access that knowledge using the internet. Some ask how non-researchers can make sense of the science. Much research is very specific, and many researchers go down to the "bottom of the test tube" for detailed understanding. They publish this detailed information. They may even write broader summaries of their findings. Those researchers may be the experts in the field, but they are usually not experts in other fields of science or knowledge. Science is too big an area to be expert in all fields. A biochemist is unlikely to know about behaviour, or the business world of food. Institutions may put together an inter-disciplinary team in a "Centre of Excellence" to try to encompass this broader view. I and others can take the information from the various diverse aspects, interpret the various and conflicting views and tell a coherent story encompassing the whole system.

Structure of This Book

This is my research on researching the science about health and diet. Diet appears to be the major contributor to our health. While we are learning every day how genetics and epigenetics are important determinants of our health and wellbeing, society has always known that what we eat (our diet) is the major determinant. The book is structured so each chapter deals with only one aspect of our health and diet. Each chapter focuses on one subject, has a "get the facts" section, expands on research, and each ends with a summary of how this relates to our diet or health.

We are complex organisms and we live in a complex society. None of these individual components can be viewed in isolation. Science often fails in communicating about diets and health because it treatd each component as separate, even when we know they are connected. I've chosen six Take-Out actions that are important and achievable for long term health. Perhaps it may be useful to read the final chapter first, but then come back and see why these six take-out actions have been chosen over other actions.

Copyright

Disclaimer

This material is not intended to be, and should not be considered, a substitute for medical advice. Treatment for some of the conditions that unwell or overweight people have is highly dependent on the individual's circumstances. And, while this material is designed to offer accurate information with respect to the subject matter covered and to be current as of the time it was written, research and knowledge about medical and health issues are constantly evolving. The publisher and author make no representation or warranties to readers, express or implied, as the accuracy or completeness of this material. The publisher and author do not accept, and expressly disclaim, any responsibility for any liability, loss or risk that may be claimed or incurred as a consequence of the use and/or application of any of the contents of this material.

CONTENTS

PROLOGUE

Bookstores house thousands of diet books and people buy them to the tune of billions of dollars each year. Yet, the public continues to get unhealthier and fatter in spite of all the diet and health information. This issue became more personal to me in my late forties and fifties when I realized I was no longer lean, but it did not concern me much until the year I was going to turn 60 years. I'd made some weight reduction over that time, and improved my fitness. Yet, over a five-year span, I was unable to effectively change my weight and clothes needed to be a size or two bigger than I remembered from my 20's or 30's. Was my weight even an issue for health? Did it matter? In fact, all I knew at the time was that skinny worms live longer than fat ones. Naturally, I knew I wanted to live a long healthy life! Who knows what worms want, other than to avoid those rampaging early birds?

I was about to turn 60 years old and I had been telling family and friends that I was going to live to 120. That is what some insurance actuaries were saying. So something needed to change if I did not want to end up dribbling in a room full of strangers in my mid-nineties. Or worse, not speaking to the intensive care unit nurse at the age of 65 due to a cardiovascular incident!

This was personal. My mother spent the last 5 years of her life living, and then dying with dementia. My father spent the last 8 of his life, frail, uncomfortable, and a quality of life that I did not want to have. Health futures became real and personal.

This book is my journey of discovery over a 2 year period. Researching the researchers. Understanding why diets fail. Defining a better and "successful" lifestyle. Understanding what changes are needed for that lifestyle. Understand the cost benefit and the change management required to implement those changes. Then using my experience and skills in science and business processes, to make those changes relevant to my lifestyle; and achieve success.

CHAPTER 1
MY STORY

My Story

I wanted to live a long and healthy life, and particularly in my latter years. There was no sense in being alive, but having poor health. Evidently, millions of others want to live a long and healthy life too. I was overweight, and assumed that I, and all the overweight people, were unhealthy. What was the relationship between weight and health, and was I overweight enough to affect my health, or would I need to be obese? In a study of formerly obese people, researchers at the University of Florida found that virtually all the participants said they would rather be blind, deaf, or have a leg amputated than be obese again. That is the extent of our desire to be slim, and yet, two-thirds of people in the UK, USA and Australia are overweight, and a quarter of these are obese. Why is reality at such odds with desire? We're told that to be slim, to achieve the thing we want more than our sight, hearing, or mobility, all we need to do is eat less and/or do more. If this information is accurate, why don't we just all follow the advice and get down to, and maintain, our optimum weight? Why is there such an obesity problem in first-world societies?

Of course, I knew that I would need to take good care of myself if longevity was to be obtained. But I also knew it may take more than just "good care", whatever that was. What specific steps? I wondered what diet and health information was based on good science, what was poor or compromised science, and what was mostly fiction. What was the current knowledge? I wondered what was written for the benefit of one who wanted to lose weight and be healthy, and what was written to "sell" something. I wanted to know what was based on recent good science, not mythology and sensationalism, and could one swing the odds to my favour? My "pedigree" or DNA seemed good with a father living to 96, paternal grandfather to 92, and mother to 89. My paternal grandmother had lived to 78, even though she smoked two packs of cigarettes a day. Were there immediate tactics that would increase my chances of living a long, healthy life? I wanted to find out what the low hanging fruit of health would be for me. Low hanging fruit is the fruit on the bottom of the tree that is easily accessible and picked without great effort, and with positive outcome. Why aim for the difficult, even if the reddest and juiciest apple taunted me from a high branch!

I know a little biochemistry with more than enough to be dangerous! With four years of undergraduate Agricultural Science and three years of PhD study in plant physiology and biochemistry, I could get my head around a few thousand compounds. At the end of my PhD, I could write down hundreds of compounds in complicated biochemical pathways from memory. I could comprehend what I read and was pretty good at reading and writing research papers. I'd published 38 science articles in peer review journals, and I have a well-developed discerning sense of what is stated in the conclusions. With six years of statistics study, 12 years in biological research and software programming statistical routines from the ground up, I knew about correlation and causation. Business numbers and trends are second nature after 20 years of looking at balance sheets, profit and losses, marketing plans, creating training resources for business products, and helping people gain understanding about the numbers. I also knew a great deal about Change Management, business process re-engineering, and how to drive change in companies, whether in sales, technology or human resources.

I also knew a little about diets. My partner and wife of 28 years had been dieting on and off for most of our life together. But diets weren't for me. I considered them only from the perspective whether or I wanted to put on weight and spend money needlessly. And I certainly had not realized there are over 660 diets, and the number of diets increases daily. Growing up, I was not particularly concerned about health or weight. I was a skinny kid and at the age of 15 wanted desperately to put on weight so I could move from the Rugby Union lightweight teams (under 133lb, 60 kg) to the open senior teams. By the age of 20, I was at 155 lb (70 kg) and 5'11" (183 cm) and there I stayed until my thirties.

By age 50, I had increased to 210 lb (95 kg, 15st) and thought it was poor diet due to a business travel lifestyle. Nonetheless, in late 1998, the doctor at an executive check-up gave me some great advice. He told me to go from full strength beer to light beer, cut out the chips, switch to salads, swap soft drinks for diet soft drinks or water, and have more fish and less steak meals. Over the next 12 months, I lost 22 lb (10 kg). I figured that if it had taken 20 years to put the weight on, 12 months was a fair time to take it off. I took it off without pain or lots of mind games. I ate more oysters, prawns, and fish. I could drink twice as much beer, but I didn't! I ate less fried chips and put the loss down to a lower fat diet. My wife was on a Weight Watchers diet, and they seemed to have some good food choice changes, few of which I followed! I just wish that doctor had known what I know now.

The weight stayed for another six years, at which stage the gym beckoned. Not for losing weight, but to build some upper chest muscle and ward off osteoporosis. I had read that weights improve bone mass. I did not have osteoporosis that I knew, but I did have the beginnings of man boobs (10% of all males have Gynecomastia) and they were a bit embarrassing to me at the beach. Kids can speak directly, and my three-year-old grandson asked why I had boobs, so it seemed like good timing to do something. Going to a gym is hard mental work, but I stuck at it three times a week, for one hour each time. I did 20 minutes of cardio (high intensity rowing and cycling) and 40 minutes of mostly upper body strengthening. Depending on business commitments, some weeks I worked out four or five days, and some weeks I did not work out at all. To my surprise, the gym actually reduced my weight slightly to about 182 lb (83 kg). My waistline trimmed down, the chest increased and boobs went. My heart rate has always been steady at 55 to 60 bpm and blood pressure 117 over 63. (Those genes!)

As I read health articles in the doctor's waiting room for my annual inspection (or proctologist for my two-year check-up), it seemed that I was not quite at optimum health. The doctor threatened to prescribe statins to bring my cholesterol down, although other risk factors such as cardiovascular or smoking were absent. My fasting sugar levels were a little high, and other measures were high. Nothing I did seemed to have any effect on that. My weight was on the high side, with a body mass index (BMI) just under 25, but everyone said, "You're okay." It did not seem okay to me, and questions remained. My father had a heart attack at 82. At ninety, he got more and more frail. Without a hip operation which was advised against due to his cardio vascular issues, he stopped walking at age 94. My mother got dementia at 82 and died at 89. Was this what I was facing if I did not get healthier? Would I have serious issues as early as mid to late nineties rather than living a healthy life to 120? I knew that it was likely I would experience what my parents experienced if I did not make some lifestyle and health changes! But what changes? Current health advice seemed complicated and ambiguous. Eggs were good in the 60's. Then in the 80's they were bad. Now they are good again!

In my work in commercializing innovative technology, I needed to get a feel for market opportunities. I reviewed popular publications such as *New Scientist, IEEE Spectrum, Science,* on-line forums, detailed medical studies, and such. I looked to identify business opportunities for colour x-rays and how to position trampolines in the market to stop kids from getting fatter. I'd seen great graphs showing the correlation between kids consuming fruit juice and increasing obesity. I listened to public health policy makers about the exploding costs of aging and obesity and many media reports on health.

Researching the Research

In the first quarter of 2013, I started a more focused journey of finding out what were the best strategies for improved health after my brother-in-law gave me a book "Sweet Poison" by David Gillespie. What was new or confirmed in medical science? In April, a friend with poor health, but sick of me always talking about health said "why not write a book of this information and what you are finding out." This book is the result. Although I thought I had the key aspects early on, I kept reading as I wrote. I became a researcher of the research! As I read more articles, and read or re-read books by others, I discovered how much I did not know. It seemed like mission impossible. What was new? What had others missed, or misinterpreted? Throughout my career in science or business there is one tenet I always tried to be faithful to: employ people smarter than yourself. While I am in the business of commercializing technology, I always try to find smarter people; people who can provide the foundation of ingenuity and creativity. I then try to create the framework for them to blossom. I found many smart people. Thus it is with this journey, this book.

My Discoveries

My conclusion (researching the research) from books, science publications, and a lifetime of business is that there is a short list of things to achieve for health. Weight management is only part of our health. The low-hanging fruit can be "picked" with little effort in the short term, but may be difficult continuing long term. It may require consistent and persistent effort to achieve these lifestyle changes. I call this lifestyle a "take-out diet." What can we *take out* of our lives to be healthier, rather than focusing on what we need to put in.

Will the current recommended healthy lifestyles remain the same over the next ten years, or will they be superseded as we gain more evidence? Much of the health advice is to put more in; to do more.

Science, pharmaceutical companies, and food companies want us to take more pills, and dieticians want us to eat more "healthy" food. Public education groups and gym owners want us to exercise more. Doctors want us to eat more healthy food and do more exercise or simplified as "eat less, move more". Prevention is always the cheapest and most effective strategy and I don't see that changing. Even though the more we discover about human biology, the less we seem to know! We actually know the important questions and answers now. Science is non-linear. As the body of science grows, and the tools we use for science become increasingly complex, we will find out more about this wonderfully intriguing area of work. I'd rather do some prevention for Alzheimer's disease than take a wonder pill in twenty years when the medical community comes up with a pill. Although I am a strong supporter for medical science, and have nothing against pills; there is no certainty that a pill will fix things and there is high probability there will be side effects. Today, we have sufficient knowledge that shows that you can prevent, or minimize, risks of ill-health in natural ways, without pills. More science may help boost confidence levels and help change existing levels of dogma. Perhaps the biggest challenge will be the entrenched commercial interests.

Change for Good

Given that the oldest verified living person is currently 122 years old, what changes are needed for the rest of us for a happy, healthy, long life? Change is very difficult: hard to start, hard to do, and hard to sustain. To change our behaviour, we need to learn the process and then do it automatically, by rote. Did you learn to ride a bike or drive a car? It took effort to get past the first 20 hours, but from then on, it only took practice to become an expert. There are some very good principles for enjoying consistently good health. Josh Kaufman, author of *The First 20 Hours,* says that the first step is to plan how you are going to learn. Then learn the principles. Consolidate. In 20 hours you can learn the skill. In just 20 hours you can learn a language, a musical instrument, a web programming language, to play a sport, to ski, to be a photographer, to ride a bike, or to drive a motor vehicle. You can't become an expert in 20 hours because that takes months or years of practice. But in 20 short hours you can learn enough to be proficient. So it is with adopting a happy, healthy diet. Stop doing what you are doing now, and plan what you will do with your health in less than 20 hours. Make a plan for the rest of your lifetime. It just might be as simple as taking out some things you currently do.

Diets are for Health

One intriguing thing I came to realize was that our current view is that diets are for losing weight. But as one researches the literature, it is easy to see that diets got hijacked in the mid-60s as a way to become healthier. The scientists thought we had to reduce the level of fat we consume because the more fat there was is in the diet, the higher the cholesterol levels were, the more difficulty there will be in managing weight, and the worse your health. While disproved, it is still current simply dogma, and many physicians still "preach" that the higher the cholesterol level, the higher the risk for heart attacks. Take on a low fat diet, you will lose weight, and you will have lower risk of heart attack. That is just plain wrong! Science shows unequivocally that diets fail. Given we all want health, and health is dependent on what we eat (our diet), where do we look, to find a diet to be successful long term? My conclusion is the cause of failure is not just from the biology but from our behaviours and our society we live in. Taken as a "whole life" approach, science and business principles *together* show us what will work to be healthier and less overweight. If only we would take notice.

CHAPTER 2
DIET AND LIFESTYLE INTERACTIONS

Get the Facts

➤ Diet and Lifestyle have at least three components: biochemistry and hormones, our behaviour from our own mind and brain and external social behaviours and lifestyle.
➤ The majority of current research focuses on the biochemistry, hormones, genetics and the microbiome we live with.
➤ Most researchers and reported studies fail to understand the interactions and complications between these factors. This confounding of research says that diets and lifestyle are complicated, whereas the principles are not.
➤ Diets / changes in lifestyles require change in each of these areas. Diets fail. Science shows us why.
➤ In understanding why diets fail, science and business principles give us direction about what to change, tactics on how to change, and how to succeed long term.

Understand the Science

Many suggest the whole food / diet / health issue is too complicated, yet others will promote a view that being healthy is as simple as 1,2,3. They will write a book and sell you the guidelines to perfect health in a few steps along with a monthly charge on your credit card.

When I started this book, I thought health and diet were mostly about biochemistry and hormonal components and excess weight was simply "eat less, move more". That's what is in the published science and that was my background and therefore my starting point. What I learnt from researching this is that these are three quite different processes. They are interconnected. The simplest way to understand this relationship is that diet and health are like a three-legged stool. If you have any of these legs "wrong" or out of alignment, the stool falls over. If your health or your weight is out of balance you need to address it as a whole system and not just one component.

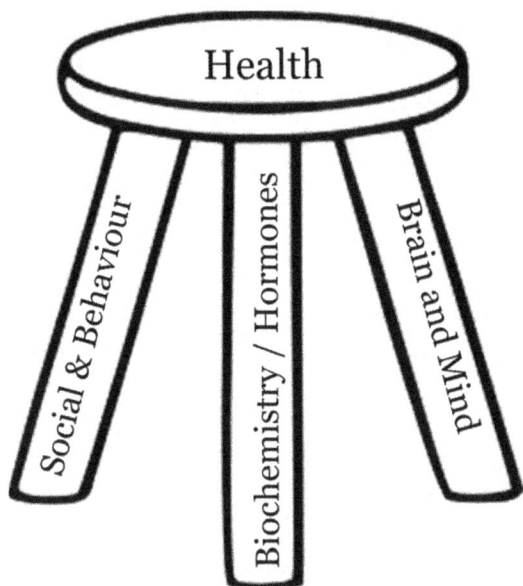

Figure 1 The Three-legged Stool of the Take-Out Diet

Science shows that all diets, and most health programs, fail in the medium to long term. Why? Eighty percent of dieters weigh more than when they started the diet two years prior. If you have dieted, and after two years still weigh less than you started, you are an anomaly! Diets are not alone in being ineffective. A recent longitudinal study in Canada followed over 5,000 patients who were aged 50 years or older. These folk had an initial diagnosis of chronic illness (heart disease, cancer, stroke, respiratory disease, and diabetes). Even after being diagnosed, and after being counselled by a health care professional on lifestyle modifications to change their condition, most people did not make major lifestyle adjustments. You would think anyone with these conditions would change, but not so.

While I was trying to understand why diets fail, I started looking for other factors. Most research is on biochemistry, endocrinology, and many of the other things that affect our appetite or metabolism seemed to be missing from this research. There are many effective short term diets. But why do people give up? Why did some diets work some of the time, but not all of the time? Experts seem to ignore this line of research, although I have seen some initiatives recently.

Why Did My Diet Work?

How did this relate to me? My personal experience may help illustrate these principles. What were the personal challenges; why

9

did I actually lose the 30 lb (14 kg) in weight? I had started this health process by going "sugar free" (*Sweet Poison* book by David Gillespie) and I combined this with the 5:2 diet (*Eat Fast Live* book by Michael Moseley and Mimi Spencer). At the same time, I was researching scholarly articles for this book, and tracked my food with MyFitnessPal (calorie logging) to see what changes I was making. These three changes in my diet effectively meant I was having a low carbohydrate high fat (LCHF) diet! It was impossible to say what was actually the most important. It became clear that keeping the weight off long-term by making "lifestyle" changes would be my challenge like most others. So I had to reconcile the science evidence into a unifying theory. Hence the three-legged stool concept. In the context of the balancing act with this stool, I started to see some of the answers about the internal behaviours, and the external societal changes too. So throughout the book we will constantly refer back to this balancing act.

Going sugar free (cutting out *added* sugar and especially the fructose component) meant that my intake of carbohydrates went way down. Why? Because sugar is added to most food products, including bread and flour-based products such as cakes and breakfast cereals. I had to change to whole foods and avoid supposedly "healthy choices" with low fat, etc. because often, when fat is reduced, sugar is added to improve taste. We know from the biochemistry and hormonal leg of the stool that lower carbohydrate diets, with no change in protein levels, makes you less hungry. Carbohydrates make you hungrier. Low carbohydrate diets increase lipogenesis (fat burning); and reduce overall calorie intake.

What was simple (avoid added sugar) became a complex event, not just from the biochemistry perspective, but also affected my behaviour and my social behaviour. To make it even more complex, a change in diet affects gut bacteria, the microbiome, and that adds another layer of complexity to the biochemistry and hormone leg. These weren't the only confounding factors.

Adopting a 5:2 diet and calorie counting (food intake, daily weighing) changed my behaviour. The more protein I consumed the less hungry I was and thus I snacked less. The 5:2 diet means average consumption over a week was reduced but the 5:2 also changes your mindset about hunger and calorie restrictions and helps manage portion size. The sugar free, lower carbohydrate and the 5:2 also confounded socializing. When I went out with friends, my food choices changed. We know eating with friends increases your food consumption. If you go to a café and get presented with a cabinet display of cookies, muffins, and bread products, it can be very difficult to snack healthier. If you go to a buffet, you will eat more. While I had plenty of willpower, I could see why the psychological components can be extremely difficult, and how these internal / external factors would cause diets to fail. It became easier for me as I was writing a book, and could look at some of these things impartially as I tried to analyze them. As I talked to others on a weight loss journey, they started to share why they failed at keeping weight off. Their stories got me looking for explanations about the other legs of the stool.

Their stories aligned with books about personal behaviour such as *Weight Loss for Food Lovers* by George Blair-West (the 2nd leg), or the book about our food producers *Salt Sugar Fat* by Michael Moss (the 3rd leg). They added to the information and gave intriguing and at the same time dismaying perspectives.

Conclusion

This three-legged stool has to be integrated into the whole area of change management. What is needed before you decide to change? What is needed to effect change? What is needed to ensure the change is effective long term? I started to see why there was so much confounded commentary out there on health. Why a program could work short term, but fail long term and why so few people actually made long term lifestyle changes. More importantly, I began to understand what the interactions were. I believe that as we understand these interactions, we can apply them for successful long term change.

References

a. Katch, V. (2013) Why is behaviour change so hard? Michigan Today. http://michigantoday.umich.edu/a8589/

CHAPTER 3
EVALUATE AND PLAN

Get the Facts

➤ Sixty-five percent or more of adults in most Western countries are overweight. Close to 30% are obese.

➤ About 50% of adults take at least one prescription medication. About 50% of seniors take at least three.

➤ For those who are normal weight, 20% will have some components of metabolic syndrome, precursor to chronic illness.

➤ It is not normal for our bodies to be sick and need medication.

➤ There are basic actions that you can take, and using the 80/20 rule (20% of what you do will give you 80% of the results), you can keep your body healthy whether fat or thin.

➤ It is never too late to start taking action for a healthy body and quality life.

➤ Health begins and ends with what you put in your mouth with few exceptions.

Understand the Science

What you eat has a significant effect on your weight and health. Do you eat a lot of processed sugar and high-carbohydrate foods? Do you eat too much food every day without ever giving your body a break from food? When you grocery shop, do you buy a lot of processed foods but only a few plants from the produce department? Do you have poor quality fats and rancid seed oils in your kitchen? Do you sit at a desk for most of the workday and sit in front of the TV after the workday ends?

Every single thing listed above significantly affects your health! There is science-based evidence behind all of it, and you'll understand the evidence as you read this book. If you answered yes to any, or especially if you answered yes to most of the questions, the bad news is that you are not doing very well at keeping yourself healthy. The good news is that these things are all low-hanging fruit issues, and that means you can easily tackle them with little effort and time! To get you started, review the checklist below.

Action You Can Take NOW

Take things out of your diet or lifestyle, rather than putting things in. Whether you call it a simpler lifestyle or diet, a low-hanging fruit approach, or an 80/20 approach, it is all about *less*. It is much easier to take stuff out than to put more stuff in. I'll call it the *take-out* diet!

- Take-out sugar from your diet. Leave in proteins and fats.

- Take-out simple carbohydrates. Leave in good food, not too much, mostly plants.

- Take-out seed oils. Leave in good fats.

- Take-out food products. Shop the perimeter of the grocery store; try to stay out of the centre aisles. Better yet, frequent farmers markets.

- Take-out food from your diet if you are overweight. I recommend the 5:2 diet as a good option because you don't need to change your social life.

- Take-out sitting down for more than 20 minutes at a time.

- Adopt a change management approach to these life style changes and be aware that your mental approach is the primary factor for a healthy body, and ultimately, a healthy weight.

You don't need to jump through a lot of hoops to live a happy, healthy life. In later chapters of this book we will go through these things in more detail and explain the rationale. Just skim these points and think about how you can implement them for weight loss and management, and good health. Or if you want to, jump ahead to the last section to where these are explained in more detail.

The next group is about things that you could do as part of a long term healthy lifestyle as there is some evidence of benefits. The last group is things you can pretty much ignore as a waste of time or money. I try to avoid getting into arguments with advocates for these behaviours: many believe in them with a religious fervor.

Some Value

- Have relationships with others. Health and well-being is associated with having good relationships. Having a partner extends life expectancy. Loneliness reduces life expectancy.

- Reduce contaminants in your life. If you have major contaminants such as smoking or drugs, get rid of those before embarking on the six things above. Health benefits are well established for quitting smoking.

- If you drink more than a 3 or 4 drinks of alcohol per week on average, you will need to adjust your lifestyle starting with alcohol. Don't bother to start the take-out diet unless you have alcohol under control. Check out the chapter on alcohol.

- You can't change your genes. Knowing your family medical history might lead to preventative strategies, or provide incentive to change.

- Trying to change your microbiome (gut bacteria) may help, but the biggest improvement to your microbiome will be taking-out sugars and simple carbohydrates and giving them a little more whole food.

- High salt consumption may be bad for you, but if you reduce your consumption of processed foods (which provides 75% of all the salt you take in) then don't bother to specifically reduce salt. Let it happen as a consequence.

- Don't try to change your meat consumption. There may be some minor risk from processed meat, but the evidence is patchy. Reducing simple carbohydrates and reducing weight provides better health outcomes.

- Exercise. While exercise is of little value in weight loss, exercise is beneficial in a range of processes, and reasonable exercise helps metabolism, improves mental state, reduces chronic illnesses, improves memory and decreases memory loss. Don't change the level of exercise as part of the 12 week program.

Of Little or No Value

All of these below fit with the 80% of effort or cost while providing less than 20% of value.

- Stop consuming vitamins and supplements. I suggest any money you spend on vitamins and supplements is put towards real food.

- Have a lifestyle that tries to eliminate toxins from your body although reducing toxins is common sense.

- Never mind buying organic food. There is little evidence it makes a difference. Organic food alone won't change your health, and don't equate organic food with healthy food. It will lighten your wallet.

- Don't worry about the low GI high GI issue. Just "take-out" eating simple carbohydrates. Complex carbohydrates are good, simple are bad.

- Don't worry about eating for your blood type.

- Don't bother to do liver cleanses and detoxifications, or any other well designed scheme to lighten your wallet. Choose to live a healthy lifestyle instead.

- Don't bother to "juice." Recycle your juicer and eat the whole fruit or vegetable.

- Don't exercise like contestants on "The Biggest Loser."

- Don't diet with any of the quick-fix programs which are designed to lighten your wallet unless you need them for social support. Results can be achieved considerably faster and cheaper with more natural steps that include eating real food. However, you may want to do these for a short period of time if you are in a mental state where you want some support and structure around an initial weigh loss program. Just don't do them long term. You will fail.

- Don't listen to your friend. Or the taxi driver. Or the health gurus. You are more likely to get inaccurate information than practical, science-based information.

- Don't listen to the conservative medical industry. Generally, they are uneducated about the latest scientific research, and many of them still support the dogma of "eat less, move more" mindset proven ineffective.

- Don't listen to, and support the big food and big pharmaceutical companies. They want your dollars at any cost. They are very good at emptying your wallet and providing little to nothing in return.

Plan Your Attack

When it comes to taking care of your body, planning is essential. I've helped many people plan their business strategies. In general, businesses are usually short on time and money, and they think they need a plan to increase money. Many want a plan to do more, but fail to see that to achieve more, you have to do less. Time is the one resource most people do not have enough of. Find time by doing less of the stuff that does not give results. Most times a plan turns out to reduce time wasted. Planning won't automatically increase wins, but it generally reduces losses. Most know enough about money to figure out how they can increase their revenue but few recognize that time may be the biggest constraint to successful business. Do fewer things for better results.

Let's use an example from business. A company has ten product lines. Pareto's Principle will say 20% of the lines (only two) give 80% of the profit, but they all take the same amount of time to manufacture. Two lines lose money and six may make a little money. If the business stopped those two loss-making product lines and just two of barely marginal products lines, the business would have 40% more time available. That time can now be used productively, either to increase production of their two profitable product lines, or take time off for leisure, or develop new products. Planning is mostly about stopping unhelpful things, not doing new things. Most are too busy doing things to start new things. Weight loss and health initiatives are no different.

In the business planning process, I get businesses to apply 80% of their time on really measuring what they are currently doing (baseline). I also insist they make no changes in the business until the planning phase is completed. I like to use the Goldratt's "Theory of Constraints" process to pinpoint what to change; what to change to, and how to cause the change. Goldratt promotes the principle there is only 1 constraint, and you need to subordinate everything to that constraint. During this planning and measuring phase, it becomes obvious what needs to be changed, but establishing the right Key Performance Indicators (KPIs) is not always straight forward. There is a saying: Measure what is important. The corollary to this is: What you measure becomes important. If you put in place a measure that does not give rise to improvement, why measure it? This measure could actually change things for the worse.

Why spend so much time on the baseline? Where you come from is usually more important than where you are going. Let's say you are planning a trip to China to see the Great Wall. If you are from an isolated farming community in Australia, speak no Mandarin, have never travelled to another culture, and only like meat and three vegetables, your experience and outcome will be quite different from that of a Chinese migrant from Australia who speaks fluent Mandarin, has travelled extensively, and loves diverse cuisine. If you come from Japan, or Italy, your journey will be much different. You might use a similar aircraft to fly in, but preparation and your experience of the journey will not be the same. Everything we see is viewed through the prism of our experience.

We will discuss change management in more detail in the upcoming section on evaluating your health. In change management you do require some key information.

- Where are you now (the Now)

- Where do you want to get to (the Where)

- What are the reasons to change (the Why)

- What processes to use (the How)

These four key issues are simple and obvious, but few actually follow them, jumping straight to the "how" and then failing.

Normal or Nearly Overweight

If you have a BMI range from 20 to 25 (normal) you probably need to start the process of health improvement. You could be thin on the outside, but fat on the inside, and have as many of the health risks as an obese person. The strategies for improving your health will also result in weight loss. There are really only two simple things to do right off the starting line, but it does take focus to make any change. So consider the changes; read the book and other information to see what actually will work for you.

If one of the goals you set yourself is feeling better about yourself, weight loss may be one of the KPIs so you will need to do all six things. If weight loss is not required as part of your goals, avoid the 5:2 diet until the other dietary patterns have changed for good. The fewer things you need to do, the higher the probability of success for a lifestyle change. Intermittent fasting does have long term health benefits, and is an effective zero-cost strategy for good quality of life when elderly. But in change management, you want to change as little as possible, to maximize the probability of success. Trying to do too much too often creates stress, and as we will see, managing your mental state is important for success. Leaving the 5:2 for three months is no big deal in a lifetime of eighty years or so.

Overweight and Obese

For the 60% plus of the population who are overweight or obese with a BMI over 25, you have a greater challenge, because your body is almost certainly physically damaged by your past diet. Those past diet and lifestyle behaviours have created a challenging environment for change. Your mind may be somewhat traumatized by past experiences, and you will have to change this thinking in order to meet your challenges for weight loss and wellness. From the physical perspective, you are likely to have many of the consequences of being obese, such as metabolic syndrome, type II diabetes, fatty liver disease, chronic kidney disease, hypertension, just to name a few. More importantly, your appetite and normal diet feedback mechanisms are probably screwed up. It takes time to get them back on track, and there is some evidence they will never get back on track. Sadly, the evidence is that if you don't want to go back to being overweight or obese, you may always have to permanently restrict your calorie intake. You will need to manage all of those legs of that 3 legged stool, and it may be more difficult for the obese than for those in the moderately overweight BMI range.

Before You Start

Spend 80% of your time in planning, and 20% in doing. Planning gives the best outcome. Understand your personal reasons for desiring change. Good health or avoidance of illness may be stronger than looks, but whatever pushes your buttons! Monitor what you eat. Keep a journal as though you are a careful scientist. Be accurate and be consistent. You can use online systems like MyFitnessPal, Lose It, Cron-O-Pal, Fitday, or any of the other dozens of sites and apps. If you can, find a buddy to monitor and check your progress and share the journey with. Not everyone's experience is the same. Understand that you need to have a twelve-week plan and will have to track your measurements and what you eat for a period of time. Don't guess! Be accurate in your record-keeping.

Read, and try to understand, as much as you can about how your body works. Compare your research with what is actually happening in your body. Keep notes. Do the exercises such as the Food Lovers sacrifice food questionnaire. Do research to find answers.

Deal with your mental state. Prepare yourself for the challenges that are associated with changing your eating style. You know your strengths and weaknesses; use them for success in your plan. Give yourself self-talks in whatever way works for you. Don't ignore your brain; it plays a huge part in your weight loss and health. You can use your brain for an edge and advantage in your program. Visualize how much better you will feel when you lose weight and diminish your risk for disease. This can be powerful motivation for adopting a healthy eating style. Hypnotherapy or other techniques may help you adopt a healthier eating and fitness style. Research in quitting smoking showed going "cold turkey" was predominately the most effective. Trying to give up smoking slowly is ineffective and it doesn't take long before you are back on the habit.

Don't Stop Before You Get Going

Twenty percent will stop a diet within two days of starting a new plan. Forty percent will have stopped within the week. Only 20% of those who start a diet will remain on it for a year. For many, this path to health is very complicated, and most of all it is about Change Management. You *must* want to make a change. Even when a change is relatively minor it can be extremely difficult. During the course of writing, and experiencing first hand, my own journey, and from my experience in the field of change management, it is pretty evident that this degree of change is very substantial. Substantial dietary change, substantial personal change, and living in a society where this degree of change has a great deal of consequences, is challenging. That's why everyone is looking for a simple solution like swallow a pill once a day and everything will work out. There are some recent diets such as No Sugar and others that have a simple message. While the message is simple, the change is complex and there's plenty of evidence that these will also fail long term.

This makes it even more important that the changes we make are as small as possible and the gains are large. Old habits can be extremely hard to change, and new habits will take effort and time; just ask a smoker. Changing food habits can be compared to alcoholism. Alcoholism is a choice, day by day. Accept that you have to make food habits that last forever. This is not about your willpower, overcoming gluttony, or being a sloth (not doing enough exercise), but because the society we live in is geared to the overweight or obese. Every shop, every restaurant, and every activity is geared to our consumptive overweight society. It is so pervasive that most just don't see it, and it may take decades to change if ever. Now that I am on this *take-out* lifestyle, I find that when I go to a coffee shop there is never food in the counters that meet my new criteria of no added sugar, no simple carbohydrates, and no seed oils. Most seem to have very little whole food. The only place I recently saw whole food was a gas station that had a bowl of apples. The apples were next to a special on chocolate bars and Coke and shelves of packaged potato crisps. The "healthy choices" displayed can be the worst offenders. Large smoothies, flavored coffee or juices are heart attacks in a glass. Coffee shops, for me, are now a place for black coffee only.

Conclusion

In conclusion, the decision to make a dietary change for a gain in health and associated weight loss is a major change management process. A dietary change has ramifications across biochemical, hormonal, mental, and social interactions. You have to know why you want to change. As well as a sense of purpose, you have to know where you are now, where and why you want to change and how to change. While some would say don't start unless you are committed to continue, I think that is defeatist. Rather, I suggest the principles in business Change Management proposes a significantly different approach and it is worth starting on some changes to get some of the benefits.

- Start with the assumption that you only will change the least amount of things in your lifestyle.

- Adopt an 80:20 approach.

- Change Management says don't try to go from Sinner to Saint. Instead of trying to do more, do less.

- Don't try to eat "healthier" but do adopt a *take-out* approach. Take-out sugar and simple carbohydrates and replace them with more of what you already eat.

- Do not add things into this change by doing extra exercise, or many of the other things advocated from doctors to charlatans.

- Take-out one thing that will make you feel better. It might be sugar. It might be the 5:2 or a kick start diet to shed some weight. Then add in some of the other take-out actions.

- It is ok to stop. You do not fail if you do the first 20 days and then stop. Change management says this approach is a valid "plan and evaluate" process. Stop. Assess. Amend the plan. Restart.

References

a. Goldratt, E. (1992) The Goal: A process of ongoing improvement. pp384 North River Press. ISBN-13: 978-0884270614

CHAPTER 4
DO WE BLAME GENETICS?

Get the Facts

➤ Genetics make a big difference to health and well-being. As understanding the complexity of DNA continues, science is beginning to understand what "good genes" may actually mean.

➤ Genetic contributions to health issues have been found for multiple diseases: cancer, cardio vascular, diabetes, and multiple behavioural issues.

➤ Lifestyle factors and diet remain more important contributors to health and weight than genetics.

➤ Obesity is a complex trait, and many genes are related to obesity.

Understand the Science

A number of genes have been identified with obesity including MC4R, MAF, NPC1 and FTO. The FTO gene is located on chromosome 16, and encodes a protein called the fat mass and obesity-associated protein (the alpha-ketoglutarate-dependent dioxygenase FTO). The relationship of the FTO gene to obesity is not proven. One study in UK showed FTO has an incidence of 16% (both copies of the DNA) and those people are 70% more likely to be obese. For one gene (incidence 49%) people are 30% more likely to be obese. The cause for the obesity appears to be a lack in the drop in hormone ghrelin after eating: they stay hungry. Other FTO studies show modest or no effect on obesity.

This example highlights why you have to be careful when reading science. There is the story in the newspaper, and then there is the science in the journals. Don't always believe the first, but neither believe the science is without shortcomings. Here is an example from studies of the FTO gene and impact on weight and diet.

The story in the Daily Mail UK seems compelling blame for genetics.

You always have room for dessert and maybe even a second helping. You are about to be handed the perfect excuse. It may be in your genes. Scientists say that millions of Britons carry a rogue stretch of DNA that stops them from feeling full and leaves them craving sugary and fatty foods. Six years after a gene called FTO was linked to obesity, researchers have shown that it probably makes people plumper by failing to dampen their hunger following meals, and by increasing the allure of mouth-watering, high-calorie foods. In the same way that people can inherit several different variants of an eye-colour gene, people can inherit two different versions of the FTO gene.

The FTO gene is carried by 49% of the population. People with two copies of one of those variants "A", or high-risk obesity, are 70% more likely to develop obesity than those who inherit two versions of the other type "TT". Even having one version of this obesity-related variant raises the risk by 30%, making FTO the gene most strongly linked with obesity.

Rachael Batterham studied 259 men that were equal in regard to education, fat levels, and body weight to try to show that the main difference was only the genes. The men with two copies of the obesity variant ranked themselves 20 to 25% hungrier over the next two hours than the non-carriers did. The concentration in their blood of ghrelin, the only hormone known to stimulate appetite, was also elevated by the same amount. But that's not all. Further experiments by the team on a different set of twenty-four men revealed that carriers of the FTO gene are more attracted to the prospect of rich food.

The FTO gene carriers do not experience a fall in ghrelin after eating as they should. Ghrelin is the hormone that causes feelings of hunger. They eat up to 200 extra calories a day and are almost 3 kg (7lb) heavier than their average counterparts. Young men with the gene find ghrelin remains high after eating, and MRI scans showed more brain activity.

Study leader Dr Rachel Batterham, of University College London, said that some of us were simply "biologically programmed to eat more". Not only do these people have higher ghrelin levels and therefore feel hungrier, their brains respond differently to ghrelin and to pictures of food. It's a double hit. We know that ghrelin, and therefore hunger, can be reduced by exercise like running or cycling or by eating a high- protein diet."

Here is the summary from a science meta-review from Peng et al who looked at the associations between FTO (obesity related gene) polymorphisms, and obesity risk across different ethnic groups. They said:

This meta-analysis investigated the associations between five FTO polymorphisms (rs9939609, rs1421085, rs8050136, rs17817449, and rs1121980) and obesity risk in 41,734 cases, and 69,837 controls from 59 studies, counting the cases and control subjects from each study only once. We found significant evidence for a modest increase in the risk of obesity associated with the five polymorphisms in various ethnic populations. However, subgroup analyses showed that in some ethnic populations, for example, rs9939609 in Hispanic and African, rs1121980 in Caucasian, and rs8050136 in Asian and African, significant associations were not found between the SNPs and obesity risk.

The UK study blames obesity on genes (70% increase), and the Daily Mail takes the research and blows it up to being the absolute truth. The sample size is small, and the behaviour from 24 men is unlikely to be representative of 60 million Britons. The meta-review of over 59 studies says you can only blame a modest increase or none. So, it is no wonder that unless you are an expert, you would be confused.

Understanding why genes and health are inter-related is a difficult but active research area. It was thought that aging is a result not so much of gene changing, but genes wearing out. Telomeres are caps that protect the tips of chromosomes when cells divide. With each generation, they wear down. So some think this is why you age. In a limited study of ten men with prostate cancer in their early sixties, researchers looked at the telomeres. The men were put on a strict healthy living regime: a meat-free diet, exercise and yoga, and they went to weekly group therapy. Telomeres grew by 10%, but the 25 men on a control group lost 3% of their telomeres. But was the effect real, or just noisy data? It was not a trial, it was an observation, but the reporting makes it sound like fact.

When you consider how many pathways and hormones are involved in hunger, and that there are more than 40 discovered so far, you can see why it is complicated. In later chapters, we will talk about how the digestive system, different parts of the brain and other organs, are all connected with a vascular system, a lymphatic system, and a nervous system.

Conclusion

Does our genetic response vary with age? We now recognize "epigenetic" effects, where the environment impacts how genes express themselves. Our current knowledge about genetics' effects on health and weight is limited. We know that genetics do impact some diseases; less so in others. We are just beginning to understand why, and how, and expect a great deal of new knowledge to be forthcoming. The ultimate goal for some research is to find a cause and create a "magic bullet" to change / turn on / turn off / reverse / modify the genetic control process. If we refer back to the 3-legged stool, two of the legs will have a genetic component. But the environment we live in does not and therefore I am pessimistic about global obesity and global health.

References

a. Daily Mail. Are you a victim of the hunger gene? It's why many diets fail and millions never feel full. http://www.dailymail.co.uk/health/article-2364156/Are-victim-hunger-gene-Its-diets-fail-millions-feel-full.html
b. Karra, E (2013) A link between FTO, ghrelin, and impaired brain food-cue responsivity. Journal of Clinical Investigation. doi:10.1172/JCI44403.
c. Ornish D, Lin J, Chan J, Epel E, Kemp C, Weidner G, Marlin M, Frenda S, Magbanua M, Daubenmier J, Estay I, Hills N, Chainani-Wu N, Carroll P, Blackburn E. (2013) Effect of comprehensive lifestyle changes on telomerase activity and telomere length in men with biopsy-proven low-risk prostate cancer: 5-year follow-up of a descriptive pilot study. The Lancet Oncology, Vol14 (11) Pages 1112 – 1120 doi:10.1016/S1470-2045(13)70366-8
d. Peng S, Zhu Y, Xu F, Ren X, Li X, Lai M. (2011) FTO gene polymorphisms and obesity risk: a meta-analysis Penget al. BMC Medicine2011,9:71 http://www.biomedcentral.com/1741-7015/9/71
e. R Bell CG, Walley AJ, Froguel P. (2005) The genetics of human obesity. Nature Reviews Genetics 6:221-234.
f. Meyre, D et al. (2009) Genome-wide association study for early-onset and morbid adult obesity identifies three new risk loci in European populations. Nat Genet 41:157-159

CHAPTER 5
BIOCHEMISTRY OF METABOLISM

Get the Facts

➢ While metabolism is seen to be complex, the overall metabolic pathways have been known for 40 plus years. Research now focuses on understanding the complexity of the control mechanisms of metabolism. Control mechanisms are constantly being revised: genetic, biota, endocrinology and psychological, in ways that continue to surprise us.

➢ Human food is only from three groups of biochemical compounds: lipids (fat), protein, and saccharides (carbohydrates). We eat them, we break them down to their smallest component, adsorb them, recombine them, and then break them back down to simple compounds to release energy.

➢ Our systems have fantastic control mechanisms to ensure we live healthy and long lives.

➢ This equilibrium is called homeostasis and provides a steady state such as constant temperate, blood glucose levels and many other factors.

➢ About 80% of the energy we use daily is just to maintain this homeostasis – body temperature and brain function; as well as constant renewal as cells die and get recreated.

Understand the Science

In the mid-nineteenth century, the French physiologist Claude Bernard said living beings are a harmonious ensemble, so all systems have to work together to ensure survival. He phrased it as "milieu interieur" and so we have a body temperature around 37 degrees Celsius (98.6 Fahrenheit),and blood sugar of 70 to 170mg/dl. This homeostasis is made possible by numerous pathways and several feedback mechanisms that are all very tightly controlled; most driven by energy use. While some suggest glucose is the common compound – it isn't. In the same way a motor vehicle requires stored energy to convert to momentum energy (using gasoline, or in the case of electric cars, electricity) our biological systems require some form of stored energy (protein, fat, or saccharide) to convert to usable energy (ATP). That usable energy powers our muscles and our nervous system. When that stops, we die.

It is astounding how complex these processes are. Yet, they tend to be the same in all life forms. The basic processes are the same whether a life form is in the bottom of the ocean, an organism in a boiling mud pool, a bacterium, fruit fly, worm, rat, monkey, dog, or human. We may vary between species: ruminants (e.g. cows) have a modification of the stomach, and some have variation on digestion, but the intestine or kidneys work basically the same. If research is done on rats, don't assume that it is not relevant to humans.

It is the control of the processes through genes, enzymes, proteins, and hormones that creates the complexity. For example, genes affect appetite. But how? Gene regulation affects some tissue in fat cells, which in turn switches on production of a hormone, in turn affecting control cells in the brain's hypothalamus, which has a whole gamut of appetite control, which in turn may control behaviour or be modified by behaviour, which may lead to additional food consumed. Complicated! At the same time, there are other control mechanisms working in opposite directions. Ongoing research will give us better understanding of these processes, but do not assume when there is some science breakthrough it will be useful for health or diet. It may be just another piece in the jigsaw puzzle of control processes. You could get a giant wall sized Roche Biochemical Pathway Wall Chart which has been in print since 1965, but it is complicated!

Metabolism Summary

Humans mostly eat protein, fats, or saccharides (carbohydrates). Bones and complex fibers are indigestible to humans, but dogs digest bones, and ruminants fiber. We break them down into their simplest component. Then we reassemble them back into proteins, fats, or saccharides! Our microbiome also plays a part. The simple diagram below shows various components. All of these carbohydrates, proteins, and fats are converted ultimately through the citric acid cycle. All of the energy we use comes from this ADP-ATP electron transport pathway, and that happens within the mitochondria within each cell. Energy is needed in every part of each process. Each of these processes can have hundreds of chemical or biological compounds involved in the sub process whether at the molecular level, the complex protein level, or at the whole body level. While most processes have been known for over 40 years, the new knowledge about control processes makes for some reassessment of the processes involved. Scientific tools today are orders of magnitude more sensitive than previously used, and every month there are new publications that enhance our understanding. Yet the core principles have remained the same.

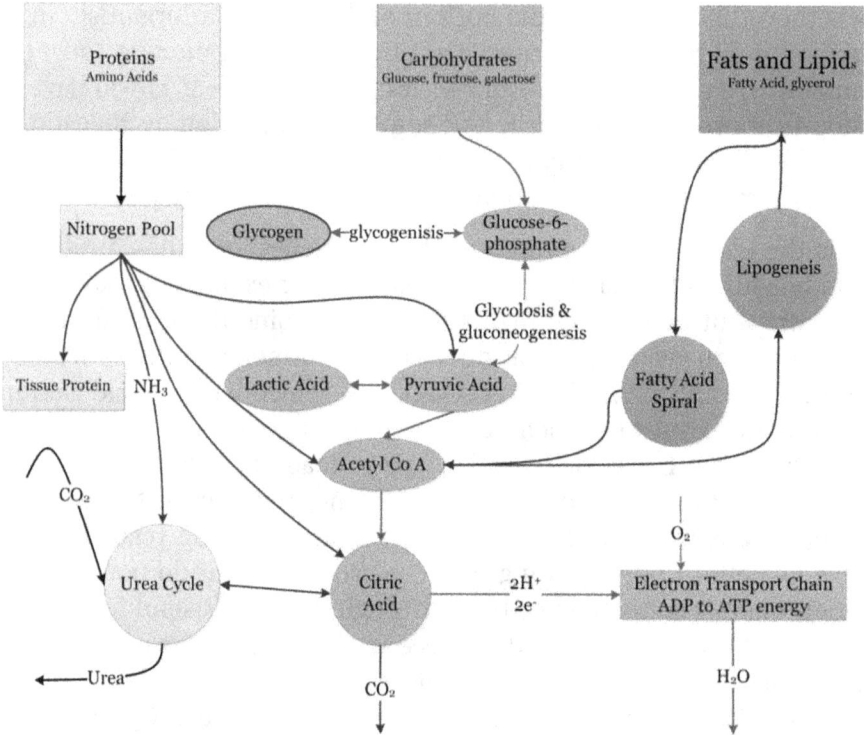

Figure 2 Metabolic Systems Overview

Energy

Energy is generally expressed in joules of energy in the SI international system. The imperial measure is a calorie which is 4.187 joules. Just to confuse things, nutrition uses Calories (capital C) which is a kilocalorie. (1,000 cal or 4,187j). (I use Calories throughout this book for consistency, although technically, a joule is the appropriate nomenclature for energy.) As an indication, a human will eat about 2000 Calories per day depending on the individual. For a small older female that may be as low as 1200 Calories, or 2500 for an active young male.

Food	Kilojoule per g	Calories per g (approx.)
Protein	17	4
Fat	37	8
Carbohydrate -Glucose	17	4
Carbohydrate (simple)	12	3
Dietary fibre (complex carbohydrate)	8	2
Alcohol	29	7

In context, 100gm of Atlantic salmon will be about 200 Calories as the flesh is a mix of protein, fat and water; and a salad of lettuce will be about 15 Calories as it is mostly water. A meal of salmon and a large serving of mixed salad will be between 300 to 350 Calories depending on what else goes into the salad. (Beware the Calories in the blue cheese salad dressing!)

This whole energy process is not simple and there are hundreds of different biochemical steps converting food into energy. We break the food down into its simplest form in our digestive system, adsorb it into our blood, and then reconstitute it back into fat and protein in our body. Some we use immediately for energy, some we store, and some we use to renew our body. It is interesting to compare the relative amounts of energy provided by various pathways in a typical 154 lb (70 kg or 11 stone) male. The free glucose in the blood is only about 4 g (1 teaspoon), and total free glucose in our whole body provides only a small energy reserve of about 40 Calories. It is just enough to maintain body functions for a few minutes. Glycogen stored in the liver and muscles after an overnight fast amounts equivalent to 600 Calories of energy. Glycogen reserves can maintain body functions for about one day without additional food. Glycogen can't be taken from muscle but it can be used by the muscle. Protein (mostly in muscle) contains a substantial energy reserve of about 25,000 Calories.

Finally, lipid reserves containing 100,000 Calories equivalent of energy can maintain human body functions without food for thirty to forty days with sufficient water. Lipids or fats represent about 24 lb (10 kg) of the body weight in a 154 lb (70 kg) male. Lipids provide the sole source of energy in hibernating animals and migrating birds. Fortunately, lipids are more energy dense than glycogen, otherwise body weight would increase approximately 110 lb (50 kg) if glycogen were to replace fat as the energy reserve.

Function of Fats

Too much fat has a bad name, obesity, but fat is essential to life as we know it. Every cell, of our billions of cells, has fat as part of the structure whether muscle tissue, brain and nervous system. Additionally, lipids or fats are stored in cells throughout the body, principally in special kinds of connective tissue called adipose tissue or depot fat. Much of the "fat" in the body is actually found as cholesterol, triglycerides, or lipoproteins (bound with proteins). Whereas most cells contain phospholipids in the bilayer cell membranes, adipose tissue cells consist of fat globules of triglycerides, which may occupy as much as 90% of the cell volume.

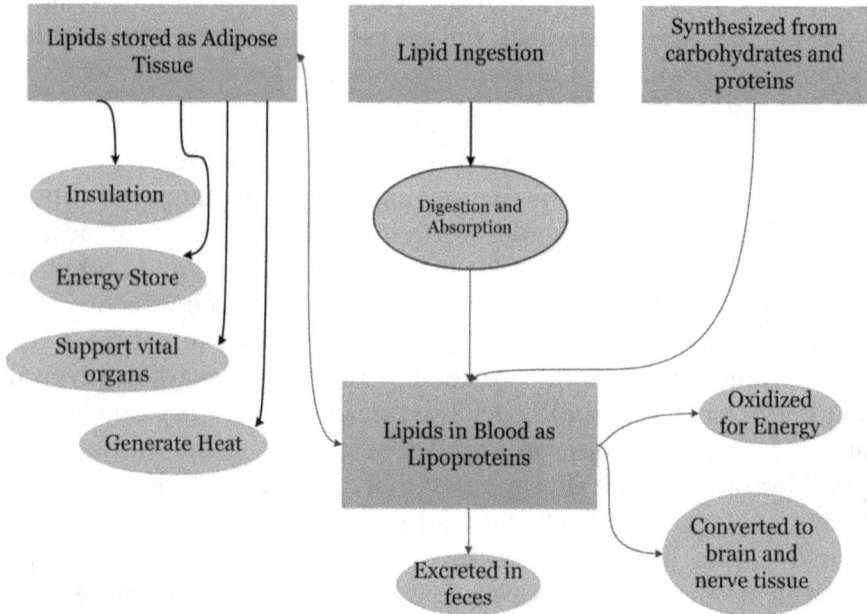

Figure 3 Lipids Metabolic Overview

By the age of two, humans have most of the fat cells they will get. From there on, the cells act like balloons. They are either empty or filled with these globules. We can grow new fat cells later in life.

So rather than visualize a fatty piece of bacon winding up as an extra dimple on your buttock ("moment on the lips – lifetime on the hips"), it is not that simple. It is more likely to be an extra saccharide (a muffin) that has been consumed as a carbohydrate and converted into a lipid.

In addition to energy storage, deposited fat provides a number of other functions. Fat serves as a protective cushion, and it provides structural support to help prevent injury to vital organs such as the heart, liver, kidneys, and spleen. Fat insulates the body from heat loss and extreme temperature changes. At the same time, fat deposits under the skin may be metabolized to generate heat in response to lower skin temperatures (brown fat) and this brown fat is thought to be beneficial, not detrimental. What does appear detrimental is visceral fat. Fats (such as cholesterol or triglycerides) are never in the blood stream as such. Oil and water don't mix. Fat is always bound up by proteins and an analogy is that the lipoprotein is a ship, and the cargo is a lipid. Or, think of a golf ball. The outside layer is the protein, and the internal bits are fat (triglycerides).

Nitrogen and Proteins

Nitrogen from proteins is recycled in the body just as carbon and oxygen are recycled in nature. Various microorganisms have the appropriate enzymes to convert elemental nitrogen from the air into ammonia, nitrate, and nitrites. Green plants use the ammonia or nitrate as raw materials for the synthesis of amino acids and proteins. Animals and humans, in turn, use the plants to supply nitrogen to make amino acids and proteins. Humans are unable to synthesize nine amino acids which must be included in the diet, and there are another nine considered "conditionally essential" as some populations can't make or get enough. Most mixed diets include sufficient amino acids in the food. Michael Pollan, in 2006, popularized this as, "Eat Food. Not too much. Mostly Plants." Finally, the nitrogen cycle is completed when plant and animal residues are decayed by microorganisms back to nitrates, nitrites, and finally nitrogen gas for the air.

The "nitrogen or amino acid pool" is a mixture of amino acids available in the cell derived from dietary sources or the degradation of protein. Since proteins and amino acids are not stored in the body, there is a constant turnover of protein. Some protein is constantly being synthesized while other protein is being degraded. For example, liver and plasma proteins have a half-life of 180 days or more, while enzymes and hormones may be recycled in a matter of minutes or hours.

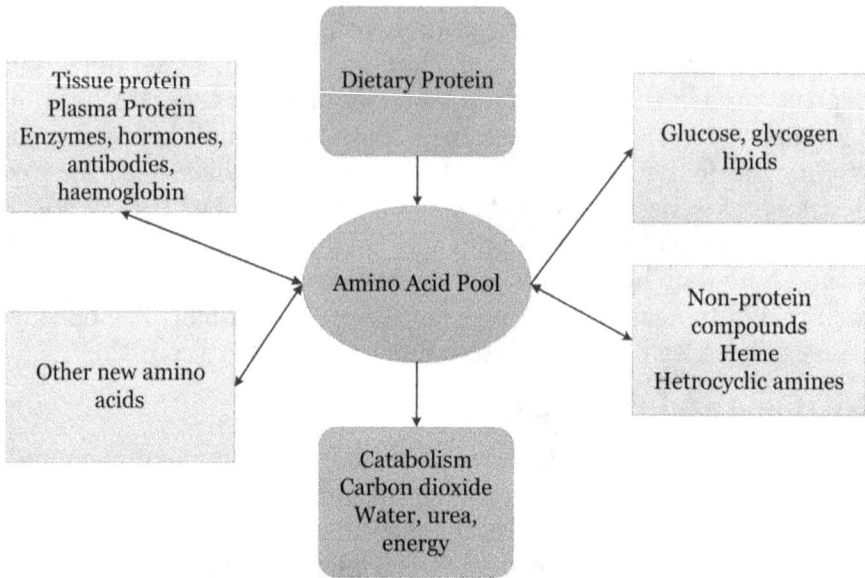

Figure 4 Protein Overview

Each day, some of the amino acids are catabolized, producing energy and ammonia. The ammonia is converted to urea and excreted from the body and represents a drain on the nitrogen pool.

A nitrogen balance is achieved by a healthy person when the dietary intake is balanced by the excretion of urea wastes. If nitrogen excretion is greater than the nitrogen content of the diet, the person is said to be in negative nitrogen balance. This is usually interpreted as an indication of tissue destruction. If the nitrogen excretion is less than the content of the diet, a positive nitrogen balance indicates the formation of protein. The dynamic balance of the nitrogen pool is summarized in the graphic above.

Conclusion

In conclusion, our energy systems are enormously complex. When you hear someone say, "My metabolism is sluggish," it will be a consequence of tens of thousands of multiple control processes in billions of cells. Interactions between these processes keeps us in homeostasis. When you hear people say "Calories In, Calories Out," as part of some diet mantra, ignore them. What is astonishing is that most humans maintain height, weight and energy balance in homeostasis through complex control mechanisms only partially understood. As part of any diet and lifestyle, we are aiming for that homeostasis. There is no concious thought to maintain our blood temperature at 37°; but we may have to think and act to maintain our weight at 175 lb (70 kg) in our modern society.

References

a. Ophardt C. E. (2003). Simple Lipids. Virtual Chembook http://www.elmhurst.edu/~chm/vchembook/620fattyacid.html
b. Michal G. (1965) Pathways Chart. http://biochemical-pathways.com/#/map/1 and 2.
c. Michal M, Schomburg D. (2012). Biochemical Pathways. An Atlas of Biochemistry and Molecular Biology (Second Edition). Hoboken, NJ: John Wiley & Sons.
d. Essential amino acids, http://en.wikipedia.org/wiki/Essential_amino_acid
e. Pollan M. (2006) The Omnivore's Dilemma: A Natural History of Four Meals, Penguin Books.

CHAPTER 6
I'M BIG BONED (BMI)

Get the Facts

➢ Weight is a mix of four different components.
➢ As people age, they get heavier, and BMI is a real issue for those aged 40 or older.
➢ Men with a waistline of 47.2" (120 cm) have twice the risk of various illnesses, than if their waist is 31.5" (80 cm).
➢ Women with a waistline of 39.4" (100 cm) have twice the risk if their waist is 25.6" (65 cm).
➢ For every 2" (5 cm) waist increase, your risk of premature death increases by 17% for men and 13% in women.
➢ There is a BMI paradox. About 20% of overweight people have minimal health issues. In normal range BMI weight, about 20% do have health issues. This "lean on the outside, fat on the inside" leads to contradictory health advice and confusion over validity of BMI and other measures.
➢ Take a minute. Measure your waist. Half your height? If it is, you're probably okay. If not, plan to do something.

Understand the Science

Body mass index (BMI) is the ratio of a person's weight in kilograms to their height squared in meters (kg/m^2). BMI can be interpreted using the following classification table (Health Canada).

BMI(kg/m^2)	Classification	Risk of developing health problems
Less than 18.5	Underweight	Increased
18.5 to 24.9	Normal	Least health issues
25.0 to 29.9	Overweight	Increased
30.0 to 34.9	Obese, Class I	High
35.0 to 39.9	Obese, Class II	Very high
40.0 and over	Obese, Class III	Extremely high

Weight is a function of four different components. BMI is often criticized for being a poor indicator, but in the absence of other measures, is a good rule of thumb. The 4 components of weight are:

- Bone mass. More bone is better. There is a high medical cost from osteoporosis and other bone loss complications.

- Muscle. Generally the more muscle, the better your health.

- External Fat. There is some advantage to having more fat. Brown fat seems important in metabolic processes.

- Visceral Fat. Fat around internal organs appears to be bad for your health, and more is worse.

I won't go into the detail of the differences between white adipose tissue (WAT), brown fat, and beige adipocytes. Beige adipocytes exist in WAT and burn fat and dissipate the energy as heat, but their abundance is diminished in obesity. Stimulating beige adipocyte development, or WAT browning, increases energy expenditure and holds potential for combating metabolic disease and obesity.

Every Western country is getting fatter. Body composition is an important indicator of the health of individuals and populations. BMI is used to identify weight-related health risks by classifying individuals as either underweight, normal weight, overweight or obese. Overweight and obesity are associated with an increased risk of numerous health problems including type 2 diabetes, hypertension, obstructive sleep apnoea, osteoarthritis, many types of cancer (including breast, colorectal, and pancreatic) and cardiovascular disease (coronary heart disease and stroke). More of this in the obesity and disease chapter. Being underweight is also associated with health problems, including osteoporosis, under-nutrition, infertility, and an increased risk of mortality.

Take the Canadians. The Canadian Health Measures Survey shows 67% of men and 54% of women aged 18 to 79 were overweight or obese. The figures are similar in other societies including UK, USA, Australia, and many others. Age is important and the older you are, the more likely you are to be obese. Adults up to 40 years old were the most likely to have a normal BMI, and significantly less likely to be overweight or obese than their counterparts aged 40 and over. Men were significantly more likely to be overweight or obese (7 out of 10) than women (5 out of 10). The figure below shows the % of males by age range, and shows the weight increases as they age.

Percent (%)

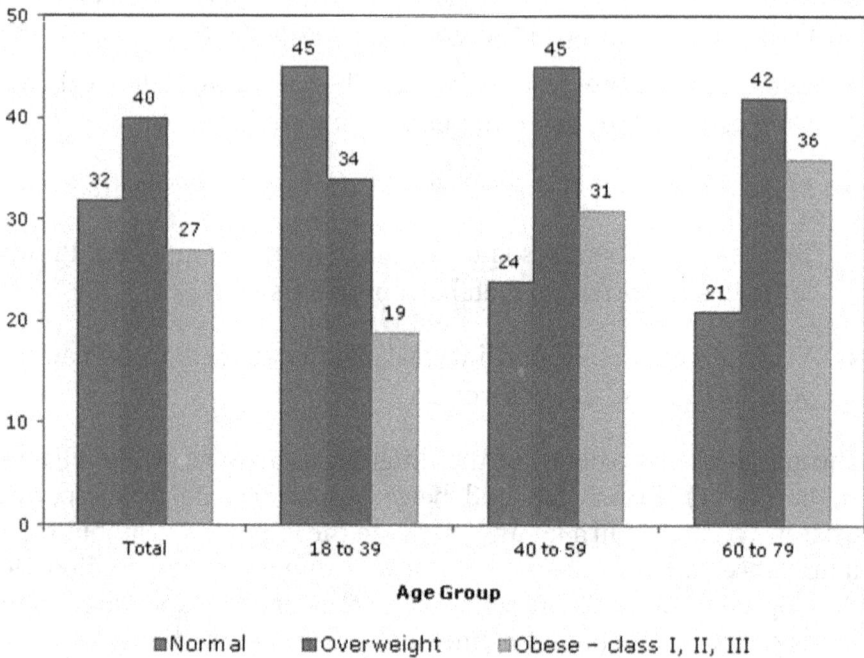

Figure 5 BMI of male Canadians

The risk is not the same for all populations. Data from Asian populations suggest higher risk of type 2 diabetes and CVD at lower BMI, and after deliberation, the WHO committee identified further potential public health action points (23.0, 27.5, 32.5, and 37.5 kg/m^2) along the continuum of BMI, and proposed methods by which countries could make decisions about the definitions of increased risk for their individual populations. If you are Asian, a BMI of 2 to 3 less, should be your goal. If you are a "big boned" Pacific Islander, two to three more. But, given 7 out of 10 Tongan females are obese even with the extra BMI, it is unsurprising about their poor health as a society.

Sports athletes, with low body fat and high muscle mass, also don't fit the normal BMI range. Endurance athletes such as marathon runners will be around 21, and most other athletes break the BMI test's grading scale since they carry more muscle mass than the average inactive person. As I have stated above, body weight is a component of four different body parts, and BMI testing doesn't differentiate between these components. That's why almost the entire USA football code (NFL) is considered severely obese! It is not why, ten years after finishing playing sport, many athletes are still obese. Fat has replaced muscle.

Waist Measurement – a Better Measure?

BMI does not provide an indication of fat distribution so the Canadians also measured waist circumference to provide an estimation of abdominal obesity. Abdominal fat can result in increased risk of health problems because excess fat around the waist and upper body is associated with greater health risks than fat located more in the hip and thigh areas. So if your waist circumference is more than 48" (102 cm) for men and 40" (88 cm) for women, you have an increased risk for developing health problems such as type 2 diabetes, coronary heart disease, and hypertension.

Percent (%)

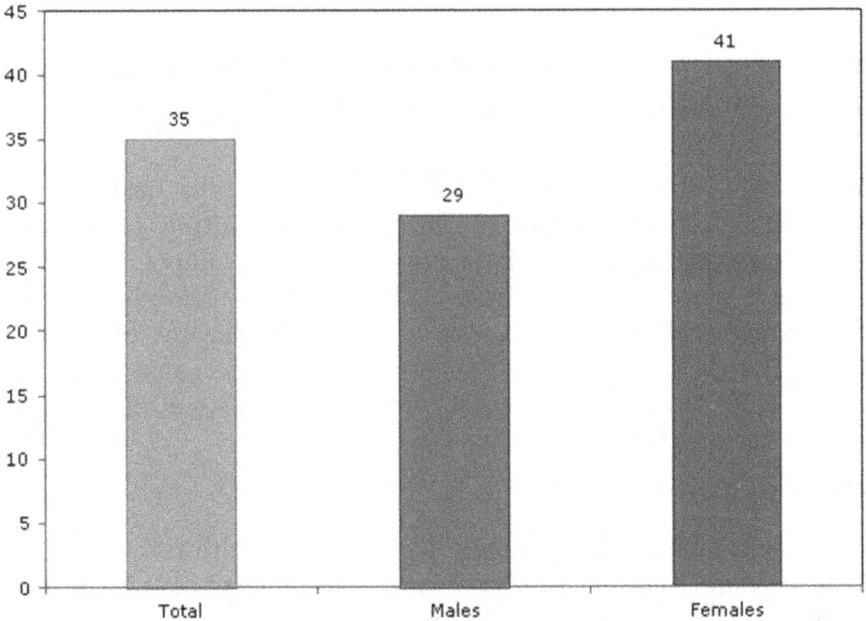

Figure 6 Health Risk % as per Waist Measure

So, how did the Canadians stack up? The average waist for all men was 95.1 cm, and for women it was 87.3 cm. Over 29% of males had a waist circumference associated with increased health risks, but over 41% of females are at risk. For males therefore either the BMI or the Waist Measure gave a good indication of health risk.

To further complicate this measure, weight is only one marker of health. There is a part of the population, a cohort, who are "lean on

37

the outside, fat on the inside." Doctors at the Mayo Clinic found that among a study of 14,000 people, those with a normal BMI, but a high waist-to-hip ratio, were the most likely to die of cardiovascular disease during the fourteen-year follow up, even more than those in obese ranges. BMI gives the same value to bone, good fat, bad fat, and muscle, and it doesn't make a lot of sense to mix all those things together.

The Europeans also have data to support the observation that a paunch poses its own particular risks, independently of fat stored elsewhere in the body. Riboli and the team looking at the EPIC study group of 366,000 Europeans reviewed the 14,723 who died over ten years. The lowest risk of death was at BMI of 25.3 for men, and 24.3 for women. However, the waist-to-hip ratio was a better measure. After controlling for factors such as overall obesity, the team found that the risk of premature death among subjects with a waist exceeding 120 cm (47.2") for men, and 100 cm (39.4") for women, was twice that for those whose waists were under 80 cm (31.5") for men and 65 cm (25.6") for women. For a given BMI, a 5 cm increase in waistline increased the risk of premature death by 17% in men and 13% in women.

Why is abdominal fat so bad? What is the generally held view of scientists? Tobias Pischon of the German Institute of Human Nutrition says, "Abdominal fat is not a mere energy depot, but it also releases messenger substances that can contribute to the development of chronic diseases. This may be the reason for the link." There are others who suggest more specific causes, but the research is still at early stages. We will discuss some more when discussing blood glucose and insulin.

Conclusion

Right now, take a minute. Check if you have a health risk. Get out a tape measure. Measure your waist at the belly button. Men: not your trouser beltline. Recent reports say that men underestimate their risk as they forget there is a stomach overhanging their trousers! Simple rule of thumb? If your waist is half your height, you have low risk of serious illness as a result of your weight. You might have higher health risk from genetics (cancer, cardiovascular), or other lifestyle behaviours (smoking, alcohol). The good news is you can do something about all those risks and improve your quality of life.

References

a. Canadian Guidelines for Body Weight Classification in Adults. Ottawa: Health Canada; 2003.

b. Obesity in Canada. Ottawa: Public Health Agency of Canada, Canadian Institute for Health Information; 2011. (see http://www.statcan.gc.ca/pub/82-625-x/2012001/article/11708-eng.htm)

c. Orpana H, Berthelot JM, Kaplan MS, Feeny DH, McFarland B, Ross NA. BMI and mortality: results from a national longitudinal study of Canadian adults. Obesity. 2010;18(1):214-8

d. BMI – should you believe your score? http://eas.com/nutrition/sports-nutrition/body-mass-index-should-you-believe-your-score

e. Shiwaku K, Anuurad E, Enkhmaa B, Kitajima K, Yamane Y. (2004) Appropriate BMI for Asian populations. The Lancet, Volume 363, Issue 9414, Page 1077, 27 doi:10.1016/S0140-6736(04)15856-X

f. Pischon T, Boeing H, Hoffman K, Bergmann M, et al (2008) General and Abdominal Adiposity and Risk of Death in Europe. N Engl J Med 2008; 359:2105-21, DOI: 10.1056/NEJMoa0801891

g. A Few Extra Pounds Won't Kill You—Really (2013) http://online.wsj.com/article/SB10001424127887323635504578215801377387088.html?mod=WSJ_hps_sections_health Journal of the American Medical Association.

h. Flegal K. (2013) Association of All-Cause Mortality With Overweight and Obesity Using Standard Body Mass Index Categories - A Systematic Review and Meta-analysis. JAMA. 2013;309(1):71-82. doi:10.1001/jama.2012.113905.

i. Robson, D (2008) Growing waistline poses weighty risk to health. http://www.newscientist.com/article/dn16028-growing-waistline-poses-weighty-risk-to-health.html#

j. Dodd G, Decherf S, Loh K, Simonds S, Wiede F, Balland E, Merry T, Münzberg H, Zhang Z, Kahn B, Neel B, Bence K, Andrews Z, Cowley M, Tiganis T. (2015) Leptin and Insulin Act on POMC Neurons to Promote the Browning of White Fat. Cell. 160 (1-2) p88-104. DOI: http://dx.doi.org/10.1016/j.cell.2014.12.022

CHAPTER 7
ABOUT THAT FAD DIET

Get the Facts

➤ Of over 660 diets out there, few have a good long term track record.

➤ Restricted calorie diets contribute to more weight gain. This is confirmed from experiments.

➤ Four out of ten regular dieters start their healthy eating regimes on Monday, but 10% have ditched it by Tuesday.

➤ Forty-percent of those who start diets on Monday have quit by the following weekend.

➤ Only 20% of those who start a diet continue for a month.

➤ Only 20% of those who start a diet continue for three months.

➤ Only 10% of those who start a diet continue for a year.

➤ After seven years – less than 8% have maintained that 10% weight loss.

➤ The Best Diet? The one you stay with!

Understand the Science

Diets have been investigated for over 100 years. The first decent trial was Benedict in 1918 from the Carnegie Institute who published data reporting on 12 men on restricted diets of 1400-2100 calories per day for a month. Researchers followed the men for three months. The outcome was hunger. At the end of the trial, the subjects had not only regained their weight, but put on 8 lb (3 kg). This type of trial has been done hundreds of times since, and the outcome is always the same. Ancel Keys did the same study with 30 male conscious objectors in 1944, to see what impact post World War II food restrictions would bring. On a 1600-calorie diet, or about half of what they were eating, they lost about 0.5 kg per week for the first three months. By the end of the rehab period, they had added 10 lb (4 kg) to their pre-diet weight, with over 50% more body fat. Not only that, but 20% dropped out for psychological reasons. These two experiments were the earliest meticulous studies with both food and behaviour measured. One lesson learned and published by Leibel in 1995 is that metabolism changes when you diet and as you age. This compensatory change means that for permanent reduction in weight, some degree of calorie reduction has to be permanent. Recent works suggest that leptin is very much involved, and at least a 200-calorie per day permanent reduction may be needed.

Gary Taubes recounts an interview with Hirsch from this Leibel work who said, "Of all the damn unsuccessful treatments, the treatment of weight reduction by diet for obese people just doesn't seem to work." Consider these calorie restrictions to popular in-vogue diets today. The popular HCG diet is 600 calories per day for three consecutive weeks, but it tries to mitigate the hunger with a homeopathic / hormonal "supplement". I know 3 people who went on this HCG diet. They all lost 15% or more of their weight, but will they keep it off after another 1 or 2 years? Science would say unlikely unless there is some change to lifestyle which avoids the weight gain.

There is a disconnect between the published policy guidelines and scientific evidence based on properly designed experiments. The USDA Dietary Guidelines for Americans suggests "eating fewer calories while increasing physical activity" and this policy is mirrored in guidelines across the world. Yet there is little or no evidence that "restricting calories" works, other than for short periods. Then you put on the weight again. Why do you think that Weight Watchers have "lifetime memberships?"

From the USDA in the 1990s, and reported in 2001/2002, the conclusion was, "*A study of diets of free-living adults in the USA showed that diets high in carbohydrate were both energy restrictive, and nutritious, and may be adopted for successful weight management.*" These studies did not look at dieting. They just looked at what people ate. Another myth that is part of the medical dogma is increasing physical activity reduces weight. There is no substantive evidence of this. You may simply eat more, due to hunger from exertion, or you may eat less because of the motivation from the exercise experience.

Size matters. People around the world are getting bigger. Today's average American male and female are about 1" (2.5 cm) taller than they were in the 1960s. (USA Centers for Disease Control data). If you are an air traveller, that means just a slight increase in thigh length, but an even bigger factor contributing to the perception that economy-class seats are less roomy than they once were is the increasing weight. An average American male aged 30 to 39 is now

41

19 lb (8.7 kg) heavier than in the 1960s. The figure for the female population is almost 24 lb (11 kg). And that is not just from obesity.

The number one thing most diets have in common is that they are not designed for people to be able to stick with them. Many of us equate the word diet with short-term deprivation, something you go "on" and ultimately go "off." In a survey, Alpro, a UK food company, found that of those who diet regularly, two out of five quit within the first seven days, one out of five last a month, and the same number — just 20% — last to the three-month mark. Just 5% last a year. Research trials can be good, but seldom measure behaviours of dieters; often they are carried out in conjunction with support throughout the research period. Most dieters don't get that support, and some actually experience negative counter-support from family or friends.

Diets are often more similar than you imagine. According to a recent Consumer Reports Magazine, these diets all had average daily calories of between 1450 and 1660 calories per day. All had about 20 to 30 g of fibre, and between 8 and 15 g of vegetables and fruits. The levels of protein are also similar. The differences are the amount of fat, saturated fat and carbohydrates. You can see that the Ornish and Jenny Craig both have high carbohydrate, whereas the Atkins (ongoing phase) is fat with a little extra protein.

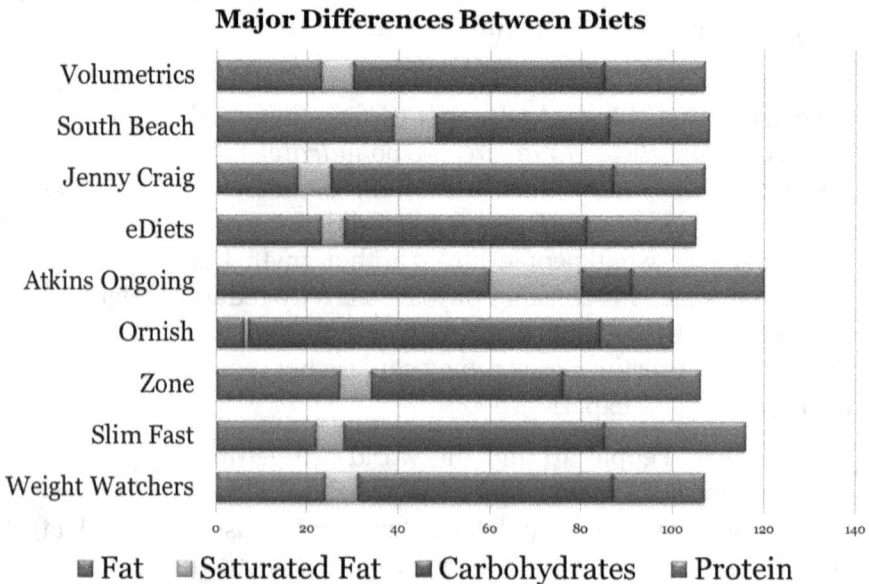

Major Differences Between Diets

■Fat ■Saturated Fat ■Carbohydrates ■Protein

Figure 7 Comparison of popular diets

42

Five Lies the Weight Industry Wants You to Believe

Dr Rick Kausman has run a weight management and eating disorder clinic for 25 years, is a director of the Butterfly Foundation, a fellow of the Australian Society for Psychological Medicine, and authored a book titled, *If Not Dieting, Then What?* His take on why diets fail is very similar, and his book is well worth a read to understand dieting from the psychological perspective.

1. *"Weight loss is a simple matter of willpower."* Weight loss is both difficult, and probably the wrong motivation for dieting. Kausman says, "Willpower is a terrific skill to have, but it's a short-term skill. You use willpower for things like studying for exams. But you wouldn't have enough willpower to force yourself to study for exams every day for the rest of your life." He makes a great point when it comes to trying to use willpower for a life-long eating plan.

2. *"You can shame other people thin."* The TV reality show, *The Biggest Loser*, takes a pretty good whack at humiliating fat people. Compassion, understanding the science, psychology, and the barriers society has put in place are a much better place to start.

3. *"Doctors and health professionals are experts in weight management."* They are competent professionals in many areas, but in my experience, medical professionals, in general, are particularly poor sources for information on weight loss issues. They merely recite the AMA or similar standard line of exercise and moderation, the drug company line, or the surgery line. I've challenged my local GP, but the dogma from the Australian Medical Association remains his line.

4. *"The weight loss industry leaders are weight loss experts."* It is astonishing that companies such as Weight Watchers have life members. What does that say, but that they know their business is about failed diets? They masquerade as health providers, but their main interest is sales, and repeat sales are usually the most profitable. People must keep in mind that these companies have a "product" they are trying to sell. Some are food production businesses (Lite and Easy). The marketing spin is great, but the outcomes are poor.

5. *"Diets lead to weight loss."* Unfortunately, weight loss programs are more likely to lead to eating disorders. The extremes that dominate most weight-loss diets can create imbalances and deficiencies in the body. In simplest of terms, extreme fad diets

can get the body off track, and that can lead to severe health issues. The Cabbage Soup Diet is a great example of nonsense.

The abstract of Mann et al, in 2007, summed it up pretty well when it talked about Medicare Policy in the USA and whether dieting is an effective treatment for obesity. They reviewed over 31 studies, which showed one-third to two-thirds of dieters regain more weight than they lost on their diets. (Mann also said these studies were probably flawed and underestimated the issue.) The studies did not provide consistent evidence that dieting results in significant health improvements, regardless of weight change. In summary, there is little support for the notion that diets lead to lasting weight loss or health benefits. This is hard for overweight people to accept. They want to believe that they can simply go on a diet and will lose the weight and everything will be fine. Nothing could be further from the truth. That is supported by much scientific research.

These are sobering conclusions, yet anyone who has been on diets over their life can attest to them. If you are one of the few people who have achieved long-term weight stability at a healthy range after using a single diet, you are the "abnormal" in Western society. It would be a great research study as to why you actually had success and did not succumb to yo-yo dieting as most do. As it turns out, researchers have looked at these very (rare) people. The National Weight Loss Control Registry out of University of Colorado has been paying attention to this since 1994. If you have lost 30 lb (13 kg) and kept it off for over one year, you are eligible to be part of their database. Common themes for those who have been successful include:

- 78% eat breakfast every day.

- 75% weigh themselves at least once a week.

- 62% watch less than ten hours of TV per week.

- 90% exercise, on average, about one hour per day.

These behaviours make sense – they tend to reflect a "lifestyle change," more so than just a fad diet. Eating breakfast, and especially protein at breakfast, has been shown to reduce food intake later in the day. Weighing is a reflection of ongoing behavioural change, and less TV watching and exercise may demonstrate the value of avoidance tactics that discourage snacking (mental and social behaviours).

Don't get me wrong. Losing weight has substantial health benefits. For every 0.45 lb (1 kg) of body mass, expect a 3 to 8% reduction in health risks. If you are overweight, a loss of 10% of your body mass halves your health risk. No pill can do that. Diets may be a good strategy either physically or emotionally to lose that 10% of your body mass quickly. Whichever diet you choose to lose weight with is less important than the strategies to maintain that weight loss for life. I advocate the 80/20 rule. What is the easiest diet and which is more sustainable long term?

Is There any Difference Between Diets?

There are few studies comparing diets that don't have gaping scientific flaws! Shai and colleagues in 2007 compared a low-fat, calorie-restricted diet to a Mediterranean, calorie-restricted diet, to a low-carbohydrate Atkins Diet, unrestricted in calories.

First flaw. This trial was confounded with a number of factors. It was held at a research centre and the main meal of the participants was a controlled meal provided at the cafeteria. Two of the diets were restricted, the Atkins was not. The authors made an attempt to assess what their subjects were eating before the trial started, and then after six, twelve, and twenty-four months.

Indicator	Low Fat	Mediterra nean	Low carbohy- drates (Atkins)
Mean Weight Loss	2.9 kg	4.4 kg	4.7 kg
Mean loss, completed	3.3 kg	4.6 kg	5.5 kg
Ratio Total cholesterol to HDL reduction	12%	15%	20%
Fasting plasma glucose (those 36 with diabetes)	No change	Better	No change
Total calorie reduction	572		535
Carbohydrate intake reduction	330		520
Fat calories reduction	170		15
Dropout rate (24 months)	10%	10%	20%

Second flaw: self-reporting in these types of studies has to be taken with a grain of salt. Most people under estimate their calories, especially those from carbohydrates. Third Flaw. The "low fat" diet was the normal food at the centre, so this group made no change to their diet! It should be called the control group. It was also mostly male (81%), and weight loss was pretty small.

The figure below is the predicted absolute mean change in body weight for participants in the low-fat and low-carbohydrate diet groups, based on a random-effects linear model. Adherence was 95% at year one, and 85% at two years, which is expected for experiments. Normally 80% give up dieting, so the difference in adherence is not statistically important.

It looks like after 24 months on the low fat diet, it was actually carbohydrate reduction that accounted for 60% of reduced calories consumed. The Atkins Diet reduced carbohydrates by 90%, but was nearly twice as effective. So should you have a low-fat or a low-carbohydrate diet?

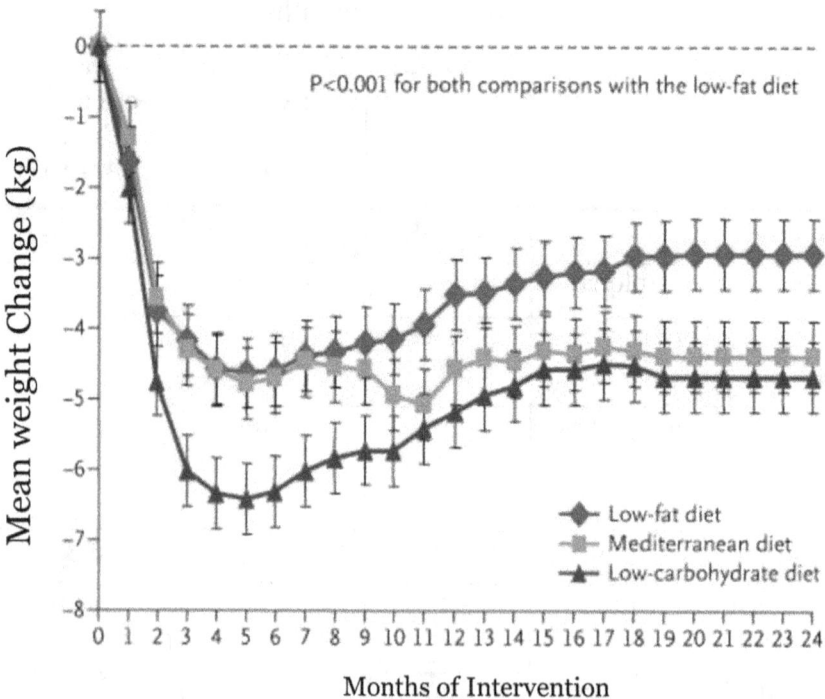

Figure 8 Comparison of diets (Shai).

The authors say, *"Mediterranean and low-carbohydrate diets are effective alternatives to low-fat diets. The more favorable effects on lipids (with the low-carbohydrate diet) and on glycaemic control (with the Mediterranean Diet) suggest that personal preferences and metabolic considerations might inform individualized tailoring of dietary interventions."*

As previously state, lopsided study had two diets calorie restricted with one not, the majority of the food was provided. The compliance rate of 80% is not what goes on in the real world. Even with these odd experimental conditions, the conclusions are clear. If you want more weight loss and good metabolic changes, go with a low-carbohydrate diet. The only group that is going to have trouble with the diet is vegetarians, as vegetarians tend to eat a lot of high-carbohydrate grains to replace meat or other protein. A follow-up study, four years later, checked 259 of those participants. Weight loss in the low-fat group was 0.6 kg, 1.7 kg in the low-carbohydrate, and 3.1 kg in the Mediterranean group. This was for men with a BMI of 31, and after 6 years. The authors of the paper claim *"long lasting favorable post-intervention effects."* Really? Who are they kidding. All these diets were good for was halting the obesity by stealth I discuss in a later chapter. It appears to me that it simply confirms diets do not work long term.

Bariatric Surgery

Why is there such an increase in laparoscopic adjustable gastric banding (LAGB) and gastric bypass surgery (RYGB)? Is it because obese people have tried and failed previous diets, or is it the only hope for morbidly obese people? The numbers and cost are becoming staggering, and only seem to be getting worse. Is this an effective strategy for the obesity pandemic?

In Australia in 2011, there were 11,950 claims on Medicare Benefit, representing 1% of the 200,000 morbidly obese citizens. Lap band procedures require adjustments, so there were a further 13,000 adjustments that year. In the USA in 2009, over 220,000 surgeries were done. A Belgium study following up 12 years after LAGB surgery found half of the bands had to be removed, and 40% had major complications. Average weight loss was about 42% of excess weight. Another study, from the Longitudinal Assessment of Bariatric Surgery (LABS) Consortium, a multicenter cohort study assessing the safety and effectiveness of USA bariatric surgical procedures tracked patients (mostly female-79%) for three years after surgery. A total of 1,738 participants underwent gastric bypass surgery and 601 laparoscopic gastric banding and the patients lost 32% and 16% median weight, respectively. Health issues also dropped. However, there is some interesting review work on the behaviour of those with surgery. Why didn't all of the patients lose weight? Why do some patients continue to eat and not see weight reductions or health improvements?

Linda Bacon and Lucy Aphramor from HAES (Health at Every Size) say we need a paradigm shift towards diets especially from the medical perspective, and *"Interventions should be constructed from a holistic perspective, where consideration is given to physical, emotional, social, occupational, intellectual, spiritual, and ecological aspects of health."*

Conclusion

In conclusion, diets are singularly ineffective long term. Bariatric surgery appears just as ineffective but costing $14,000 upwards, is a pretty drastic alternative. Health complications when patients are morbidly obese are also extremely costly, and death from morbid obesity is singularly unattractive. Many in the world are prepared to spend lots of money on cosmetic surgery. Is there a simple solution? What can change the dismal results from dieting? I would suggest we have to frame the obesity problem differently, and use a holistic approach. I suggest the simple 3 legged stool is a good starting position.

References

a. Shai I, Schwarzfuchs D, Henkin Y, Shahar D, Witkow S, Greenberg I, Golan R, et al, for the Dietary Intervention Randomized Controlled Trial (DIRECT) Group. (2008) /NEJMoa0708681.Weight loss with a low-carbohydrate, Mediterranean, or low-fat diet. N Engl J Med. 2008 Jul 17; 359(3):229-41. doi: 10.1056/NEJMoa0708681.
b. Schwarzfuchs D, Golan R. (2012) Four-Year Follow-up after Two-Year Dietary Interventions. N Engl J Med 367:1373-1374 DOI: 10.1056/NEJMc1204792
c. Bacon L, Aphramor L. (2011) Weight Science: Evaluating the Evidence for a Paradigm Shift. Nutrition Journal 10:9 doi:10.1186/1475-2891-10-9
d. Sass C. (2013) 5 Reasons Most Diets Fail Within 7 Days www.huffingtonpost.com/2013/09/24/why-diets-dont-work_n_3975610.html

e. Leibel R, Rosenbaum M, Hirsch J. (1995) Changes in Energy Expenditure Resulting from Altered Body Weight N Engl J Med 1995; 332:621-628 doi: 10.1056/NEJM199503093321001

f. Kennedy E, Bowman S, Spence J, Freedman M, King J. (2001) Popular diets: correlation to health, nutrition, and obesity. J Am Diet Assoc. Vol 101(4):411-20 PMID:11320946

g. Bowman S, Spence J. (2002) A comparison of low-carbohydrate vs. high-carbohydrate diets: energy restriction, nutrient quality and correlation to body mass index. J Am Coll Nutr. 2002 Jun;21(3):268-74. PMID: 12074255

h. Himpens J, Cadière GB, Bazi M, Vouche M, Cadière B, Dapri G. (2011) Long-term Outcomes of Laparoscopic Adjustable Gastric Banding Arch Surg. 2011;146(7):802-807. doi:10.1001/archsurg.2011.45.

i. Courcoulas A; et al. (2013) Weight Change and Health Outcomes at 3 Years After Bariatric Surgery Among Individuals With Severe Obesity. JAMA. Online doi:10.1001/jama.2013.280928. Ref 1

j. Mann T, Tomiyama A.J, Westling E, Lew A, Samuels B, Chatman J. (2007) Medicare's search for effective obesity treatments: diets are not the answer. Am Psychol. 62(3):220-33. PMID:17469900

k. National Weight Control Registry. Research Findings. http://www.nwcr.ws/Research/published%20research.htm

CHAPTER 8
WESTERN DIET VERSUS NATIVE DIETS

Get the Facts:

➤ When populations that live on coconut and fish get sugar and flour, they develop Western diseases, such as high levels of diabetes, gout, osteoarthritis, and associated weight gain.

➤ The side effect of the SAD (Standard American Diet) is most likely a global pandemic of metabolic syndrome and resultant obesity crisis.

Understand the Science

Gary Taubes is a science writer. For many years his specialty was particle physics, but since early 2000 he has focused on writing science books and articles about nutrition. His work is illuminative about how science can be overridden by dogma, and poor or compromised science. In *The Diet Delusion*, he details the work of Captain T.L. (Peter) Cleave and George Campbell and concludes they had it right with their thoughts about "saccharine disease." He says modern nutritionists who are proponents of the low-fat diet have it wrong.

Cleave and Campbell published *Diabetes, Coronary Thrombosis and the Saccharine Disease* in 1966. They argued that all common chronic diseases of the Western societies, including heart disease, obesity, diabetes, peptic ulcers, and appendicitis were manifestations of a single primary disorder defined as "refined-carbohydrate disease," and they opted to call it "saccharine disease" (related to sugar). This saccharine disease took up to two decades or more to show up in the general population of various locations, and also was dependent on what sort of carbohydrates, and how quickly sugar went from a 6 kg or so per person per year, to the Western level of 40 kg (about 88 lb) or more. These meticulously documented observational studies were based on thousands (60,000 up to 600,000) of hospital patients.

It is a simple and reasonable conclusion. If the primary change in traditional diets with Westernization was the addition of sugar, flour, and white rice, and this in turn occurred shortly before the appearance of chronic disease, then the most likely explanation was those processed, refined carbohydrates were the cause of the disease.

I would suggest if these carbohydrates were added to any diet, no matter how replete with the essential protein, vitamins, minerals, and fatty acids, it would lead to these diseases. This would explain why the same diseases appeared after Westernization in cultures that lived almost exclusively on animal products: the Inuit, Masai and Samburu nomads, Australian Aborigines, or Native Americans of the Great Plains, as well as in primarily agrarian cultures such as the Hunza in the Himalayas or the Kikuyu in Kenya.

Regrettably, during this same period, other researchers in the USA were well into the doctrine, that the rise in cardio vascular disease was due to dietary fat and cholesterol, and the argument that chronic illness was due to fat and meat consumption and not excess sugar and refined carbohydrate consumption.

Recent scientific research in mice and short lived animals is conclusive: when sugar is added to animal diets, it causes these diseases. The complication for humans is we are longer lived animals. Adding sugar to human diets may take decades for disease to show up. However, removing sugar from diet reduces weight and improves metabolic health rapidly and can have profound short term value. If you look at CRON communities (Calorie Restricted Optimal Nutrition) whom I discuss elsewhere in the book, or Paleo dieters, much of that anecdotal evidence may now be found.

About the same time that Cleave and Campbell published their book, Ian Prior, a young epidemiologist from New Zealand, went to Tokelau in 1967. He followed their work and used their techniques to track changing lifestyles and diets of Tokelauans. He tracked them both in Tokelau and also in New Zealand, as over 70% of the Tokelauans migrated to NZ. He had two communities – those who stayed, and those who migrated to Auckland, New Zealand. Additionally, other studies compared two populations of Polynesians living on atolls near the equator, and the relative effects of saturated fat and dietary cholesterol. Coconut is their chief source of energy with up to 63% of their energy. Vascular disease was uncommon, and there was no evidence of the high saturated fat intake having a harmful effect in these populations. It appears that the Tokelauans were similar to other Polynesian communities.

The community that stayed in Tokelau showed sugar consumption rose from 3 kg sugar per person, per year in 1960 to 30 kg by 1980. Flour went from 5 kg per year to 25 kg. The community that migrated from Tokelau to New Zealand had a bigger dietary change. Fat consumption went down, and carbohydrate intake went up from 202 g/day to over 251 g/day, and cholesterol levels rose from 112 to 350mg. What was the outcome from 30 years of increased flour and sugar consumption? Exceptionally high incidence of diabetes, gout, osteoarthritis, and associated weight gain was the result! The data from this extended study mirrors that of Cleave's study and are consistent throughout most societies that have, over the past 50 years, adopted the Western diet, which is high in simple carbohydrates and sugar.

China and India are further examples of how the Western diet and its consequences have infiltrated the world. Obesity is no longer solely a Western epidemic. It is a disease of civilization. In 2011, over 1.3 million Chinese, and 0.98 million Indians died from related causes of type 2 diabetes. Qatar leads the world with one in four of its citizens afflicted with diabetes. In India, nationwide prevalence is at 9%, but more than doubles to 20% in its more prosperous southern cities.

There is absolutely no doubt that refined carbohydrates and sugar have a significant impact on disease.

However, the question remains whether the increase in disease is primarily brought on by the consumption of sugar or by the consumption of refined carbohydrates such as flour or rice. It is difficult to separate the two since both increased with the adoption of the Western diet. We can conclude that since fat and protein consumption have remained unchanged or declined with the advent of the SAD (Standard American Diet) diet, they have not played a role in the increase of disease.

The Inuit Studies

If the work presented by Cleave and Campbell, or Prior, is to be dismissed as anthropological, and not medically based, there are other well-documented cases as well. The Danes have excellent health records, and tracked the Inuit closely for over 100 years. Friborg writes:

Inuit (or Eskimos) inhabit the circumpolar region, with most living in Alaska, northwest Canada, and Greenland. Although malignant diseases were believed to be almost non-existent in Inuit populations during the beginning of the 20th century, the increasing life expectancy within these populations showed a distinct pattern, characterized by a high risk of Epstein-Barr virus-associated carcinomas of the nasopharynx and salivary glands, and a low risk of tumours common in white populations, including cancer of the prostate, testis, and haemopoietic system. Both genetic and environmental factors seem to be responsible for this pattern. During the second half of the 20th century, Inuit societies underwent major changes in lifestyle and living conditions, and the risk of lifestyle-associated tumours, especially cancers of the lung, colon, and breast, increased considerably after changes in smoking, diet, and reproductive factors.

The high incidence of these "traditional" types of cancer among the Inuit is hypothesized to have a strong genetic basis. (Friborg)

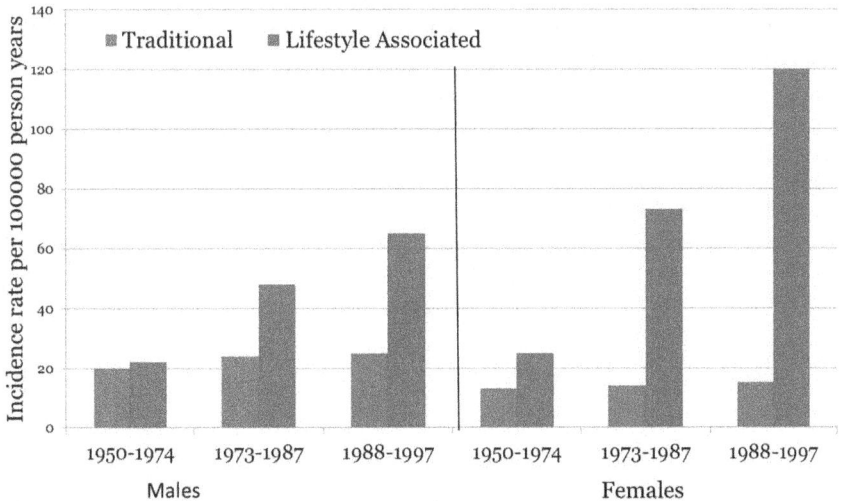

Figure 9 Traditional and lifestyle-associated cancers

Nevertheless, some also believe these cancers to be associated with practices that were arguably not common among the ancestral Inuit, such as preservation of fish and meat with salt. Genetic markers in the present-day Inuit population show a shared Asian heritage, which is consistent with the higher incidence of similar types of cancer among Asians, particularly those consuming large amounts of salt-preserved foods. The Inuit are believed to originate from East Asia, having crossed the Bering Strait about 5,000 years ago. To grasp the changes that have occurred in Inuit disease and health, look at the chart from Friborg. The "traditional cancers" are nasopharynx, salivary gland, and oesophageal, and the "life-style" associated cancers include lung, colon, rectum, and female breast cancers. The incidence of traditional cancers has not increased for both sexes. However, lifestyle cancers doubled for males and increased four to five times for females. What are the lifestyle changes in the Westernized diet and culture? One is increased consumption of tobacco. The other is a shift from animal protein and fat to refined carbohydrates as the main source of energy.

Conclusion

In conclusion, while these studies are observational studies, they are measures on the whole population and not just a subset of the population. There are few statistical "adjustments" needed. While correlation does not mean causation, it is hard to draw any other conclusion that the SAD (Standard American Diet) must be a major factor in the decrease of health. Health issues such as Cardio Vascular Disease, Cancer, diabetes and poor dental health. Furthermore, none of these communities with high saturated fat diets appeared to cause health issues. The introduction of simple carbohydrates appears the most likely cause.

References

a. Cleave and Campbell (1966): The Saccharine Disease. Conditions caused by the Taking of Refined Carbohydrates, such as Sugar and White Flour. Wright & Sons, 1974 pp 6– 13. ISBN 0 7236 0368 5 http://www.hcvsociety.org/files/Diet/The-Saccharine-Disease.pdf
b. Taubes, Gary (2009). The Diet Delusion. Pub. Vermillion. 640pp. ISBN-13: 978-0091924287
c. Prior, I, (1981) Cholesterol, coconuts, and diet on Polynesian atolls: a natural experiment: the Pukapuka and Tokelau island studies. Am J Clin Nutr. 1981 Aug; 34(8):1552-61.
d. Hooper, A. et al. (1992) Migration and Health in a Small Society: The Case of Tokelau (Research Monographs on Human Population Biology) Oxford University Press pp468 ISBN-13: 978-0198542629
e. Friborg JT, Melbye M. (2008) Cancer patterns in Inuit populations. The Lancet Oncology. 2008; 9:892-900. doi:10.1016/S1470-2045(08)70231-6

CHAPTER 9
BIGGEST LOSER TV FAIL

Get the Facts

➤ In an environment where stigma surrounds obesity, people do not do well with weight loss and do not succeed in keeping off any weight that they lose.
➤ Watching TV shows such as The Biggest Loser makes our attitude more anti-fat.
➤ The show encourages viewers to think that weight control is all about willpower and personal behaviour.
➤ People who are concerned about their own weight watch more episodes of the show and are more affected by the show.

Understand the Science

Dr Jina Yoo, an associate professor of communication at the University of Missouri, St. Louis, believes that shows such as *The Biggest Loser* encourage anti-fat attitudes by leading viewers to believe weight control comes down to the willpower of individuals. She also believes that they encourage unhealthy weight loss practices and increase the stigma surrounding obesity. People who watch reality weight-loss shows are more likely to have fattist attitudes. Also, people who are more concerned with their own weight watch more episodes of the program. Dr Yoo goes on to claim that this negative perception is fuelled by viewers repeatedly watching obese contestants lose up to 100 lb (45kg) in three months. Yoo says the show frames obesity as a matter of personal responsibility and behavioural solutions, ignoring societal or environmental contributors.

The contestants are bound by legal agreements so getting data out is difficult. It may be the only clear winners in this unrealistic entertainment are the sponsors and advertisers of supplements, fitness gyms and personal trainers, and the diet industry. All are beneficiaries of the dogma that weight reduction is a matter of overcoming gluttony and slothfulness. It perpetuates the myth that exercise will reduce weight.

References

a. Yoo JH. (2013). No clear winner: Effects of The Biggest Loser on the stigmatization of obese persons. Health Communication, 28, 294-303.

CHAPTER 10
PALEO DIET – NEARLY RIGHT

Get the Facts

➤ Not since Palaeolithic times has it been so fashionable to eat like a hunter-gatherer. The Paleo Diet is more a lifestyle than a diet, per se. The Paleo Diet, which is also called "Caveman" or "Stone Age" Diet, advocates eating pre-agrarian foods. If our hunter-gatherer ancestors didn't eat it, Paleo eaters don't want to eat it either.

➤ This diet requires dieters to avoid nutrient–sparse food, and the consequences are that sugar and processed food are removed from the diet. No bread, no added sugar, no potatoes, no rice, and no processed foods. Some Paleo dieters even avoid alcohol.

➤ Paleo eaters choose grass-fed beef and lamb, pastured chicken, fish, fruit and vegetables. Many avoid solanum genus vegetables such as eggplant and tomato.

➤ In an ideal Paleo diet, food would be wild animals, which have less fat and saturated fat than farmed animals, and plants would be those that you can forage or grow yourself. This might be difficult in our modern society.

➤ It is easy to see the appeal of following this diet. The list of forbidden foods closely resembles the foods Harvard Medical School counsels patients to avoid! It is whole food, grain-free although somewhat meat-heavy.

➤ The food critics say the Paleo Diet is complicated, a fad diet and hard to follow, but most adherents say it is simple and makes good common sense.

Understand the Science

The Paleo Diet comes from Loren Cordain, professor emeritus at Colorado State University, and in his 7th book comes out in early 2015.

There are both pros and cons to consider about the Paleo Diet. Cavemen did not appear to have a short life. Their average lifespan

57

was estimated at about 72 years, and short life was probably mostly due to the other hazards such as poisonous food and accidents or serious trauma. Other pros about the diet are:

- Avoid Processed foods. There is no arguing that this is a very good thing when it comes to enjoying good health.

- The Paleo Diet encourages participants to pair exercise with diet to stay strong, lean, and muscular. The encouraged exercise is often the SIT or HIT exercise (see the chapter on High Intensity Workouts), or the Cross-Fit which is a more natural form of exercise than gym work.

- Paleo Diet discourages use of heavy salt, with no processed food.

- Paleo Diet encourages eating good fats, and to avoid manufactured fats such as canola.

- To eat a true Paleo Diet (or close to it) most of the time, you have to cook for yourself, although it is becoming more common to find Paleo-type foods in restaurants and stores. Cooking one's own food further helps with avoiding any unknown chemicals and additives common to store-bought or restaurant food.

- Paleo Dieters don't count calories. They eat as much as they want of lean meat, vegetables, fruit, and good fat, and yet, those on the Paleo Diet reduce their body fat.

- The diet omits legume vegetables such as beans and the story is that legumes are "toxic poisons" and legumes are inferior foods. While they are lower in zinc and iron than meat, most vegetarians and communities get by quite happily with a legume based diet. It may be that legumes gave Cordain digestive upset and gas, and hence his recommendation to avoid legumes. I have an allergy to raw legumes such as peanuts, peas, and beans. I have tracked it down to a protein most likely. If the legume is cooked, I have no reaction.

The ten principles espoused by Mark Sisson from the Daily Apple website outlines the main principles of the Paleo Diet. As you look through these 10 items, diet is only one of the lifestyle changes advocated.

1. Eat lots of animals, insects, and seasonal plants (random, nonlinear varied diet).
2. Move a lot at a slow pace I.e. a low aerobic pace.
3. Lift heavy things to build muscle.
4. Run really fast every once in a while to build fast twitch muscle.
5. Get lots of sleep.
6. Play to build social bonds and to reduce stress.
7. Get some sunlight every day for vitamin D.
8. Avoid trauma.
9. Avoid poisonous things, and that includes legumes and beans.
10. Use your mind.

In one small randomized cross-over study of 29 subjects with type 2 diabetes, over a three-month study period, a Palaeolithic Diet improved glycaemic control and several cardiovascular risk factors, compared to a diabetes diet. A Palaeolithic Diet was more satiating per calorie than a Mediterranean Diet. Men have touted the Paleo Diet as one that is finally right for them because the diet encourages eating lots of meat rather than just salads for every meal. (Just like the Atkins.)

Sisson, from the Daily Apple, also espouses an 80/20 rule, allowing one day a week to eat anything you like to help ensure long-term adherence to the Paleo Diet. The Paleo Diet is excellent for the purpose of eliminating excess sugar and simple carbohydrates from the diet with the exception of occasional raw honey or pure maple syrup, and sugar naturally within whole fruit.

Conclusion

In conclusion, and with a cynic's viewpoint, I suggest the Paleo diet story is mostly fabricated. We don't actually know what our ancestors ate; including whether they ate grain, nuts, seeds and legumes. What they ate more likely depended on their locale and climate. Our agriculture has been transformed over the past 100 years. Someone from the early 1900's, let alone our 30,000-year-old ancestor, would not recognize the plants in the fruit and vegetable bins of our food stores. It seems to encourage people to purchase "Paleo" meals and (surprise!) supplements. Not everything is wrong with this diet, and I make an exception and purchase a Paleo mayonnaise which has none of the normal fructose / canola / vegetable oils / fillers that regular mayonnaise has. However, given that the focus on the diet is to eat whole foods and avoid the pitfalls of SAD (Standard American Diet), it probably achieves the desired outcomes, if only explained by a great imagination. If it works for you and results come in, great. Those ten principles from Sisson have a good basis in evidence based science.

A trendy diet which makes one feel special could also be part of its popularity. Anything that helps behavioural changes, or that second leg of the 3-legged stool has value.

References

a. Loren Cordain (2010). The Paleo Diet: Lose Weight and Get Healthy by Eating the Foods You Were Designed to Eat. Wiley. Pp 272 ISBN-13: 978-0471413905

b. Mark Sisson. (2013) The Primal Blueprint: Reprogram your genes for effortless weight loss, vibrant health, and boundless energy Primal Nutrition. PP 360 ISBN-13: 978-0982207789 http://www.marksdailyapple.com/

c. Mark Sisson. (2013). A Metabolic Paradigm Shift, or Why Fat is the Preferred Fuel for Human Metabolism. http://www.marksdailyapple.com/a-metabolic-paradigm-shift-fat-carbs-human-body-metabolism

d. John Durant (2013) The Paleo Manifesto: Ancient Wisdom for Lifelong Health. Harmony. PP 368. ISBN-13: 978-0307889171

e. Jönsson T, Granfeldt Y, Ahrén B, Branell UC, Pålsson G, Hansson A, Söderström M, Lindeberg S. (2009) Beneficial effects of a Palaeolithic diet on cardiovascular risk factors in type 2 diabetes: a randomized cross-over pilot study. Cardiovascular Diabetology 2009, 8:35 doi:10.1186/1475-2840-8-35

f. 6 Health Lessons From The Paleo Diet (2013). http://www.huffingtonpost.com/2013/09/13/healthy-paleo-diet-tips_n_3900690.html

g. Nichols G, Hillier T, Brown J. (2008) Normal Fasting Plasma Glucose and Risk of Type 2 Diabetes Diagnosis. The American Journal of Medicine. 121 (6), P 519-524 doi:10.1016/j.amjmed.2008.02.026

CHAPTER 11
ATKINS DIET – CLOSE, BUT NOT EXACTLY

Get the Facts

➢ Atkins Diet is a low-carbohydrate diet, with a plan, cookbooks, pre-packaged products, and a large number of followers.

➢ Atkins claimed most people can lose up to 2 lb (1 kg) per week at the start, slowing to 1 lb (0.5 kg) towards the final or maintenance phase.

➢ Dieters reduce their total carbohydrates from the average 150 to 200g per day in the Standard American Diet (SAD) to less than 20g during the diet, and no more than 50g during maintenance. Dieters count carbohydrates rather than calories.

➢ Why the diet succeeds has been variously, and incorrectly, explained. Was it due to the magical properties of ketosis; or the extra fat consumption; or the higher protein. From recent studies, the diet works the same as low carbohydrate diets. When you stop feeding yourself carbohydrates, your body does what it is designed to do and your appetite reduces. You eat less.

➢ The Atkins Diet focuses on weight loss, not health. It assumes lowered weight equals better health. Weight management definitely contributes to better health, so you can't go wrong there, as long as all health issues are addressed and not just the weight loss.

➢ Dieters achieve better weight reduction and longer term compliance (twice as much) compared with low calorie diets.

➢ If this diet works for you – use it. Other diets, including low carbohydrate, or a sugar free diet, achieves the same outcomes and for the same reasons.

Understand the Science

Unless you've been living on Mars, chances are you've heard of the Atkins Diet, and you probably know someone who has tried it, if you haven't done so yourself. (One in eleven Americans were on it in

2003/2004.) After all, it's a diet that sounds too good to be true. Start the day with bacon and eggs, snack on chunks of cheese, top coffee with cream, and feast on steaks fried in butter. The hardest thing for many Atkins Dieters is giving up toast with that bacon and eggs, crackers with that cheese, or sugar in their coffee.

The brief history is that in 1958, Robert Atkins, a cardiologist and an obese, failed dieter, read Pennington's Weight Reduction paper. He had tried various diets to control his obesity without success. Atkins may have even read Leith's 1961 paper where patients lost weight on the "liberal" Pennington diet. The Pennington diet worked for Atkins, and he began to put his own patients on this diet, and it worked for them as well. Shunned by the establishment, his book, *The Atkins Diet*, and his "fad" diet were adopted by a huge following. The diet is officially called the Atkins Nutritional Approach and is a low-carbohydrate diet. Atkins wrote a number of books, and since his death from slipping on an icy street and suffering a brain injury in 2003, others have carried on with *The New Atkins for a New You* in 2010, and a cookbook in 2011. There is some controversy about Atkins death. The coroner's report was leaked, and Atkins was 117 kg (258 lb). Some from within the Atkins Foundation said he was 88 kg (195 lb) on admission to hospital, and gained fluid. Either way, it appears Atkins was overweight and had high blood pressure.

Atkins believed one needed to keep up essential nutrients, and got into the business of pre-packaged foods and nutrients. They are not exactly the typical foods you'd find on the shopping lists of most slim people who had grown up with the idea that a low-fat diet is the best way to lose weight. The catch is that filling up on high-fat foods needs to be balanced by giving up most carbohydrates, including bread, potatoes, pasta, rice, chocolate, crisps, biscuits, cake, and even fruit, milk, and some starchy vegetables in the early stages of the diet. Despite millions having tried it, nutrition experts aren't absolutely convinced that it's a sound diet that works for the long-term. Studies over the past ten years have shown it is probably better than most diets, and not as bad as others.

The A to Z Weight Loss Study (2007, Stanford University Medical School) compared the Atkins Diet with the Zone, Ornish, and LEARN diets in a randomized group of 311 obese premenopausal women over a period of 12 months. They had weekly instruction for two months, then a follow-up at ten months. Weight loss (10 lb, 4.7 kg) was twice as high for the Atkins Diet compared to the other three diets (5 lb, 2 kg). Secondary factors such as HDL-C, triglyceride levels, and systolic blood pressure, were also found to have improved to greater levels compared to the other diets. Twenty percent of patients dropped out of the diet. Other studies have shown similar results.

Concluding remarks from this study are below, but you can see the bias in the conclusion. They do say though that diets need to be easier to adhere to.

> *"The main findings of this weight loss study, presented in a previous report, indicated that while all three diet groups lost modest amounts of weight, the Atkins group at 12 months lost approximately twice the weight of the other groups. The findings presented here indicate that weight loss in the lowest tertile [third] of adherence was negligible in all three diet groups, and more pronounced in the highest tertile of adherence for each diet group. It appears that substantial differences in proportions of dietary macronutrients play only a modest role in weight loss success, and that success is possible on any of these diets provided there is adequate adherence. Getting individuals to adhere to whatever diet they choose to follow deserves more emphasis. It remains to be determined to what extent there is a need for dietary weight loss programs that are easier to adhere to vs identifying and addressing individual barriers to adherence, or both."*

What's the Atkins Theory?

The Atkins Diet is a high-protein, low-carbohydrate diet. When you cut out carbohydrates, your body is forced into burning fat stores to provide it with energy. (See the chapter on energy and lipogenesis.) It was thought that you burn more calories when your body burns fat compared with carbohydrates (ketosis). (It isn't the reason.) Then it was thought it was the higher protein consumption that caused the weight loss and protein was excreted or burned off in preference. (Not that either.) It comes back to the evidence seen in other research that the change in diet to a higher percentage of protein and fat reduces appetite and therefore prevents overeating.

The Four Phases of the Atkins Diet

Induction. For the duration of two weeks, limit your intake of carbohydrates to 20g a day (the AMA recommendation is about 45% of our diet, which is about 250 g a day). That means no biscuits, cakes, chocolate, crisps, soft drinks, fruit drinks, croissants, pastries, bread, potatoes, pasta, rice, milk, fruit, and most high-carbohydrate vegetables from the menu. But you can eat unlimited amounts of red meat, chicken, fish, cheese, eggs, mayo, cream, and butter. The Atkins sales pitch says this is to switch from burning carbohydrates to burning fat so blood sugar levels stabilize, which they do, and therefore hunger patterns will change, as will eating habits.

Ongoing Weight Loss. Slowly, slightly increase carbohydrates intake by 5g daily for a week at a time, until you find your Critical Carbohydrate Level for Losing Weight. This is the maximum amount of carbohydrate grams you can eat each day to lose between 1 to 3 lb (0.5 and 1.2 kg) a week. This ranges from 25 g to 50 g of carbohydrates. It really only allows for the introduction of a few more veggies, fruits, nuts, and seeds. Bread, potatoes, rice, pasta and breakfast cereals are still off limits!

Pre-maintenance. The Pre-maintenance phase is when you have 5 to 10 lb (2 to 4 kg) left to lose. Increase carbohydrate intake by 10 g each day for a week at a time. Slow down your weight loss to no more than 1 lb (0.5 kg) a week in an effort to prepare your body for the final phase, which is weight maintenance. Introduce tiny amounts of traditional starchy foods such as porridge, bread, and pasta. Just to give a bit of perspective, 40 g cooked brown rice or 30 g cooked pasta each provide 10 g of carbohydrates!

Lifetime Maintenance. Most people need to limit carbohydrates to less than 90g a day, about a third of what current nutritionists recommend for a balanced diet. In summary, Atkins expects losses of 5-10 lb (2 kg to 4 kg) in the first two weeks of Induction, slowing to 1 to 3 lb (0.5 to 1.2 kg) in the Ongoing Weight Loss Phase, and during the final Pre-maintenance less than 1 lb (0.5 kg) a week.

The Atkins Diet is about mid-range in expense. It is less expensive than Jenny Craig, and it is more expensive than Weight Watchers, which also includes more carbohydrates, and you have to consider that most high carbohydrate foods are very cheap compared to most high-protein food. Many find the Atkins Diet costly due to the high cost of meats and cheeses.

Why Does the Atkins Diet Work?

Over the past 20 years, researchers have tried to figure out why the Atkins Diet works:

- It was thought that adsorption of fat was less efficient than carbohydrates. Nope.

- It was suggested that you excreted more calories in the form of nitrogen, mostly through urine. Nope.

- Protein is more filling than carbohydrate. Astrup, from Sweden, conducted a study comparing a group of people on a high protein diet to another group on a high carbohydrate diet. The group eating more protein lost almost double the weight because protein is more filling, and thus members of that group consumed fewer calories, even though they had free access to whatever food they wanted. Astrup has been looking for genetic markers but has yet to find a genetic basis for weight loss.

- Interestingly, the Induction changes that occur in the first two weeks of the Atkins Diet mirror those symptoms reported from elimination of fructose (added sugar) diets. It may be that some of the benefits from the Atkins Diet are a result of fructose reduction. Because so much prepared foods have added sugar, eliminating "carbohydrates" will also eliminate added fructose. As discussed elsewhere, we know fructose increases appetite.

- Long-term compliance is better for those on the Atkins Diet than low calorie diets. So, what you eat is less important than how long the eating change persists. This was the conclusion from Gardener et al.

Gary Taubes, a science writer in the USA, says in a commentary in 2010 that this research and that by Foster is flawed.

> "But if you read this article carefully, you'd have noticed that there was another significant difference between the low-fat and low-carbohydrate diets. The low fat diet was a low-calorie diet also. "A low-fat diet consisted of limited energy intake (1200 to 1800kcal/d; less than or equal to 30% calories from fat)," the authors explained. The low-carbohydrate diet was not calorie-restricted. And if Foster and his colleagues were being either intellectually honest or good scientists, they would've defined the two diets to make this clear. Not low-fat vs. low-carbohydrate, but low-fat, calorie-restricted vs. low-carbohydrate, calorie-unrestricted. In other words they'd have acknowledged that there was at least one other variable that was different between the two experiments and had to be taken into account when interpreting the results — the amount of

calories the subjects were instructed to consume. As we'll see, there were also other variables that were changing, but this one — how much food can be consumed if desired — is a whopper.

It's a whopper because it begs this question: is it the total calories consumed that is the variable determining weight loss? And, by the same token, is it the calories consumed (or expended) that determines how much weight we gain?"

So this research on the Atkins Diet has not really focused on what is the cause of Atkins being "nearly right." Is it that people eat fewer calories, or is it because they eat the same calories but consume fewer carbohydrates? The data is now pretty clear. **People eat less on an Atkins diet than on low-calorie diets**.

As in all science, there are some "wrinkles," and one wrinkle is confounding with Insulin intolerance. A few years after the Atkins vs. Ornish diet was published, the researchers went back and did some further measurements. (From Volek). They re-examined the data from the A to Z Study (Gardner). When they divided the women into tertiles based on insulin resistance, the weight loss at 12 months show that insulin resistance strongly influences how we respond to different diets.

Weight loss by insulin resistance	Low carbohydrate Diet	Low Fat Diet
Insulin resistant	-5.4 kg	-1.5 kg
Insulin sensitive	-5.3 kg	-4.1 kg

Simply put: if you have insulin resistance (e.g. you are overweight and you have metabolic syndrome or type 2 diabetes) a low carbohydrate diet such as the Atkins is a better diet than any low-calorie diet.

Over the years, as my friends and family went on the Atkins, it seemed like it was a fad diet. But reviewing the evidence, and understanding what I know now, it seems clear that Atkins got many things right. Is it a fad diet? The low carbohydrate diet that Atkins based it on has been around since 1850s. He might have got the reasons why it worked wrong. Advances in biochemistry, endocrinology and behavioural studies provide more understanding of what is going on with this type of diet, and I suggest that the Atkins is a reasonable diet for these reasons:

66

- Biochemistry. The biochemistry is good and matches what we now know. The diet does not promote excessive consumption of protein. High levels of protein do spike insulin, so when you drop the carbohydrates, you probably may need to increase the fat component rather than the protein, which is what most dieters do. They eat the chicken with the skin on, or change from low fat to full fat dairy products.

- Health is improved. Serum cholesterol factors improve. This improvement may be due to the carbohydrate reduction but it is still a win.

- The diet reduces fructose consumption and sugar and candy have no part in this diet!

- The diet focuses on whole foods, not refined foods.

- Endocrinology works. Insulin levels are reduced, and remain more stable under this diet.

- For many the best part is that there is no "dieting" per se. No psychological denial. It is that 2nd leg of that three-legged stool we began with. You are given permission to eat as much as you want. The slight increase in protein, and the major reduction in insulin means you are less hungry. It sounds counter intuitive, but take-out simple carbohydrates and you are less hungry!

- Some find the Atkins boring with too few carbohydrates although complex carbohydrates are permitted. The new Atkins 40 even allows some toast with the eggs for breakfast!

- This is a social friendly diet. That 3rd leg of the stool. When you go out to eat, you only have to say "hold the carbohydrates!" Even then it is only the simple carbohydrates you have to avoid.

The lead nutritionist at Atkins, Colette Heimowitz, has just released the new "Atkins 40", which doubles the allowed carbohydrates at the start of the program, includes a mandatory level of vegetable intake, and allows for 25 g of additional carbohydrates. Sugars are still off the list.

Conclusion

Do you need to go on an Atkins diet? I don't believe so. It is detailed and prescriptive, but I recognise many may need that detail. Cookbooks and food products make for an easy change. There is good evidence that this diet fails like most others over time. Even the good doctor himself was overweight at his death. The diet I went on is similar to the lifetime phase of an Atkins, or even the new Atkins. My low carbohydrate, sugar free, and a 5:2 diet resulted in more than 1 kg per week weight loss. Furthermore, my diet addressed other components of that 3 legged stool, giving permission to indulge in more expensive whole food, maintain my social lifestyle, and on a lower food budget.

References

a. Atkins Diet. (2013). http://en.wikipedia.org/wiki/Atkins_diet
b. Kellow J. (2013) The Atkins Diet Under the Spotlight. http://www.weightlossresources.co.uk/diet/atkins_diet/atkins. htm
c. Pennington A. (1958) Weight Reduction. JAMA 166(17):2214-2215. doi:10.1001/jama.1958.02990170112033
d. Leith W. (1961) Experiences with the Pennington Diet in the Management of Obesity Can Med Assoc J. Jun 24, 1961; 84(25): 1411–1414 PMCID: PMC1848046
e. Gardner C, Kiazand A, Alhassan S, Kim S, Stafford R, Balise R, Kraemer H, King A. (2007). Comparison of the Atkins Zone, Ornish, and LEARN Diets for Change in Weight and Related Risk Factors Among Overweight Premenopausal Women. The A TO Z Weight Loss Study: A Randomized Trial. Journal of the American Medical Association 297 (9): 969–977. doi:10.1001/jama.297.9.969
f. Volek J. (2011). A Calorie is a Calorie... Or is it. http://www.cce.csus.edu/conferences/childobesity/11/uploads/ VOLEK,%20Jeff.pdf
g. Alhassan S, Kim S, Bersamin A, King AC, Gardner D. (2008) Dietary adherence and weight loss success among overweight women: results from the A TO Z weight loss study. Int J Obes (Lond). 2008 Jun;32(6):985-91. doi: 10.1038/ijo.2008.8.
h. Skov A, Toubro S, Holm L, Astrup A. (1999) Randomized trial on protein vs carbohydrate in ad libitum fat reduced diet for the treatment of obesity. J Obesity. Vol 23 (5) P 528-536
i. Uncovering the Atkins Diet Secret (2004) http://news.bbc.co.uk/2/hi/health/3416637.stm

j. Taubes G (2010) Calories fat or carbohydrates? Why diets work (when they do) http://garytaubes.com/2010/12/calories-fat-or-carbohydrates/

k. Foster G, Wyatt H, Hill. J, Makris A, Rosenbaum L, Brill C, Stein R, Mohammed B, Miller B, Rader D, Zemel B, Wadden T, Tenhave T, Newcomb C, Klein S. (2010) Weight and metabolic outcomes after 2 years on a low-carbohydrate versus low-fat diet: a randomized trial. Ann Intern Med. 2010 Aug 3;153(3):147-57. doi: 10.7326/0003-4819-153-3-201008030-00005.

CHAPTER 12
BLOOD TYPE DIET – NONSENSE BUT RIGHT

Get the Facts

➤ The Blood Type Diet is a nutritional diet advocated by Peter D'Adamo, outlined in his book Eat Right 4 Your Type. D'Adamo claims that the ABO blood type is the most important factor in determining a healthy diet, and he recommends distinct diets for each blood type.

➤ The justification for eliminating certain foods from these diets, is that the lectin found in them, trigger agglutination (clumping) of the red blood cells, when consumed by someone with the wrong blood type.

➤ There is no scientific data to substantiate the diet. Furthermore, there is no data to support the lectin theory; and the limited data tends to contradict it.

➤ Intriguingly there is some interesting relationship between disease and blood type, e.g. malaria resistance, but not food.

➤ In some ways, the Blood Type Diet is similar to Paleo, Atkins, and LCHF. Many people say they feel better and have lost weight on the diet. So if you want to spend the money and buy the book, and follow the diet, do so. Better still, cut out added sugar, simple carbohydrates, and eat whole foods.

Understand the Science

There is not much science to back up the Blood Type Diet, and what is available is widely disputed. It is an interesting theory, and clearly people believe it, but the consensus from dieticians, physicians, and scientists is that there is no provable science showing that the diet works on the basis of blood type. I suspect that the reason there are some good results from the diet is because the food on the diet is not made up of high-carbohydrate, processed food. Anyone will lose weight if they cut out high-carbohydrate processed foods.

Blood types are inherited and represent contributions from both parents. A total of 33 human blood group systems are now recognized by the International Society of Blood Transfusion. The two most important ones are ABO and the RhD antigen; they determine someone's blood type (A, B, AB and O, with + and - denoting RhD status. Other antigens include Kell, MNS & Le). The blood type is actually the antigen on a red blood cell, and these antigens might be proteins, carbohydrates, glycoproteins, or glycolipids.

D'Adamo's premise is that blood type is a key to the human body's ability to differentiate self from non-self. Lectins in foods, he asserts, react differently with each ABO blood type, and to a lesser extent, with an individual's secretor status. In "Lectins: The Diet Connection" and subsequent chapters *of Eat Right 4 Your Type*, lectins, which interact with the different ABO type antigens, are described as incompatible and harmful, and that the selection of different foods for A, AB, B, and O types is therefore important in minimizing reactions with these lectins.

D'Adamo got some of the anthropology mixed up. He got the lectin story wrong and does not make any difference, but the diet seems to work, so there are vocal supporters of the diet. There is also some interesting evidence that blood types are associated with different rates of certain diseases.

The proposed diets all tend to be decent, whole foods-based ways of eating, and they're all better than the SAD (Standard American Diet) of industrial processed junk. Here is the basic breakdown of all four blood type diets:

- Type O: The hunter or "original" blood type and the oldest one. D'Adamo claimed it evolved among hunter-gatherers in response to their diet of animals and plants. Eat more meat, fish, and certain fruits and vegetables. Limit starches and omit grains (especially wheat), beans, legumes, and dairy. If you like to eat just meat, this diet is for you. It's also pretty much what the Paleo Diet advocates.
- Type A: The agrarian or cultivator (agricultural) blood type is claimed to have surfaced after the advent of agriculture. People with this blood type do best on vegetables, fruits, grains, beans, legumes, and limited fish. Avoid meat, wheat, and dairy. It's basically a vegetarian, or more properly, a "piscatorial" diet.
- Type B: The "nomad" type, proponents claim it arose amongst pastoralists raising animals for meat and milk. D'Adamo states that this blood type is associated with a strong immune system and a flexible digestive system, and those with Type B blood do

best with lamb, mutton, rabbit, and most other meats (except for chicken and pork), dairy, beans, and vegetables. They should avoid wheat, olives, tomatoes, and corn. D'Adamo got it really wrong with this group by asserting that people of blood type B are the only people able to thrive on dairy products. Most people with blood type B tend to be from Asia (specifically, China or India) and most have lactose intolerance!

- Type AB: The enigma, or "generalist" blood type. D'Adamo treats these as an intermediate between A and AB. People with this blood type can eat many meats, some seafood, dairy, beans, grains, and fruit, but they should limit kidney beans, lima beans, seeds, corn, beef, chicken, and buckwheat.

The removal of grains from many of these diets is one of the confounding factors. Wheat allergy and gluten allergy are two completely different problems with similar, but not identical, treatments. Researchers have actually identified 27 different potential wheat allergens including gluten intolerance, so it is not surprising that some find the diet good. That's the problem with confounding factors in diet. What are the causes?

Conclusion

It appears that the blood type diet "works" because it eliminates processed food regardless of blood type. Furthermore it removes wheat from the diets of people with blood types A, B, and O (which takes care of the vast majority of the population of the world), and recommends that most people (type O is the most common blood type) eat a diet based on meat and plants with little to no grains, beans, sugar, and legumes. Sound familiar?

This just goes to show that wrong assumptions about "cause" can still wind up with a diet that is essentially a low carbohydrate, whole food diet. Don't knock it: just smile and support those who believe it and manage to lose the weight. If all it achieves is effective change management about life style, then it works!

References

a. D'Adamo, P. (1997). *Eat Right 4 Your Type*. Putnam Adult. ISBN 978-0399142550.
b. Blood Type Diet http://en.wikipedia.org/wiki/Blood_type_diet
c. Sissan, M. (2013) Does Your Blood Type Determine Your Optimal Diet? www.marksdailyapple.com/blood-type-diet

CHAPTER 13
THE LEPTIN DIET – AND OTHERS

Get the Facts

➢ The Leptin Diet / lifestyle has five simple rules for healthy weight loss, but the reasons promoted have no scientific basis.

➢ The Leptin Diet, the Rosedale Diet, the Fat Resistant Diet are all promoted around control of leptin.

➢ The diet recommendations mirror those of a low carbohydrate, high fat diet. The cutting out of added sugars, reduction in simple carbohydrates, increases in protein, and restriction of calories to 1200 to 1800 calories per day, will achieve weight loss.

➢ Believe it if you must. It seems to help some people achieve their goals. Placebos work!

Understand the Science

Fat cells produce the hormone leptin, which is part of the complicated hormonal process for metabolism, weight management, and hormone balance. With hundreds of research articles on leptin and appetite control, the diet writers stepped up to the challenge of a new diet. The late Byron Richards was a prolific writer against Big Pharma. He used some of the leptin research to devise his diet plan. His Wellness Institute sells books and supplements and condenses it into five basic rules:

- Never eat after dinner. Finish eating dinner at least three hours before bed.
- Eat three meals a day. Allow five to six hours between meals. Do not snack!
- Do not eat large meals. Finish a meal when you are slightly less than full.
- Eat a high protein breakfast.
- Reduce the amount of carbohydrates eaten.

Other leptin diets include the Rosedale Diet by Dr Ron Rosedale, which explores dietary solutions to correct leptin imbalances. The Fat Resistant Diet by Leo Galland, focuses on an anti-inflammatory diet that addresses leptin. These diets are pretty general, and because they advocate eliminating SSB (sugar sweetened beverages), soy foods and drinks, permit no snacks, increase protein, and restrict food to three meals of 400 to 600 calories, (i.e. diet of 1200 to 1800 calories per day), these diets will work because they are aligned with what is now known about successful weight loss using LCHF diets. Further, Richards advocates the following: don't be calorie obsessed or calorie ignorant; know the content of the foods you usually eat. Keep each meal between 400 and 600 calories with general ratios of 40% fat, 30% protein, and 30% carbohydrates. He advocates some exercise, but he focuses his marketing on thyroid complications as well.

Should you buy the extra supplements? If it is part of the psychology of dieting and helps people maintain their commitment to change, then it probably does not do any harm to anything more than the wallet. It is just unlikely to have much more effect than a placebo effect.

Conclusion

Just like many other diets, the leptin-styled diets will work, just not necessarily for the reasons promoted. Generally, a major outcome will be thinning down your wallet. The diet is a restrictive diet and involves some "will power," and as we have discussed elsewhere that is likely to result in long term failure. They will work short term because the biochemistry and endocrinology are in line with the 1st leg of the stool. But they fail to address the 2nd leg (internal behaviour) or the 3rd leg (society).

References

a. Richards, Bryon J. (2012) *The Leptin Diet: How fit is your fat.* Wellness Resources.
b. Richards, Bryon J. (2002) Mastering Leptin: The Leptin Diet, Solving Obesity and Preventing Disease. Wellness Resources. 3rd Ed.
c. Galland L. (2006) The Fat Resistance Diet: Unlock the Secret of the Hormone Leptin to: Eliminate Cravings, Supercharge Your Metabolism, Fight Inflammation, Lose Weight & Reprogram Your Body to Stay Thin pp368 ISBN 978-0767920537

d. Rosedale R. (2005) *The Rosedale Diet. Turn off your hunger switch.* pp335 ISBN006056573X http://www.drrosedale.com/

CHAPTER 14
ENERGY USE AND LIPOGENESIS

Get the Facts

➤ We use a range of interchangeable sources for energy including glucose, fatty acids, proteins, and ketone bodies.

➤ The adage *"Calories in / Calories out"* is actually true, but we are not simple mechanical machines.

➤ If we eat more calories than we use, we store them in our fat reserves. When we eat fewer calories than we use, we start using body fat reserves.

➤ The body is brilliant at "homeostasis" – delicately balancing processes with intricate feedback processes to keep things stable.

➤ When we eat, we break everything down to its simplest form. We then re-assemble the simple compounds back into complex forms in our own system.

➤ Our primary energy source is fat and protein, not simple carbohydrates.

➤ Disrupt the endocrine (hormone) control mechanisms or some of the other external control mechanisms, and the "homeostasis" fails, and we become too fat or too thin.

➤ View insulin as the primary control hormone of this storing / using calorie system.

➤ View fat as the body's protection mechanism against glucose (from simple carbohydrates such as sugar and starch).

Understand the Science

It can be very confusing to know what diet advice to take, and what to ignore. You find what you think is solid information that is backed by science and research that says do this, or do that, and in 5 years' time the advice is the other way around. How are you supposed to know what to do? How do you interpret the research and advice in a constructive framework? It seems like a jigsaw puzzle with all the pieces of evidence. I am not even sure I am dealing with one puzzle or with multiple puzzles!

This is not a novel where you are left hanging in suspense until the last page. It took six months of reading before I said, "Ah ha, I think I've got it!" With a clear framework, it was simpler to see the underlying unifying processes and I explain it with the 3 legged stool model.

- Why is there conflicting research?

- Why do some diets work for some, but not for others?

- What are the tactics to improve health outcomes?

- Why do "alternative therapies" work in part?

My understanding was framed in the biochemistry and endocrinology leg of that 3 legged stool. Within the biochemistry leg, I had trouble to understand why a low carbohydrate diet appeared to work the best of the various diets and lifestyles. Others may frame their views within the other legs of the stool such as the mind. Others may frame this in the 3rd leg of the context of our society.

What Energy Do We Use?

Glucose is often thought of as the only energy we use. Many people are unaware of our primary energy source: fatty acids. When they are *not attached* to proteins, they are called *free* fatty acids. When fatty acids are metabolized, they release lots of energy. The heart and muscle actually prefer fatty acids. The brain can also use fatty acids. That's not all. We also use protein and ketone bodies for energy. The only thing in our body that has to use glucose is our red blood cells. The glucose needed comes from fat, protein, and not just from carbohydrates. So when someone says "fat burns in the fire of carbohydrates" or "ketones are dangerous," close that book, and read a novel. At least the novel is truthful about itself!

I've concluded that many people fail to understand the process that takes place when we eat fat, including the policy makers who said dietary fat increases the risk of heart attack. If you hear a nutritionist advocating eating less and moving more, they probably do not understand the processes. Eating less and moving more is overly simplistic. And I shake my head at those who believe in the mantra of Calories in, Calories out as the way to lose weight. Just as we break down all carbohydrates (saccharides) into simple sugars, we also break down dietary fat into free fatty acids. As shown in the biochemistry of metabolism, these things work in cycles. Too much energy in the food we consume, and we store it as fat, in cells. Energy demand can be met with eating, or taking fat from storage cells. If the process was one way, obese people would surely continue to get fatter and fatter. But they do not. Most diets work initially as the fat cells shrink.

Our stores of energy are fat, protein, glycogen, and glucose. We can't store glucose as it is too toxic, but glycogen (complex glucose) is stored in the liver and in some cells. We have about eight hours' worth of glycogen stored.

Muscle protein is generally not useful for energy, but fat is a huge reservoir of energy. People do not get fat from accumulation of glycogen storage, or muscle build up. What is the cause of the fat build up? Saying it is because we eat too much is a pointless circular discussion.

The key question remains: what is the control mechanism? How do we move to homeostasis with our food intake so we don't get our fat store increasing? We want this to be part of unconscious homeostasis, and not have to use conscious thoughts. We most certainly do not want to use willpower to restrict food. We want a normal lifestyle. This book is principally about this control process of appetite.

Appetite is why people eat more, or less, and if we manage the factors that affect appetite, we are on the way to self-regulate our weight.

In the section on biochemistry of metabolism we discussed that when we eat saccharides, we break them down to the mono-saccharides. We adsorb them into our blood. Glucose in our blood is used and/or stored. Fructose is converted into other products in the liver. We want that energy balance to work in homeostasis. Although we may over consume, we want to under consume at other times so we don't accumulate energy and pack on the kilos/pounds in storage.

Understanding Glucose Homeostasis

Many of us know someone who has diabetes, and diabetes is a disease where normal blood glucose regulation through insulin is faulty. One of the things that has surprised me, is how little people know about glucose. I asked two simple questions.

- Firstly, how much blood do you have in your body? The answers range from 2 to 20 l. It is about 5.5 l or 1.5 gallons.

- Secondly, how much glucose is in your blood? The answers range from a cup to one 1/3rd of your blood. Serum blood glucose is about 4.2g total, or less than 1 teaspoon in the whole of our blood. Normal levels in our blood are 80mg/dl, or 3.8mol/l. We turn it over perhaps 60 times a day.

Glucose is highly active and poisonous. If the glucose blood level rises by three times, we are probably diabetic (over 200mg/dl). More, and we go into a coma (ask a diabetic). Too little (under 2.2 mmol/L), and we pass out and get a trip to the emergency department. That's not much range for a so-called "preferred" fuel, is it? Our blood glucose level is part of our "homeostasis" or a process which relies on keeping levels pretty well constant.

Glucose regulation is robust. A loaf of bread is 800 g (UK definition), and as a hungry teenager, I could eat ½ a loaf of bread in just a few minutes smothered in butter and jam. Within 20 minutes all of that would be blood glucose, if it were not for the remarkable homeostasis, and capacity of insulin and the body to deal with this toxic level of sugar, and push it off to glycogen or fat. In contrast, this sort of glucose loading would see a diabetic in a coma if it were not for additional insulin by injection.

Eating a lot of bread as an active teenager playing a lot of sport might be okay, but what if you did this day in, day out? What about a "healthy" breakfast cereal with toast, jam, and a large fruit juice? How does your system cope with 30 teaspoons of sugar gulped down in a few minutes?

So what is the minimum level of saccharides (carbohydrates) for living? Do you need any carbohydrates? Several studies have shown that under normal low metabolic conditions (at rest or moderate levels of activity such as walking and easy work) the body only needs about five grams of glucose an hour. And that's for people who aren't fat-adapted, or keto-adapted. The brain is the major consumer of glucose, needing 120 g a day in people who aren't on a low carbohydrate eating program. Low carbohydrate eating reduces the brain's glucose requirements considerably, and those who are very low carbohydrate (VLC) and keto-adapted may only require about 30 g of glucose per day to fuel the brain (and little-to-none) to fuel the muscles at <75% max efforts. Most of us are not athletes, and never come close to that level of exercise. Twenty of those grams can come from glycerol (a by-product of fat metabolism) and the balance from gluconeogenesis in the liver. A healthy liver can actually make up to a whopping 150 g glycerol per day. If you have metabolically damaged the liver with non-alcoholic fatty liver disease (NAFLD) through fructose overdosing and obesity, it might be asking a bit much of it!

The bottom line is that unless you are a physical labourer or are exercising vigorously on a daily basis, once you become fat-adapted, you probably won't ever need to consume more than 150 grams of dietary carbohydrates. That level is for the associated vitamins and minerals and fiber for your gut health, and you can probably thrive on far less. Many low-carbohydrate dieters do very well (including working out) on 30-70 grams a day. We will come back to the issue of carbohydrates later in the book.

Fat Homeostasis

What about fat? Fatty acid digestion, absorption, levels, and transport are more complicated, and dependent on the particular fatty acid size. (Check out the chapter on Biochemistry of Fats and oils for more details.) Short and medium fatty acids are absorbed directly into the blood system, but some larger ones are absorbed, coated with cholesterol and protein (chylomicron), and transported via the lymphatic system. They are eventually emptied into the blood stream near the heart and then carried to tissue and used by the body. Regulation, like that of glucose, is a very well defined and controlled process. If 100 people were measured, they all have much the same levels, most of the time. Even eating a big meal will not raise the fatty acid levels by 10%. Just think about cholesterol tests you have done as part of any medical check-up. Levels are expressed as mg/dl in the USA and mmol/l the rest of the world. Most fall in a very limited range from 150 to 300 mg/dl) (4 to 8 mmol/L). Desirable range is below 200 mg/dl (5.2 mmol/dl), and a high range is above 240 mg/dl (6.2 mmol/l). In many respects our fatty acid levels are even more in homeostasis than glucose levels.

We need energy all the time for our brain. If the glucose level falls, we need to raise it again, and have four things we can do to increase "available energy". Behaviour and appetite are integrated as we discuss in the chapter Leptin and Ghrelin. We can eat, have a drink, or ignore. If we ignore, then within a few minutes that "hunger" dissipates as we convert our reserves to glucose.

- Use the glucose in our blood and tissues. (Takes only a few minutes.)

- Eat and digest food and that can take 20 minutes or less.

- Use some of the glycogen in our liver and muscle. (Immediate)

- Convert some of the fat stored in our body. (Immediate)

Lipogenesis Cycle and Regulation

Lipogenesis is a central part of how we regulate our energy balance. As we have seen, lipids make up the bulk of our energy reserves and it is important to understand how we move energy into storage, and then move it back out. A bit of simple biochemistry is needed before we go through the whole process. For more information on the biochemistry of fats, check out that chapter. But for now, stick with me here; it's important.

Lipogenesis is the process of how sugar converts into fat. Simple sugars such as glucose are converted to fatty acids, and then to triglycerides. Lipogenesis encompasses the whole process of fatty acid synthesis and subsequent triglyceride synthesis, but I'll only look at the overview, not the very complex biochemistry. We won't even look at the first part of how glucose gets into the fatty acids. Remember that carbohydrates can turn into fat! Live on a diet of white bread and sugar, and you can get very fat, very quickly!

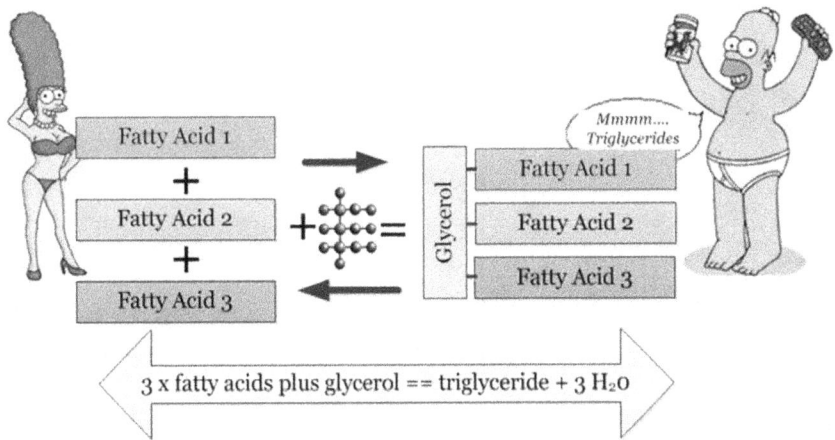

Figure 10 Triglycerides and fatty acids

Fat can be in various forms – principally either a free fatty acid or a triglyceride. In figure 10 above, on the left, we have free fatty acids, and each is a single long chain compound. There are many types of fatty acids as discussed in the fat biochemistry chapter. We don't need to know what specific fatty acid or triglyceride in this energy discussion as there are many different variations. The symbol is glycerol. On the right is a triglyceride which is a compound shaped a bit like the letter "E" with a glucose-like compound (glycerol phosphate) joined with three free fatty acids. This process (from fatty acids plus glycerol to triglyceride, or the reverse) requires energy. This process is dynamic, complex and controlled by many things. Think of it this way: the more triglycerides, the more you will look like Homer Simpson! With fewer triglycerides, you will look more like Marge.

Let's go through figure 11 below with this energy balance within our blood vessels. Our brain is monitoring blood pretty closely, and it has a number of tactics to maintain homeostasis of the energy available in the blood.

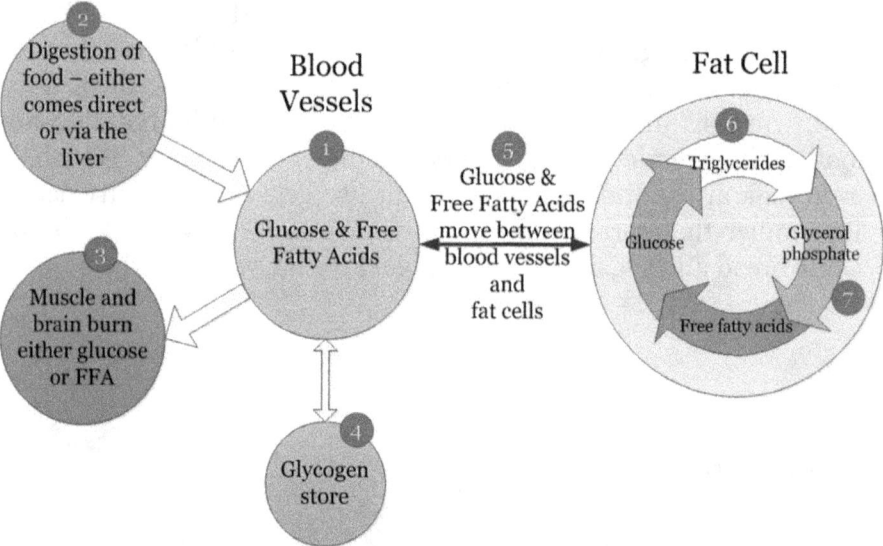

Figure 11 Lipogenesis Overview

Firstly, when energy levels change in our blood vessels, our primary response is to eat. We become conscious of this process when we get hunger pains and want to replenish by eating. The blood vessels (number 1 in the figure) holds both serum glucose, and free fatty acids. There are also other things in our blood such as lipoproteins which transport cholesterol in the blood. Cholesterol is not in the blood (remember, oil does not mix with water) so we can ignore this as part of this energy discussion. These concentrations of glucose and free fatty acids are in homeostasis and constantly added to or taken away. It is not static. Energy is used by muscle or brain (3). Muscle has its own reserves, but the brain very little. Energy can be replenished from glycogen in the liver (4); from additional food (2); or can move in and out of fat cells (5,6,7).

The second simplest short-term response to a change in serum glucose is conversion of glucose to glycogen (step 4), or vice versa. Only the liver can store or release glycogen back to serum glucose and glycogen that gets stored in muscles cannot be re-exported. Muscle glycogen gets used when needed, but only in that muscle. We will use the glycogen in the liver, but as pointed out there is not much, so it is a short-term store only (1 days' worth of energy). The third source of energy replenishment in the blood is replenishment from fat cells. Step (5) is the complicated process between the blood vessel and the fat cell. Steps 6 and 7 are the processes within that fat cell. Fat cells are not like empty milk jugs where you pour in the fat or pour it out. It is a complicated process moving glucose and free fatty acids into the fat cells and the reverse. We'll explore this in more detail, but stay at the overview level and not at the very complex biochemical and physiology detail in these processes. There is much research going on at this "bottom of the test tube" level. While glucose and free fatty acids can move between the blood vessel and the fat cell; triglycerides cannot, as the compound is too big for the cellular membranes. We will now explore two different energy states: fat burning, and fat storing.

What Happens With Low Blood Sugar Levels (Fat Burning)?

When you have low blood sugar, refer to figure 12 for the various steps in this process. This process moves energy from the fat cell back into the bloodstream.

- Serum blood sugar (glucose) levels fall (step a).

- Less glucose goes into the fat cell (step b), so fat glucose is lower (step c).

- With less glucose available in the fat cell, there is also less glycerol phosphate (step d).

- With less glycerol phosphate available, there is less conversion of free fatty acids to triglycerides (step e).

- Therefore more free fatty acids go back to the blood (step f).

- Net result – have MORE ENERGY in the blood – (free fatty acids- step g) supplying energy to the brain and muscle AND

- Most importantly, have reduced fat cell size (Woo hoo!)

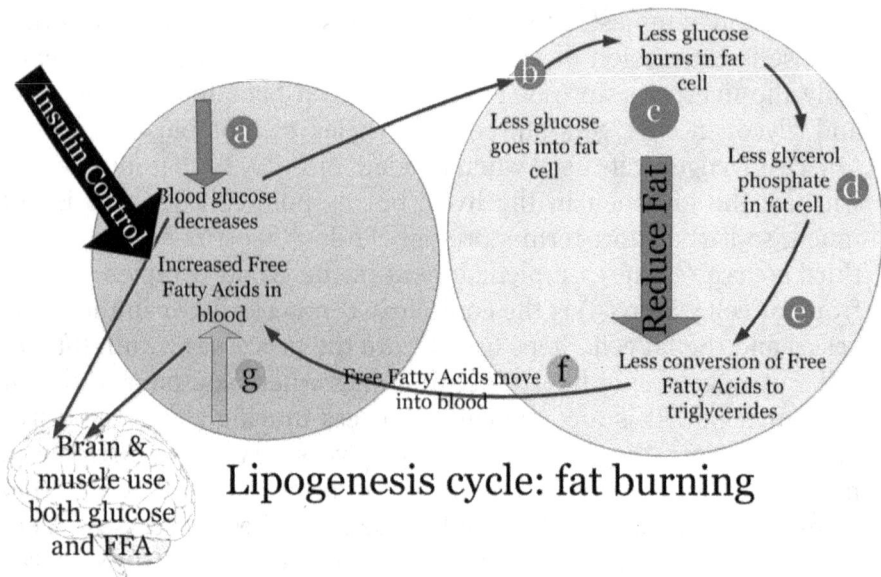

Figure 12 Lipogenesis with Low Blood Sugar

What Happens With High Blood Sugar Levels (Fat Deposit)?

Almost the converse of the fat burning process happens with high blood sugar. The body has to get rid of the glucose or you get glucose poisoning. So the process stores the energy as fat and we wind up with bigger fat cells.

- Serum blood sugar (glucose) levels rise (Step a).

- More glucose goes into the fat cell, so fat glucose is higher (step b).

- With more glucose available (step c), there is more glycerol phosphate (step d).

- This higher level accelerates the conversion of free fatty acids to triglycerides (step e).

- Therefore, less free fatty acids go back to the blood. (Step f, remember, triglycerides cannot get through the fat cell membrane.)

- The net effect is there is LESS ENERGY in the form of lower free fatty acids in the blood (step g) AND most importantly

84

- Glucose has been reduced but now the fat cells are bigger (Darn!)

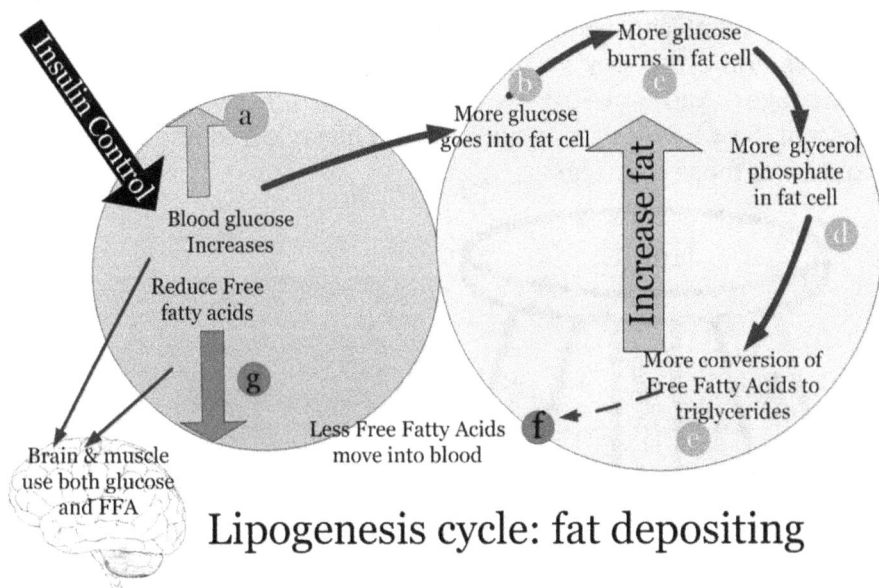

Insulin Control

a — Blood glucose Increases

Reduce Free fatty acids

g

Brain & muscle use both glucose and FFA

More glucose goes into fat cell

b

More glucose burns in fat cell — c

More glycerol phosphate in fat cell — d

Increase fat

More conversion of Free Fatty Acids to triglycerides — e

Less Free Fatty Acids move into blood — f

Lipogenesis cycle: fat depositing

Figure 13 Lipogenesis with High Blood Sugar

This complex process is actually very simple in principle. If our blood glucose levels rise, we have to store the excess glucose, and we convert it to fat. If our blood sugar falls, we start to burn fat. Therefore we should avoid simple carbohydrates to reduce fat in fat cells and to make sure we do not make any more fat cells. Is that what all weight loss diets are about? I would suggest it is a cornerstone of understanding why low carbohydrate diets work. The theory of lipogenesis is this simple. There are complications because fats have higher energy content than simple carbohydrates, and what we eat affects our appetite differently. We will discuss some of these complications elsewhere. Most are just consequences of these processes.

Control of This Process

The hormonal and genetic control of lipogenesis is clearly very complex, but there are some principles. You should be able to imagine how things we do in daily life can affect this process. In the diagrams above, you will notice insulin. Insulin helps regulate this process, but insulin has impacts more than just on these processes. It affects more than just biochemistry and endocrinology. It is also about the other two legs of the stool – brain, mind, behaviours, and social interactions. What happens when we eat? What food do we eat to minimize the process to store fat and drive the cycle the other way to reduce fat? Does it matter *when* we eat? Do genetics affect this process? What can we do with the hormonal control to keep the process going the way we want? Can we modify this cycle to our advantage? And how? If we go back to this three-legged stool concept, how do we modify our diet and lifestyle and understand the context of those changes?

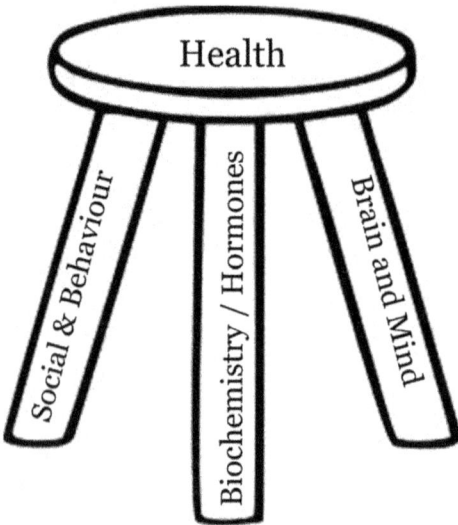

Figure 14 Three-legged Stool

With so many control mechanisms in this process, biochemical explanations are not enough in themselves. We eat differently, different things, different times, and in different places. And it is the things we eat that have the majority (80%) of effect. It is never straightforward. Insulin is part of this process. Leptin is part of this process. What we eat and where we eat has a role in how much and what type of food we eat. Our eating is not just physical. It is affected by our moods, our mind, our company, and social behaviours. I think the reason that "diets" and health are thought to be complicated is that our health is not just biochemistry and hormonal / genetic. I would further suggest that research is often poorly executed because the researchers have ignored these other complicating factors. For example, insulin does not just control the rate of conversion of glucose by the cells. It has differential effects within the fat cells and changes our appetite. Cellular biochemists tend to ignore social and behavioural interactions.

Insulin has a major effect on appetite. When we sit down for a meal, we may start to salivate as our digestive system starts getting ready for food. But as well, our blood glucose drops because insulin production goes up in anticipation of getting more energy. Have you ever wondered why the best meal, and the most hunger, is felt as we get ready for a meal? We feel hungrier. That's the insulin dropping our blood glucose, and raising our appetite. Within 20 minutes or so, our hunger has gone as other appetite suppressing hormones get to work. If we have a couple of cookies (simple carbohydrates and sugar), we stop the process of fat burning. Glucose levels go up. Fat is deposited. However, if we eat fat or protein, we don't get that blood glucose spike and raised insulin levels to dampen down the glucose loading. And we keep on reducing the fat from the cells. A very simple example is eating cheese and crackers (biscuits). Crackers are 100% simple carbohydrates (refined white flour or rice) so within a few minutes they have elevated our glucose levels, and we go into the fat depositing mode. If we eat cheese without crackers, we remain in burning fat mode, as the fat takes longer to digest, and other hormones kick in to dampen down our appetite.

Conclusion

We now understand that carbohydrates have some serious effects on the disruption of homeostasis.

- We have a sophisticated control processes for glucose regulation. Glucose is highly toxic, and we have to control levels rapidly to avoid serious toxicity.

- Simple carbohydrates stop the process of fat burning, and turn excess glucose into fat quickly.

- Carbohydrates make us hungrier through insulin levels changes. We eat more. The consequence is we put on fat.

Appetite control is critical because it will change the amount of food and energy we consume and therefore store. This is almost certainly why low carbohydrate diets (Atkins, Paleo, LCHF, Mediterranean) work better, both short-term and long-term, than any calorie-restricted diet. As well, as discussed in the section on Atkins Diet, a low carbohydrate diet is more effective when you have insulin resistance. Lastly, these diets tend to have different social implications, and adherents tend to stick to the diets for a longer period. As we look at the 5:2 Diet or intermittent fasting regimes or exercise, or whole food programs, we begin to understand why science says that these may work better in the long term, rather than just the calorie restriction diets. It also raises the question why some nutritionists still say "fat burns in the fire of carbohydrates". How wrong can they be?

References

The information in this chapter is taken from other chapters, so I have not duplicated the references. You can find detailed information of lipogenesis on Wikipedia, and most biochemistry books.

a. Lipogenesis.   Wikipedia.
   http://en.wikipedia.org/wiki/Lipogenesis

CHAPTER 15
DURING PREGNANCY

Get the Facts

➤ Prenatal and post natal dietary lifestyles appear to set up obesity for life. Society needs to help pregnant females maintain a reasonable weight increase over their pregnancy.

➤ Drinking sodas during pregnancy can increase risk of type 2 diabetes, miscarriage and death of newborn, and obesity or diabetes in children.

➤ Reasonable weight gain can be difficult to achieve due to women's hormonal changes and social and political implications.

Understand the Science

Gestational diabetes mellitus (GDM), defined as glucose intolerance with onset, or first recognition, during pregnancy, is one of the most common pregnancy complications. Women with GDM are at increased risk of pregnancy complications, type 2 diabetes in the years after pregnancy, and prenatal morbidity. Prenatal morbidity is miscarriages after 24 weeks pregnancy through to deaths within the first week after birth.gyly The UK rate is 8 per 1000. Offspring of women with GDM have increased risk of obesity, glucose intolerance, and diabetes in childhood and early adulthood.

Dr Chen and researchers found that drinking more than five servings of sugar-sweetened cola a week prior to pregnancy increased risk of developing diabetes during pregnancy by 22%. This was compared to those who had less than one can per month. The research was based upon a group of 13,475 women from the Nurses' Health Study II. During ten years of follow-up, 860 GDM cases were identified. This was after adjustments for known risk factors for GDM, including: age, family history of diabetes, parity, physical activity, smoking status, sugar-sweetened beverage intake, alcohol intake, pre-pregnancy BMI, and Western dietary patterns. In this study, no significant association was found for other sugar-sweetened beverages or diet beverages, but only for the sugar-sweetened cola. So a question remains: was it the cola or the sugar component?

Given that other studies don't show significant differences between any of the sugar-sweetened beverages on weight and other metabolic syndromes, it would be prudent not to drink any sweetened beverages.

Fat Children = Adult Metabolic Disease

There is both epidemiological evidence and animal studies that show a direct relationship between foetal and early postnatal growth patterns, and an increased risk of adult metabolic disease. Maternal health and nutrition are key determinants in influencing infant growth, but the precise molecular mechanisms underlying this relationship are unclear. There are critical time windows when these effects are important.

Using animals, researchers can reverse this "fat child = diseased adult" scenario. You can intervene, either through the mother or directly with the child using orally administered peptides which are absorbed intact by the new born. Intervention would be possible by providing supplemental leptin as drops or in milk, and this may be a means of reducing, or reversing, the obesity and type 2 diabetes epidemic. The ethical and political environment would be tough to change!

Conclusion

In conclusion, pregnancy is a critical time in human development and the impacts of poor lifestyle last throughout the lifetime of the offspring. I was fortunate in my generation not to have much of the western diet. Pregnancy was normal and uneventful. Most food eaten in early life was from whole food.

References

a. Chen L, Hu F, Yeung E, Willett W, Zhang C. (2009) Prospective Study of Pre-Gravid Sugar-Sweetened Beverage Consumption and the Risk of Gestational Diabetes Mellitus. Diabetes Care. 32(12): 2236–2241. doi: 10.2337/dc09-0866

CHAPTER 16
CHANGE MANAGEMENT

Get the Facts

- ➢ Change management is a well-defined business process.
- ➢ Components include reasons for change, planning processes, phases to go through, and tactics to improve likelihood of change.
- ➢ Changing a diet for improved lifestyle should use all components of change management, to improve outcomes.

Understand the Science

For the past 30 years, I have focused on change management, even before change management became an area of expertise. As I looked at health and weight management, it struck me that this whole area of health is about how to effect change. Why change? What drives people to change? What are some of the principles we can take from the formal study, and use to apply them to health and wellbeing? Fifteen years ago, I was talking to a Canadian engineer, and he said something that has always stuck with me. He said people in business only change for one of three reasons, and he put it in monetary terms:

- You make money, i.e. a benefit.
- You lose money, i.e. a loss.
- It's the law, i.e. you have to.

The benefit or loss does not necessarily have to be monetary. It might be a friendship, reward, feeling good about yourself, or a personal loss. We tend to connect it to money because we can put a specific value on it. If we want to lose some weight, we know one benefit is that we will feel better. This might cause us to monitor calories in hope of going down a dress or pant size so that we look better. If you're a salesperson, looking better might translate to more sales/more revenue.

So what is your reason to change? Mine was simple. A loss. Firstly I saw my mother spend her last five years with increasing severe Alzheimer's, becoming muddled, losing her laughter, and her connectedness to people and life. What did I need to do to prevent that from happening to me? I did not want to accept that my risk of Alzheimer's increased because my mother had it. Secondly, my father spent his last 10 years with a diminishing quality of life due to cardio vascular disease and complications. I did not want to take three or four medications, lose mobility, suffer pain, and be very restricted on lifestyle.

Sometimes people change because they want to increase self-worth. Others change because of fear. I don't see society changing the law anytime soon, although the ideas of a soda tax or some form of fat tax have been raised as strategies, and then defeated by the "my right to choose" activists in conjunction with food companies. Whatever the reason, something has to happen within an individual to make them want to change. People have to be motivated to change. What is your motivation?

As an aside, I believe economic change tactics are legitimate. Everyone is paying for increased health care costs through their taxes or medical insurance. Why should I pay for the consequences of others' poor diet choices?

You need to have a reason to start your diet and continue it. If you're going to be one of the 19 out of 20 who gives up the diet within a year, why bother starting it? Don't start unless there is a strong reason to start; a reason compelling enough to stick with it. Only you will know the real reason why you want to lose weight and be healthy. What is important to you? Is it important to you to look great? (Maybe you're looking for a partner!) Is it important to you to be healthy and fit enough to play with your children? Do you feel your excess weight is holding back your career goals? Have you lost self-respect because you are undisciplined in your eating habits? Understand *why* you want to change and set a goal to endure what it takes to make the change that you want to make. Your motivation must be more muscular than the lure of that cupcake!

Psychologically we have a problem as taste is more important than health, as reported by Sullivan in 2014. So you need strong drivers for change.

To meet your goal, create a reasonable plan that is broken down into daily steps that are doable for you. If your goal and plan are not feasible, or are too ambitious, you will be inclined to give up before you build any momentum. Momentum builds momentum. Start out with a plan that allows you gain enough momentum to help propel you for the rest of the journey.

One of the best examples of nationwide change is to do with people quitting smoking. To stop people smoking, the only effective way has been a combination of some loss and some laws. The government tried to tell us we would have better health by quitting. No one stopped. They tried to educate us by saying "if you smoke you will die of lung cancer." Only a few more stopped. But when they raised the price of cigarettes, people stopped smoking. The high cost of smoking hit people where it hurts: the wallet. Tobacco company documents provide clear evidence of the impact of cigarette prices on cigarette smoking, describing how tax related, and other price increases, led to significant reductions in smoking, particularly among young persons. That is why Australia has a 63% tax on cigarettes, the USA 43%, and most of Europe around 79%. Indonesia has a 46% tax rate. So what's the best strategy for governments who hope to reduce smoking? An Australian meta-analysis from 2011 found that ads hammering the negative health impacts were most effective in getting smokers to kick the habit (Loss). The 2003 study from the WHO advocates an approach composed of a combination of bans, educational campaigns, and restrictions, but it also highlights the effectiveness of price increases. For every 10% increase, the WHO says smoking drops by 2.5 to 5% in the short run, and 10% in the long run, leading to 500,000 to 2 million fewer deaths per year from smoking in high-income countries. This change is simply not going to happen for food and food products. No government is going to bring in food taxes on junk food, without a very strong mandate and deep pockets for court cases. So any change will have to be by the individual. It is unlikely there will be much support from the government at least for the short term. Even hospitals are struggling to get unhealthy food out of canteens and vending machines on their campuses.

The Planning Phases

Create a baseline of your health and weight. It is important for change management. In addition, you'll be encouraged when you start to reduce your waist and other fatty areas of the body. Get a medical check-up that will indicate physical measures such as weight, height, circumference, fat level; and metabolic indicators such as blood pressure, cholesterol, fasting sugar, and insulin levels.

This provides the baseline to help keep you motivated. The principles in business change management are simple.

- Have a goal. What do you want to achieve? For me, the primary goal was health. For most, especially the overweight and obese, a major goal will be about image and self-worth. While weight is a symptom of poor health, that is all it is except for the obese where mechanical stress will be a direct consequence. For lean people, without any weight issues, 20% will have some form of health issues, and so the only goal will be better health.

- Know your starting position.

- Understand the reasons to change.

- Keep the time to a manageable period. This plan is a twelve week plan. Even large projects should be broken into manageable 12 week projects. Bigger, and the risk of failure is higher. Smaller, and the management time is too high. Twelve weeks is a good length of time so you can see results.

- Use the first 21 days (3 weeks) to learn the skills of healthy living

- Use the balance of the 12 weeks to practice, refine the process, gain the benefits, and cement them into "the way we operate".

As in business, it may not be important if the process fails during the introduction phase. The loss is time but the gains are knowledge about the challenges and hurdles of the change. Most don't doubt the overall value of the change. So good businesses reassess what they learned, make some process changes, or even change their approach to the issue, and when, ready for the change again, have another go.

The Phases

When I implement change in a business environment there are three phases. For example, let's say we are going to implement a new phone system in a business. Critical in this, is that the new phone system is going to have some benefits. Perhaps the benefits are that the phone system is easy to answer, calls are directed to the right person without intervention by a telephonist, customers don't stay on hold as long, and sales will increase with improved customer service.

- Explain. Go to your staff and customers and tell them why the new phone system will be installed. What are the reasons for change? What is expected? Why will it be better? What will go wrong? What training do they need?

- Pain. The new system is in. But it does not work the way it used to work and you used to work with "Hey, Joe, pick up line one". There is no line one. Now, everything is automated!

- Gain. Customers get answered more quickly, it is better for them and easier for staff.

Here is a graph of what happens to expectations over time with a new phone system deployment. You start off in a project highlighting the benefits. As implementation draws closer, do not oversell the benefits too much. Transition to the new change happens. Day One: it is sort of okay. Day Two: why doesn't the phone system work the way it used to? Day Three: this phone system sucks. Day Ten: this phone system works okay. Day Twenty: the new phone system is really great!

There are two things that make for a good change. Firstly, after you make a change try to reduce the time before the gains kick in. Secondly, try to have some big quick wins after you make the changes. Both of these decrease any negativity and keep people encouraged so they don't give up.

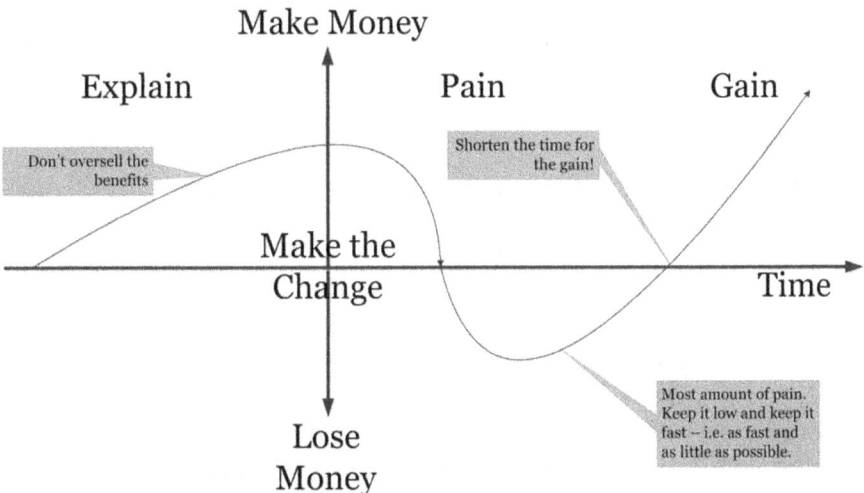

Figure 15 Change Management Cycle

Many of you will have experienced this in the businesses you work in. Many will also have experienced poor change management. Don't oversell. Under promise, and over deliver.

The same process happens with a diet. You psych yourself up. Yep. Going to be great to be 45 lb (20 kg) lighter. Day One: Whoops. Don't like this. Day Two: I cannot think over my stomach rumbling. Day Five: forget it.

A UK food company found that of those who diet regularly, 10% quit on day two and 40% have quit by day seven; 20% last a month, and just 20% make it to the three-month mark. Another 20% last six months, and only 5% lasted a year. Why?

- Body rebellion (pain). Drastic or too-strict diets can trigger mood swings, headaches, physical and mental fatigue, irritability, upset digestion and brain fog.

- Feeling hungry (pain).

- Cravings (pain). Trying to be "perfect" week after week typically leads to feelings of deprivation, resentment, even anger or depression, and culminates in either binge eating, or diet abandonment.

- Social pressure (pain). One recent study found that friends who eat together consume more food than those paired with strangers. Friends give each other "permission" to overeat. "Try it, it's delicious!"

- Emotions. We're practically programmed from birth to use food emotionally. Guilt: "Mom made it just for you."

Set Goals

Whether you are building a house, tending the back garden, writing a business plan, or doing anything where you want an outcome, start with creating some goals. There is no right way or wrong way to set goals. There are hundreds of planning tools available online and otherwise for anyone who wants to use them. Some coaches don't like goals and put them in context of life values. In my business and personal life I use a simple one-page outline. I only set a maximum of three goals at a time – one business goal, and two personal goals. An acronym for this type of planning is SMART goals.

Goals must be:

- Stated. If you can't write it down, then it is not a goal, but a dream.

- Measureable. What is relevant to measure? Blood pressure? Waist size? Dress size? Fitness level?

- Achievable. Reduce from BMI of 32 to BMI of 24.

- Relevant. My health is at risk, and I want to be around for my grandkids.

- Timely. Lose 2 lb (1 kg) per week for the first six weeks, reducing to 0.5 lb (0.25kg) per month for the next 11 months.

I also encourage people to adhere to the **Four Ls**. They are:

- Live: you have to maintain a life so these goals have to be liveable and enjoyable.

- Love: for many the goals have to be compatible with your loves such as relationships with friends, spouses, and children.

- Learn: some goals are about satisfying your learning desires.

- Legacy: depending on your stage of life, you may want to give back to others.

Depending on where you are emotionally, financially and spiritually, these 4-Ls need to be addressed, or you are unlikely to reach your goals.

The "Take Out" Strategies In Action

William, a middle aged friend who exercises three times a week, and was in the 183lb/92kg weight range, decided to make some changes to his health. He had heard David Gillespie speak and read David's *Sweet Poison*. Before he started looking into weight reduction, I got him onto MyFitnessPal to monitor what he was eating. He works from his home office, and when working at home, he goes upstairs to the kitchen for a cup of tea or coffee three to four times a day. Each time he went for coffee or tea, he grabbed a handful of nuts. (Nuts are healthy, right?). Through monitoring what he was eating at MyFitnessPal, he learned that each time he grabbed a handful of nuts, he was consuming well over 100 calories. He was scoffing down an extra 400-600 calories per day with the nut snacks! Since learning this, the salty mixed nuts have gone. In their place is a jar of nutrient-dense, whole macadamia nuts. For William to have one of those delicious nuts, he first has to crack it. In the time that it takes for his tea or coffee to brew, he can only crack five or six of the nuts and pop them in his mouth. So, he only consumes 50 calories or less. With one small change, he is reducing his calorie count of each snack by 50% or more! Over a week's time, he is eating thousands of calories less without feeling deprived. He didn't have to completely cut out his tea time snack, he just needed to make an adjustment. When we completely cut out all snacks, we set ourselves up for failure. Total deprivation rarely works for anyone.

Joseph, age 63, was overweight and had been on a diet under the supervision of a hospital dietician to control his high blood pressure. He went from 230 lb (105kg) down to 198 lb (90kg) on the 1200-calorie a day plan. He finished the program, but six months later, he was back up to 100kg, and over 108kg a year later. The diet didn't work long term for Joseph. Why? He followed a diet, but he didn't make lifestyle changes. Temporary portion control weight-loss diets don't work!

When we discussed what he was eating, he said that he ate anywhere from about six to ten slices of bread a day. A cup of tea and some toast early, toast and jam for breakfast, and his lunch could consist of three or four slices of bread spread with peanut butter. At dinner, he'd have bread roll. That's a whole lot of bread and calories. While he said he wanted to make some changes in his health, there weren't strong drivers for change. He was reluctant to go on a 5:2 Diet because his doctor had informed him that it would interfere with his blood pressure medication. In a discussion about my book, I helped him understand the tactics for keeping in high value foods and that he could reduce his weight and make improvements to his health just by reducing bread intake to maybe half a slice of toast, but increasing protein. A key part of any diet is to ensure you do not get hungry, and a moderate protein increase, and a carbohydrate decrease helps decrease appetite and hunger. Five weeks later he was down 9 lb (4 kg) without any particular diet. He "took-out" the excessive amounts of bread he was consuming. Eight months on and slow and surely his weight is further down, his blood pressure back to normal, and his diet is sustainable for the long term.

A photographer I know was in the habit of going for a morning coffee, but always had a muffin to go along with it. His change: purchase of a home coffee machine. After eight weeks he had dropped 22 lb (10 kg). He "took-out" the trip to the tempting café and cut out the snacks between meals.

Conclusion

If your enthusiasm or driver for change is small, you need to find a "take-out" strategy for yourself. You have to have a reason for change commensurate with the degree of change you want to achieve, and take out something from your lifestyle (choose something you can do without much change) as the change should be minimal for the mind, but substantial for the outcome. (Less pain, more gain!) Changing the balance of the diet (not even reducing the calories specifically) may allow the normal regulatory mechanisms of the body to make that subtle, gradual and yet permanent change.

References

a. Chaloupka FJ, Cummings K, Morley CP, Horan JK. (2002) Tax, price and cigarette smoking: evidence from the tobacco documents and implications for tobacco company marketing strategies. Tobacco Control 2002;11(Suppl I):i62–i72 see http://www.ncbi.nlm.nih.gov/pmc/articles/PMC1766067/pdf/v011p00i62.pdf

b. Daily Mail. (2013) http://www.dailymail.co.uk/news/article-2421737/Diet-starts-today--ends-Friday-How-quickly-slip-bad-eating-habits-days.html

c. Gregoire, C. (2014) Why We Make Bad Food Decisions, Even When We Know Better. The Huffington Post http://huff.to/1wFhPFR

d. Sullivan N, Hutcherson C, Harris A, Rangel A. (2014) Dietary Self-Control Is Related to the Speed With Which Attributes of Healthfulness and Tastiness Are Processed. Psychological Science . ISSN 0956-7976 http://dx.doi.org/10.1177/0956797614559543

CHAPTER 17
MENTAL PREP FOR HEALTHY LIVING

Get the Facts

➤ The psychology of weight loss and health is an absolutely necessary aspect of why diets fail, and why they can succeed. It needs to match the other strategies of biochemistry, and the social behaviours of the dieters.

➤ The subconscious plays a part in weight loss. Conscious mismatch is very real. It is important to deal with this as part of your health and diet process. While you may consciously want to be healthier and/or more attractive, your subconscious may have a completely different agenda.

➤ What if the whole goal of eating, is a reward to make us feel better emotionally? One of the reasons the subconscious *always* wins is that we may not even realize we are in a battle. It is common for a person to battle addiction, and depression, among other things.

➤ People struggle with obesity and self-worth. We hold onto unhealthy perceptions and worry about what others think of us, particularly when overweight or obese.

➤ Understand what works for a balanced, long-term eating plan.

Understand the Science

As I researched the biochemistry and endocrinology of health, what became glaringly obvious was that the mental state of the humans, in the study, was a major confounder of the research. It's a bit easier with animal studies. With animals, we have the ability to control their food intake. In some nutrition studies, the researchers could even manipulate the food intake by force feeding animals. Therefore, they could determine if their appetite or their metabolism was a result of the food or other behaviours. It is a little trickier with humans. We have self-control and self-abandonment!

There is a genre of books out there that actually deal with the mental state of dieting. I had come to a conclusion that the mental state was one of the primary determinants of any change in weight and health as part of the second leg of that stool. I came across Dr George Blair-West's work in his book, *Weight Loss for Food Lovers* as I searched for authors who had looked at this area of dieting. His series provides practical and sound information from his work as both a doctor and psychotherapist. As a point of reference, I am very concerned about the rigidity of any diet including *Sweet Poison* and the anti-sugar theme. I have strong willpower. I am often called the food Nazi by those who know me but I, like many others, cannot stop at one piece of chocolate offered after dinner. Blair-West describes three behaviours that he calls the "Last Supper Effect," the "What the Hell Effect," and the "Restraint Theory." Blair-West says these three behaviours cause diet failure, because they result in "mini-binges". These mini-binges cause diets to fail. He instead uses terms include "High Sacrifice Foods" and "Low Sacrifice Foods". We will come back to some of these tactics as part of this mental process later in the chapter.

What also puzzled me was how books on self-help or hypnotherapy also seemed to contribute to success. What was the interaction? Could these various components be brought together for a successful weight loss program? While not achieving 100% long term success, could the success rate be doubled from 20% to 40%? That would make a huge difference to people who really want to lose weight and be healthy.

Success is not only about the internal state of how we feel. Low levels of social connectedness also adversely affect the body, lowering the immune response and affecting heart health. One study demonstrated that first-year college students who mixed with fewer people, or felt lonely, had a lower immune response to influenza vaccinations than their more gregarious or socially contented classmates did. According to Sarah Pressman, a health psychologist at Carnegie Mellon University, Pittsburgh, USA, a second study suggests that men who are socially isolated have elevated levels of a blood marker for inflammation, which has a role in atherosclerosis. It was known that isolation has detrimental effects on heart health, and the study gives clues as to how this is mediated. Surprisingly, the effects were independent of one another. "Loneliness is the *perception* of being alone," she explains, whereas social networks can be counted objectively as the number of people with whom a person has contact. Pressman acknowledges that there is no easy or obvious way to remedy a person's feelings of loneliness. But she notes that simply keeping in touch with social contacts like family and friends would have a protective effect. People who have good support systems in place seem to be healthier and happier, even if the social interaction is not frequent. "You can have very few friends but still not feel lonely. Alternatively, you can have many friends yet feel lonely," says Pressman. It seems, in this instance, that quality outweighs quantity.

Poor mental health translates to poorer physical health and the Mental Illness Fellowship of Australia data shows:

- Schizophrenics are 50% more likely to have a stroke, and subsequently, more than twice as likely to die as non-schizophrenic people.

- Schizophrenics are 20% more likely to get cancer.

- Schizophrenics have a one in three chance of developing diabetes.

- 40% of all the smokers who continue to smoke in Australia are people with some form of mental illness.

- If you have a mental illness, you will have worse oral health. You are 3.4 times more likely to have lost all your teeth, and to have six times worse decayed, filled, or missing teeth.

Sexual abuse reputedly involves one in four girls and one in six boys in the general population. In very obese people who applied for stomach surgery for weight loss, one in three had a history of sexual abuse. Do these people use being overweight as a mechanism to be less attractive? There's the subconscious again! In partnerships, it may be that sabotage of the diet, by the other partner, is a very real issue. Partners who do not want their significant other to be "attractive enough" to catch the attention of another may consciously or subconsciously encourage their partner to eat too much and eat foods that can help put on excess weight.

Diet Sabotage Behaviours

We will look at Blair-West's three behaviours which we can all relate to. The consequence of these behaviours is a "mini-binge," and this mini-binge does two things: it negates the reduced calorie intake from the diet, that dieters try to stick to; and psychologically it undermines and undoes the willpower of the dieter.

- The "Last Supper Effect." Research shows that if you know you are going to restrict calories in the future, you compensate by overeating. You stock up as though you are preparing for some sort of famine in the land. If you know that chocolate bars are going to become a forbidden item, you may gorge on three or four chocolate bars. Or eat more the day before you start a diet.

- The "What the Hell Effect." You are doing well on your diet, but then you have a treat such as a chocolate cookie. (A TimTam biscuit for Australians). But you don't stop at just one. No! You have two, and then it is "What the Hell," and you eat the whole packet.

- The "Restraint Theory." In practice, if you give up too many foods, you eventually rebel, and say "What the Hell." It is human nature to desire what should not, or cannot, be had. If you feel like your choices in food are severely limited to the point that you can barely eat anything, you feel the restraint is too great and will give up. You might follow it with a "Last Supper," go back on the diet, and then repeat the "What the Hell."

Blair-West suggests the solution to these behaviours is the "Low Sacrifice Diet." Analyze your foods and put them into three different groups. Fattening foods that are *high sacrifice* and you do not want to give them up; fattening foods that you are happy to give up (*low sacrifice*); and healthy foods. Then drop just the low sacrifice foods. I.e. Take-out only the low sacrifice foods. Note: Don't cheat by listing foods you *dislike* on the low sacrifice list just to make yourself feel better!

He gives the example that a high sacrifice food for him was chocolate cookies. His tactic was to have them midmorning, after a big protein breakfast, when he was still full. He could stop at two, and not the whole packet. But if he ate them at afternoon snack time, he would be hungry, have a couple and the "What the Hell" effect kicked in, and he ate the whole packet. He says that deprivation of high sacrifice foods is probably the major reason why diets fail. You don't fail a diet if you do a "What the Hell" on healthy foods!

A friend of mine loves his bread, and it falls in the high sacrifice food group for him. At lunch, when hungry, he could easily consume four slices or more (that's 400 calories plus). So the tactic for him was to have one slice of bread at breakfast, with high protein bacon and eggs. At lunchtime, he ate high protein chicken instead of a few sandwiches that required so much bread. Less calories and no "What the Hell" effect. He would be full and satisfied without the bread, yet it was not a banned food. You have to work out the delicate balance of sticking to a low simple carbohydrate diet yet having tactics for high value foods.

I love Christmas cake (fruitcake). For six months, I avoided it and asked my family not to buy or bake me one. It was tough salivating as I went past the market stalls where the rich cakes were temptingly displayed. I knew it was impossible to stop at one slice, and five slices add up to 1000 calories and more sugar and fructose than I wanted to eat. I learnt from my research that the fructose had its own serious health issues. Reading Blair-West's book provided understanding. I recognized that fruit cake is a high sacrifice food for me. I went to boarding school, and the fruit cakes provided by my mother every few weeks were more than just food – they were a high comfort food that softened home-sickness. Denial created restraint, and then a 'What the Hell" moment. I now have one small slice at mid-morning with a coffee, and I savor that piece. I'm not hungry at that time of day due to a big breakfast, and I can stop at the one slice (200 calories) and adjust my daily intake. However, I don't have that cake at 4:00 in the afternoon with a cup of tea and when I am hungry. (Low glucose levels.) It always seemed I needed 2 pieces for the cup of tea, and then another couple with the second cup of tea. When I realized this complexity, I accepted a cake the neighbour provided, and I could have a piece, or none for a few days. My addiction had gone. The willpower required for this tactic is minimal especially as I no longer felt deprived.

Conclusion

To sum up the mental prep required for healthy living, it is your mind, the 2nd leg of the stool, which is another major reason for diet failure. You have to understand why you like food, and what it means on both conscious and subconscious levels. You will need strategies and tactics on how you are going to overcome habits and beliefs. Losing weight on a diet is undone by mini-binges. You have to accept everyone has them, and plan for counter measures, such as Blair-West's exercise, the 5:2 diet, and taking-out simple carbohydrates from your diet. You have to do things smarter, not work harder.

Spend some time to do Blair-West's exercise. Take a sheet of paper, turn it landscape and rule across the middle, and then divide the top into 2 columns. That makes 3 boxes. High value "unhealthy" on the left top, low value "unhealthy" foods on the right top, and "healthy foods" for the half page on the bottom. Write down a dozen foods or more in each box. Then, take-out of your diet those low value unhealthy foods in the top right hand box. Keep the high value foods. Have as much healthy food as you want. Buy his book. I found it excellent. While I am not really a food lover his approach works for me but more importantly for those who love their food. He has much more detailed information to help.

References

a. Dr George Blair-West. (2010) Weight Loss for Food Lovers: Understanding our minds and why we sabotage our weight loss. Alclare. Pp240 ASIN: B004Q9U4ZM
b. Pressman SD, Cohen S, Miller GE, Barkin A, Rabin BS, Treanor JJ. (2005) Loneliness, Social Network Size, and Immune Response to Influenza Vaccination in College. Health Psychol 24(4) 297-306 DOI: 10.1037/0278-6133.24.3.000
c. MIFA (2011) The Physical Health of People Living With a Mental Illness - Literature Review, Programs Overview & Recommendations. http://www.mifa.org.au/index.php/media-alias/physical-health-and-wellbeing
d. Fergusson D, Mullen P. (1999) Childhood Sexual Abuse. An Evidence Based Perspective. Sage. pp144 ISBN 9781452221526

CHAPTER 18
TAKE OUT SUGAR

Get the Facts

➢ Take-Out added sugar and fructose from your diet is the first and most important step for health.
➢ Understand the difference between sugar and carbohydrates.
➢ Consuming sugar prevents weight loss and makes it difficult to manage your weight.
➢ View added sugar in your diet to be as detrimental as alcohol to your health, whether you are fat or thin.
➢ Even though there are other factors involved, the kind of food you eat affects your weight.
➢ You need a plan that is simple and doable so that you will turn the plan into a life-time of healthy living.

Understand the Science

Back in 1825, Jean Anthelme Brillat-Savarin in The Physiology of Taste knew the causes of obesity were flour and sugar.

"Since it has been proved that fatty congestion is simply due to flour and starch, it may be inferred that a more or less strict abstinence from all floury or starchy foods leads to a diminution of flesh."

Sugar is the new tobacco. It seems there is a new book out on the topic of sugar every week! What is it with this sugar thing? To understand what the hype is about, we have to be very clear about what the issues are, and where to start. The biochemistry of saccharides is in the next chapter. Here are five things about sugar and carbohydrates that you need to remember. Sugar is a simple saccharide; carbohydrates are more complex ones, so you have to be precise about which one you are consuming.

• Glucose is essential to life, but if it is too low or too high, levels are toxic. At any one time you only have about 5 g of glucose in your blood, but it is a dynamic and precise cycle. Glucose is only one of the simple sugars.

- Another simple sugar, fructose, should be viewed as similar to alcohol. There is no "safe level" of added fructose in your diet, and added fructose should be eliminated for health reasons alone. Just as a glass of wine is okay, but a bottle every day will kill you; fructose will kill you slowly and just as surely.

- Simple carbohydrates (which include sugars) in the Western diet are the primary causes for fatness and obesity. Carbohydrates are eaten, converted to glucose, and either get used or deposited as fat. For effective weight reduction and management of obesity, cut out all added sugars and all simple carbohydrates (potatoes, rice, and flour products) to get your normal appetite processes under control.

- Sugars and/or simple carbohydrates (white flour, rice) are the major contributors to chronic illnesses including cardiovascular disease, diabetes, fatty liver disease, chronic kidney disease, cancer, and dementia.

- Dietary fat is not the problem.

Questions we need to ask are:
- Is the problem sugar, refined carbohydrates, or both?
- Is one more important in dieting than the other?

You can't avoid sugars completely (especially fructose) as it is in fruit and vegetables. Small amounts won't kill you. Complex carbohydrates such as green leafy vegetables appear to be excellent, but avoid added sugar like the plague. Global food companies know that sugar and fat sell more food because people's taste buds have adjusted to the taste. People like/love the way sugar makes food taste. Many medical professionals are not up to date with the compelling studies on sugar consumption. It takes decades for human studies to lead to concrete conclusions. Can you afford not to act until the studies on humans are all in? No, of course not! There is no argument about sugar with animal studies. The question that remains is to what level is sugar safe for consumption? Is there any "safe" consumption level?

Prof Lustig certainly does not dabble in shades of grey. He emphatically says that sugar is not just an empty calorie. He says that its effect on humans is much more insidious. "It's not about the calories," he says. "It has nothing to do with the calories. It's a poison by itself."

Tips to Reduce Sugar

So what can you do practically?

- Stop adding sugar to any food or drink.

- Do not eat any food product more than about 3% sugar. Check the label and if more than 3 g per 100 g eat something else.

- Do not eat more than two or three pieces of fruit per day.

- You can eat as many complex carbohydrates (green leafy vegetables) as you want.

If you are overweight, and you go sugar free, you probably will lose weight. Some may choose a diet program with some form of intermittent fasting as part of the change process to accelerate the weight loss and for other change management reasons. I suggest the 5:2 diet as a tactic to counter the mini-binge (as per the Mental Prep chapter). When you change from high levels of sugar consumption (e.g. chocoholics or have a "sweet tooth") to being sugar free, you will have relapses when you have those "what the hell moments."

Read and study more. This is not a new issue, and it has been going on for the past 170 years. Regrettably, the nutritionists have focused on low-fat diets as part of a reduction in heart disease, and in doing so, have created a global pandemic of obesity. Poor science and dogma have dismissed low-carbohydrate and zero-fructose diets to societies' detriment, and probably to you as well. This is far less complicated than many make it out to be. When it comes to simple carbohydrates and sugars, "drop the fork." To what level is the question. Completely or some.

Take-out the sugar from your diet. It is hard! We look at this in the mental prep for healthy eating section and elsewhere. Humans have dieted for centuries. The standard approach for losing weight was to eliminate carbohydrates such as starch, potatoes, and flour in all forms. But in the mid-50s and 60s the emphasis switched to reducing heart disease. For a very good and detailed science-based treatise on this read Gary Taubes' 2012 book *The Diet Delusion*.

Taubes reported a conversation with a professor of Public Policy for the USA Government on Obesity Today who stated, *"Maybe America has gone too far. It is going to take us a long time to get back on track because the marketing, the money, and the patterns have been deeply established. My hope is that the developing nations see what we have done and don't follow our lead.*" In 1990, China had little to no known cases of obesity. Today, one in three people are overweight or obese. It is too late. Australia is fattening up: 63% of the population is overweight or obese. The obesity issue is no longer a Western problem anymore.

The populist move against added sugar and carbohydrates has been going on for decades. It is not new. Recent books by science writers such as Gary Taubes have been around for five years or more. There has been tremendous populist understanding created by Prof Robert Lustig, UC Berkley, with a video in 2010, and subsequent books. The popularization of the anti-fructose movement has been extended by writers such as David Gillespie, author of *Sweet Poison*. Gillespie assessed the information and provided much needed simplicity to the science articles. Some of the other books have the same type of information, but not as easy reading. They have detailed articles and reviews, but do not necessarily capture the simple message. The information can be found in science literature, but again, the obvious truth about how sugar directly and adversely affects real people on a daily basis is not emphasized. This rejection of the low dietary fat argument and the proponent of low carbohydrate diets has been with us from the early 1820s right through to now. In the mid-1960s, Cleave said the Westernization of diet into other cultures generated a "saccharine disease," and elevated levels of diabetes, chronic illnesses including coronary heart disease and cancer. Countries went from negligible illnesses to levels approaching or exceeding the highest Western levels.

It was only in the latter part of the 1970s that the rising rate of obesity and increasing diabetes created what is now termed Metabolic Syndrome (MetS). MetS is a combination of medical disorders that, when occurring together, increases the risk of developing diabetes and heart disease. It is estimated that 25% of the USA has MetS. Symptoms include abdominal obesity (BMI >30 or waist >94 cm male or 84 cm female), high blood pressure (over 140/90 mmHg), high cholesterol (>150mg/dl), insulin resistance (fasting plasma glucose >6 mmol/l), and urinary albumin excretion (creatinine >30). The best marker is the presence of visceral fat. If you have visceral fat, you are very likely to have MetS, which is why waist measurement is a pretty good indicator.

Fructose is demonstrated to not only cause MetS, but cause directly or indirectly these six diseases:

- Cardio vascular disease

- Cancer

- Diabetes

- Chronic kidney disease

- Liver disease

- Dementia

Each of these "diseases" may have a large number of specific diseases, but the symptoms are similar. Prognosis is individual to each disease. For example, there are dozens of cancers. Each may have a different cause, but exhibit similar outcomes. Treatment can be variable and prognosis different. As the disease is better understood, treatments and prevention, may also be better understood. These metabolic diseases probably reduce our lifespan, and our lifestyle quality, even when a person is not overweight. So what role does being overweight play in these diseases? The role of fructose as a contributor to being overweight is shown in the next diagram.

What Effect Does Sugar Have?

We can review animal studies to see what effect sugar and various types of sugars cause. Researchers at the University of Utah fed mice a daily diet of 25% extra sugar, which is the equivalent of a healthy human diet plus three cans of soda. They found that female mice were twice as likely to die, or have fewer babies, than those on a diet without the added sugar. Males were 25% less likely to present normal territorial behaviour and reproduce. Despite this, the mice didn't become obese or demonstrate significant metabolic symptoms. The effects the researchers did see, however, were just as harmful to the mice's health as being the inbred offspring of two cousins. The study's senior author, biology professor Wayne Potts, stressed the relevancy of the study to humans. "*Our results provide evidence that added sugar consumed at concentrations currently considered safe exerts dramatic adverse impacts on mammalian health,*" Potts said in a press release. "*I have reduced refined sugar intake and encouraged my family to do the same.*" The study contrasts with previous research work that involved feeding mice exceedingly large quantities of sugar disproportionate to levels seen in human diets. What is "dramatic adverse impact"? The clinical defects of fructose/glucose-fed mice were decreased glucose clearance and increased fasting cholesterol, both linked to MetS, diabetes and cardiovascular disease.

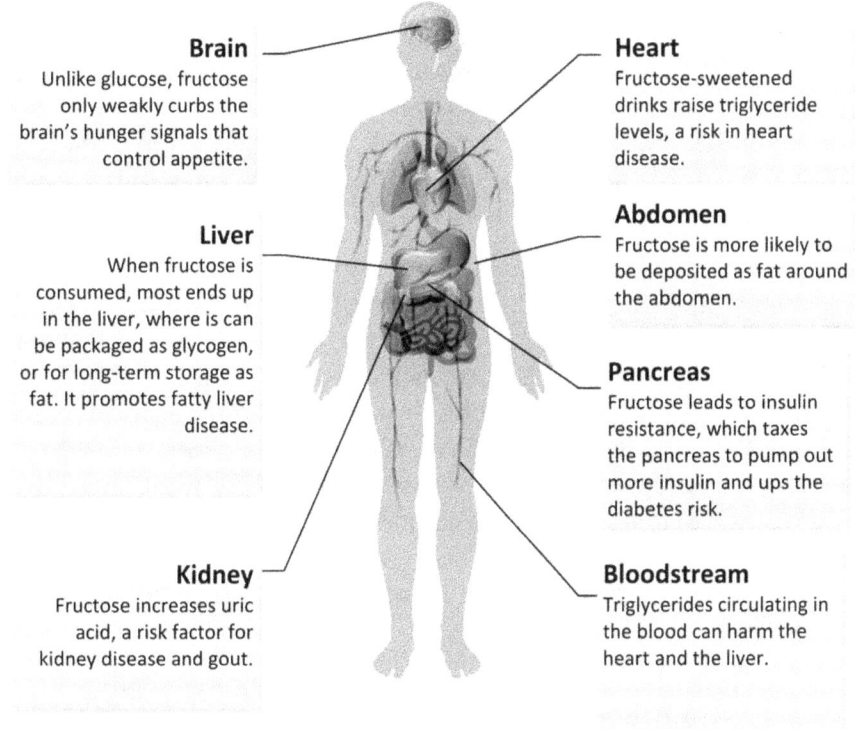

Brain
Unlike glucose, fructose only weakly curbs the brain's hunger signals that control appetite.

Heart
Fructose-sweetened drinks raise triglyceride levels, a risk in heart disease.

Liver
When fructose is consumed, most ends up in the liver, where is can be packaged as glycogen, or for long-term storage as fat. It promotes fatty liver disease.

Abdomen
Fructose is more likely to be deposited as fat around the abdomen.

Pancreas
Fructose leads to insulin resistance, which taxes the pancreas to pump out more insulin and ups the diabetes risk.

Kidney
Fructose increases uric acid, a risk factor for kidney disease and gout.

Bloodstream
Triglycerides circulating in the blood can harm the heart and the liver.

Figure 16 Fructose effects in the body

How much sugar do you actually have? Elsewhere we have discussed the total amount of glucose dissolved in the bloodstream of a healthy non-diabetic is equivalent to 5 g (1 teaspoon). More than that is toxic, and less than that can cause you to pass out, and the control of that homeostasis is complex. Several studies have shown that under normal low metabolic conditions (at rest or low-to mid-levels of activity such as walking and easy work) the body only needs about 5 g/hr. The brain is the major consumer of glucose, needing maybe 120 g/day. Low-carbohydrate eating reduces the brain's glucose requirements considerably, and those who are very low carbohydrate (VLC) and keto-adapted may only require about 30 grams of glucose per day to fuel the brain (and little-to-none, to fuel the muscles at <75% max efforts). Twenty of those grams can come from glycerol (a by-product of fat metabolism) and the balance from gluconeogenesis in the liver (which can actually make up to a whopping 150 grams a day if you haven't metabolically damaged it with NAFLD through fructose overdosing). You probably don't ever need to consume more than 150 grams of dietary carbohydrates, and you can thrive on far less.

Fructose or Carbohydrate – the Evil One?

One of the real difficulties that I have in making sense of the "sugar is evil" concept, is finding research that clearly differentiates between glucose, fructose, sugars, and carbohydrates. All carbohydrates must be hydrolyzed to monosaccharides prior to absorption in the small intestine. Some carbohydrates that are not adsorbed, move to the large intestine. It is a quick process.

There are not even very good epidemiological studies. A long term study may start out to measure some variables, data may not be collected, or the results confounded by a range of factors. By their very nature, they never provide causation. The gold standard for science is randomized double blind placebo based trials and there is an example in the Science and Studies chapter. It is impossible to do this type of study with food because people know what treatment they have. When studies are done, patients exercise free will. Some stop the diet. Some cheat. There are research examples where patients eat different food under supervision, and then go home and binge on other food.

Animal studies can be better controlled, and rat studies show that added sugar (at the levels that society consumes) puts on weight, and is a direct cause of obesity, metabolic syndrome diseases, and dementia. But humans are not rats (prejudices aside). When people cut out added sugar, they cut out more than just sugar. Because of food products in our society, they will also cut out other simple carbohydrates (starch) as well as glucose and fructose. Simple carbohydrate products from flour or rice that are in buns, donuts, cakes, breads, and other prepared foods, all go when you cut out "added sugar." They also are removed because food products often have added sugar, so when you reduce added sugar, you also remove those simple carbohydrates as well. Diets become more restrictive and they have to eat more whole food. Without acknowledging it, they have changed to a low carbohydrate diet. So are the benefits and results they get from this diet caused by the lowering of glucose, lowering of fructose, lowering consumption of simple carbohydrates, or a combination of all three factors?

Anyone on an Atkins Diet will eliminate fructose, glucose, and 90% of their carbohydrates. Paleo Dieters will likewise eliminate fructose and most simple carbohydrates, as will those on the South Beach Diet. With higher protein and fat, dieters simply eat less simple carbohydrates.

As I was doing the 5:2 Diet and tracking my food intake, I realized that I had cut out 70% of my carbohydrates. On the two days of low calories (600 calories), my strategy was no simple carbohydrates and more protein and unlimited leafy green vegetables. No alcohol such as beer or wine. No bread, potatoes, rice, or pasta. If it was a choice between 100 gm of protein or a slice of bread, it was no contest! Protein is more satisfying.

The common element of this is insulin. Insulin controls glucose levels in the blood and is a major determinant in the hunger and appetite process.

Remove Added Sugar

Science is getting clearer about added sugar in the diet. Take it out! Anyone who argues added sugar should remain in the diet is basing their conclusions on poor and old research. With new understandings, and what was promoted as the "hard facts" have become less "hard," or even proven incorrect. There is immense vested interest from food and drug companies to maintain consumption of simple carbohydrates. The pharmaceutical companies keep a tight lid on what serves them best. To make things worse, the science community is slow to change. Not all research is published. Nil results and adverse results are often not made public, so practices that have no benefit continue to be promoted.

Another reason for removal of sugar and simple carbohydrates from our diet is that their impacts take a long time to show up. A researcher might do a study for three months or maybe even a year, but the metabolic effect may not show up for 5 or even 20 years. Reviews of Westernization of indigenous communities by Cleave and Campbell, suggest a decade or two will lapse between the diet change and the rise of chronic health diseases that result from the diet change. Dementia might show up after 40 or more years. So the time-frame between ingestion and disease onset can be pretty tenuous. That is why most studies have been done in shorter lived species such as mice. Then the counter argument is raised that the studies were "small animal" and should be discounted.

Further Reading

This is not a book like Gary Taubes' *The Diet Delusion*, *Sweet Poison* by David Gillespie, Robert Lustig's *Fat Chance* or Michael Moss' *Salt, Sugar, Fat: How the food giants hooked us,* and other books. Those authors provide a wealth of knowledge and base their conclusions on the way they see it. They focused particularly on the role of excess sugars (fructose and glucose), simple carbohydrates, and fat in our diet.

Excess glucose and simple carbohydrates make us fat. Fructose makes us fat and sick.

Conclusion

If you hate big companies or love them, if you're pro-science or anti-science, then there is enough reading material out there by well-informed and excellent authors. In particular, if you want to be informed and get concerned about un-ethical behaviour, Moss's book on the food companies is a compelling and disconcerting read.

This book is about trying to have a balanced and rational approach to gain and maintain better health. It's not about a specific diet or ideal lifestyle. As with all biological systems, there is seldom a single best approach. The anti-sugar diet is ridiculed by the sugar producers and food companies and some dieticians as being too extreme and restrictive. I have not found it so, but sugar is not a high sacrifice value food for me. Health, not weight reduction, was my primary goal.

My conclusion is that to improve health, there are two simple actions, and there is sufficient evidence-based science to support these actions.

- Take-out added fructose from your diet. No exceptions. Note this is added fructose and naturally present fructose in fruit and in dairy products is ok in small quantities.

- Take-out simple carbohydrates from your diet. The more the better for both health and weight outcomes. Do it to a level you can sustain long-term.

The risk to long term health is simply too great not to address these two actions.

References

a. Lustig, Dr Robert H M.D., (2012) Fat Chance. The Bitter truth about Sugar. Harper Collins ISBN 978-000-7514-137

b. Gary Taubes (2008) The Diet Delusion p288 Reprint 2011 ISBN-13: 978-0307474254 ASIN: B0031RS9S4

c. Michael Moss (2013) Salt Sugar, Fat. How the Food Giants hooked us. Epub. ISBN 978-1-4481-3387-1 Random House

d. Gillespie, David (2013). Sweet Poison. Why Sugar makes us fat. Viking. Pp208 ISBN-13: 978-0670072477

e. Gillespie, David (2012) Big Fat Lies. How the diet industry is making you sick, fat and poor. Penguin ISBN 978-1-74253-482-4

f. Wilson, Sarah (2012). I Quit Sugar ISBN-13: 978-1-4566-0700-5

g. Ruff J.S, Suchy A, Hugentobler S, Sosa M, Schwartz B, Morrison L, Gieng S, Shigenaga M, Pottset W. (2013) Human-relevant levels of added sugar consumption increase female mortality and lower male fitness in mice. Nature Communications 4, Article number: 2245 doi:10.1038/ncomms3245

h. Mark Sisson (2103) A Metabolic Paradigm Shift, or Why Fat is the Preferred Fuel for Human Metabolism. http://www.marksdailyapple.com/a-metabolic-paradigm-shift-fat-carbs-human-body-metabolism

i. Taubes, G. (2012). Is Sugar Toxic. http://www.nytimes.com/2011/04/17/magazine/mag-17Sugar-t.html

j. Van Den Bergh AJ, Houtman S, Heerschap A, Rehrer NJ, Van Den Boogert HJ, Oeseburg B, Hopman MTE: (1996) Muscle glycogen recovery after exercise during glucose and fructose intake monitored by13C-NMR. J. Appl. Physiol. 81(4): 1495–1500.

k. Conlee RK, Lawler RM, Ross PE. (1987) Effects of glucose or fructose feeding on glycogen repletion in muscle and liver after exercise or fasting. Ann Nutr Metab. 31(2):126-32.

CHAPTER 19
BIOCHEMISTRY OF CARBOHYDRATES

Get the Facts

➢ A sugar is a type of carbohydrate.
➢ Reduction of simple carbohydrates is primarily about reduction of obesity.
➢ Obesity is only one indicator of poor health.
➢ Reduction of fructose is primarily about health.

Understand the Science

Homer Simpson of the famous *The Simpsons* TV show once said, "In America, first you get the sugar, then you get the women, then you get the power" on an episode where a truck carrying sugar overturned, and Homer decided to salvage and sell the sugar. Sugar is everywhere in our modern society.

What's the difference between sugars (saccharides) and carbohydrates? Nothing. Just a little chemistry and a name. A carbohydrate is a synonym of "saccharide." Carbohydrates or saccharides are divided into four chemical groupings: monosaccharides, disaccharides, oligosaccharides, and polysaccharides. In general, the monosaccharides and disaccharides, which are smaller carbohydrates, are commonly referred to as sugars. Carbohydrates all have a generic formula of $C_m(H_2O)_n$ – the hydrogen : oxygen ratio the same as water (2:1). So it is important in science to spell out what saccharide is being studied, and the difficulty is that saccharides are in everything, from the cube of sucrose, the leaf of lettuce, the floret of broccoli, or a potato chip!

Monosaccharide sugars (glucose, fructose, galactose) have the formula $C_6H_{12}O_6$ and differ only by geometry; disaccharide sugars have 2 of these monosaccharides joined as one and include sucrose (glucose + fructose), lactose (glucose + galactose), maltose (glucose + glucose). Complex sugars (e.g. xylitol) or carbohydrates (e.g. starch) are the same structure, but many more molecules joined together.

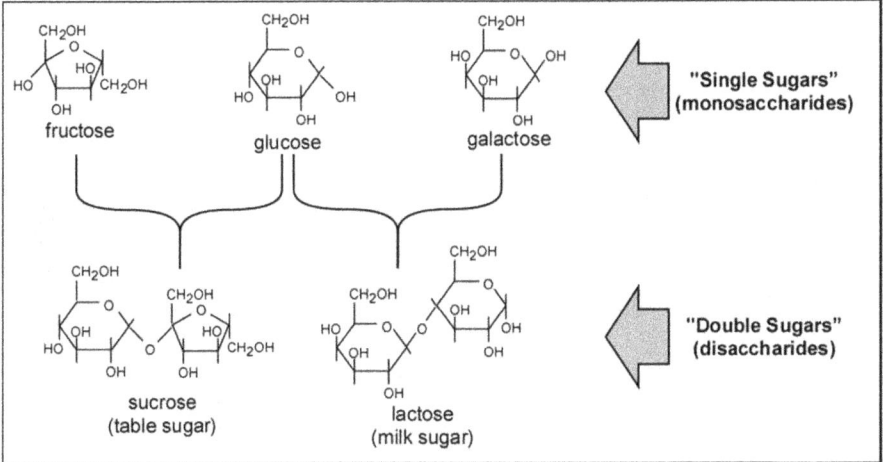

Figure 17 Chemical Structure of sugar

Humans break starch into simple glucose with the enzyme amylase, but not cellulose.

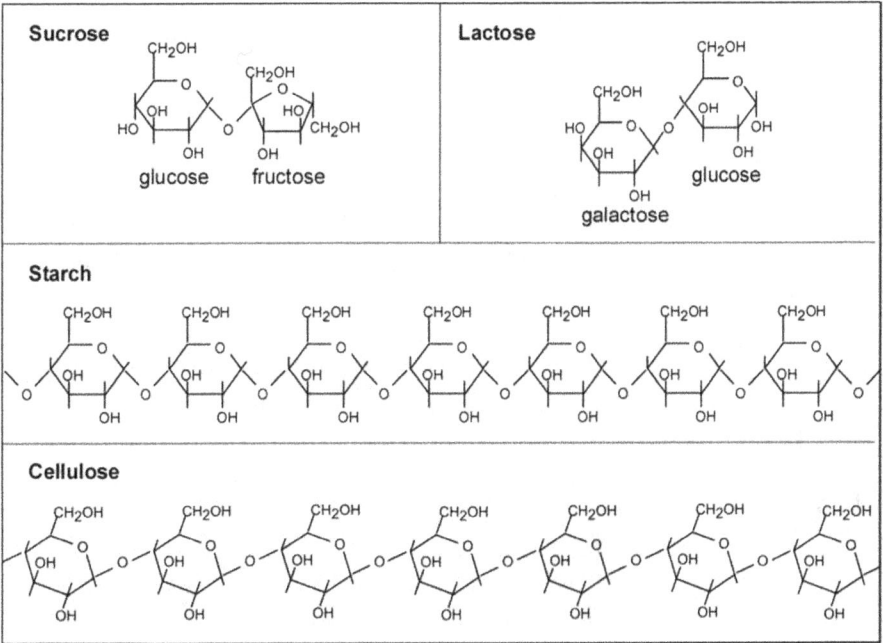

Figure 18 Starch and Cellulose Chemical Structure

Ruminants such as cows do use cellulose via their bacteria in the rumen. In humans the cellulose passes through to our lower intestine, and our bacteria break most of it down into the simple sugars.

Glucose is often quoted as being essential for life, but it is not that simple. We do have within every cell small bodies called mitochondria, and within these there are complex energy processes. The complex process involves a chemical called ATP (Adenosine triphosphate) often called the "molecular unit of currency" of intracellular energy transfer. All energy goes through the ATP processes. Glucose, fats and proteins are converted and the energy from those various reactions is then used. It is complex and comprehensive, and manages our energy balance "just right". There is general misunderstanding glucose is the only source of energy, and nothing is further from reality. There are no "essential" carbohydrates, simple or complex. There are other chemical compounds within plants such as vitamins and minerals but most of those we synthesize ourselves. If we eat some vegetables, or a little fruit that is about it. Governments around the world exhort people to eat 3 to 5 serves of vegetables and a couple of serves of fruit per day, but we certainly do not need cups of sugar or platefuls of pasta. We will discuss this more elsewhere.

Why is Fructose of Concern?

Fructose is 60% sweeter than either glucose or sucrose. In fruit, it serves as a marker for foods that are nutritionally rich. However, in soft drinks and other sweets, fructose serves to reward our desire for sweet tasting food associated with calories, often without much else in the way of nutrition. Fructose enables a higher bliss point, as does fat and salt. The intake of soft drinks containing high-fructose corn syrup (HFCS) or sucrose has risen in parallel with the epidemic of obesity (correlation, not causation). Excessive intake of fructose may induce fatty liver, insulin resistance, dyslipidaemia, hypertension, and kidney disease. Excessive intake of fructose might have an etiologic role in the epidemic of obesity, diabetes, and cardio renal disease. High-fructose corn syrup (HFCS) is a commercial liquid product consisting of fructose and glucose in varying proportions, and in soft drinks is usually 55% fructose and 45% glucose. It is similar to sucrose which is 50/50, but glucose and fructose are separate compounds in the HFCS, and unlike sucrose is not split apart when we consume the food product or beverage.

Fructose Uptake And Metabolism

This section is a little technical for while glucose and fructose are the same chemical structure, there are major differences on how we deal with them. In summary fructose is very similar to alcohol.

Glucose	Fructose
Adsorbed by small intestine	Adsorbed by small intestine, but if too much goes into large intestine, it causes gut issues such as irritable bowel. Fructose also competes with glucose adsorption. (Glut-5 specific transporter)
Glucose passes through liver into bloodstream, and 80% winds up in the rest of the body, converting to glycogen, mostly in muscle.	Majority (80%) goes to liver and only 20% into the bloodstream. Too much fructose gives rise to non-alcoholic fatty liver disease.
Any cell can use glucose.	The liver is the primary site. Kidneys are especially sensitive.
Metabolized anywhere in the body.	Metabolized in the liver cells (hepatocyte). Fructose is phosphorylated to fructose-1-phosphate by fructokinase.
Good feedback mechanism. See previous chapter on metabolism	This reaction has no negative feedback system. If sufficient fructose is present, intracellular phosphate and ATP depletion can transiently occur. This results in the generation of AMP which is metabolized by AMP deaminase to inosine mono-phosphate and eventually to uric acid

Fructose has some other issues. With transient ATP depletion (has some similarities to ischemia), it can result in arrest of protein synthesis with the induction of oxidative stress and inflammation. Circulating fructose is taken up by a variety of cell types, including endothelial cells, but also is excreted into the urine where it is absorbed via the Glut-5 transporter into the S3 segment of the proximal tubule. This cell also expresses fructokinase; as such, the metabolism of fructose by this proximal tubular cell can also lead to local oxidative stress and inflammation.

Fructose is a serious inflammatory compound, and leads to liver function damage, uric acid production which has flow on effects for the kidney, is a cause of gout, disrupts digestion, and has inflammatory actions. Glucose, also inflammatory, has very good feedback mechanisms. Next time you empty a couple of teaspoons of sugar or honey into your coffee, drink a can of soft drink, have a glass of fruit juice, imagine what's going on. Frightening.

How much fructose do we consume? The graph shows over the past 40 years consumption of sugar has climbed from 55 to 70 kg (150lb) per person, but more importantly most of that has been with sucrose and HFCS. That's one major change in diet! Most blame this rise in sugar for rises in obesity and for worsening health.

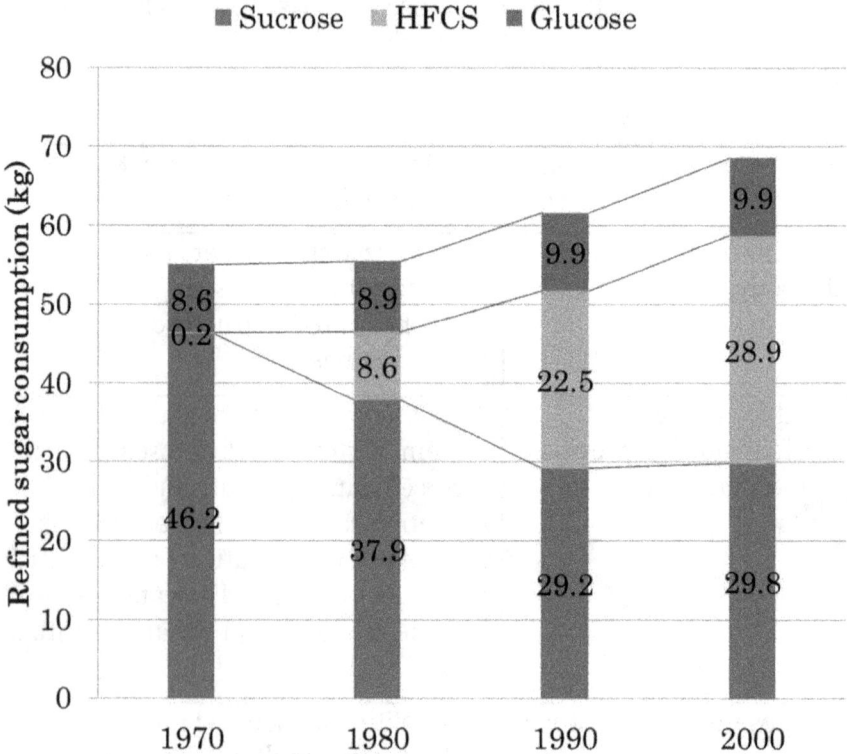

Figure 19 Sugar Consumption USA- data from USDA

Carbohydrates

Carbohydrates have received some negative press, but not the bad press that sugars have. There is a whole genre of Low GI, High GI, *Eat Food, Not too Much, Mostly Plants* type books on the market. Ultimately, polysaccharides and oligosaccharides are digested and broken down into glucose. Sweet fruit will have moderate levels of fructose, but to its credit, fruit also has fiber. Pure digestible carbohydrates have about 4 calories/g.

Carbohydrates are not essential for the synthesis of other molecules.

Humans are able to obtain 100% of their energy requirement from protein and fats.

All carbohydrates, from sugars to broccoli are broken down to monosaccharides.

Health professionals recommend 45-60% of our energy from carbohydrates, but diets such as Atkins recommend almost none. A diet of very low amounts of daily carbohydrate for several days will usually result in higher levels of blood ketone bodies. Higher carbon carbohydrates, such as cellulose, are indigestible to humans (not ruminants), but the cellulose is an important part of dietary fiber, which helps the passage of food through the gut.

The simple, versus complex, carbohydrate distinction has little value for determining the nutritional quality of carbohydrates. Some simple carbohydrates (e.g. fructose) raise blood glucose slowly, while some complex carbohydrates (starches), especially if processed, raise blood sugar rapidly. The speed of digestion is determined by a variety of factors, including which other nutrients are consumed with the carbohydrate, how the food is prepared, individual differences in metabolism, and the chemistry of the carbohydrate.

Digestion of Carbohydrates

All dietary carbohydrates, from simple sugars to oligosaccharides found in complex fibrous vegetables, need to be broken down to monosaccharides (simple sugars) before they can be adsorbed. The process is well explained in Wikipedia or any elementary biology or science book. Starches and complex sugars all get broken down to simpler carbohydrates, then to disaccharides, and eventually to monosaccharides. While the saliva does some breakdown, most is done in the small intestine. These three steps are:

- For starch breakdown, amylase from the pancreas hydrolyzes starch to alpha-dextrin, which in turn is digested by gluco-amylase (alpha-dextrinases) to maltose and maltotriose. The products of digestion of alpha-amylase and alpha-dextrinase, along with dietary disaccharides, are hydrolyzed to their corresponding monosaccharides.

- Enzymes break disaccharides (sucrose, maltose, lactose) and the products of digestion of the starches into monosaccharides. These enzymes have name endings such as "-ase": maltase, isomaltase, sucrase, and lactase.

- Eventually, the products of the digested food – the three main monosaccharides (glucose, fructose, and galactose) are absorbed. They are absorbed in the intestine through the brush border of the epithelium covering the villi (small hair-like structures). It is not a simple diffusion of substances, but is active, and requires energy use by the epithelial cells.

In the typical Western diet, digestion and absorption of carbohydrates is fast, and takes place usually in the upper small intestine. However, when the diet contains carbohydrates that are not easily digestible, digestion and absorption take place mainly at the end of the small intestine (the ileum).

Not every carbohydrate is digested and absorbed in the small intestine. Starchy foods such as potatoes, beans, oats, and wheat flour go through to the large intestine where the bacterial flora metabolize these compounds. It is anaerobic, and gases such as hydrogen, carbon dioxide, and methane, and short-chain fatty acids (acetate, propionate, and butyrate) are absorbed and breathed out or cause flatulence. Hence the expression fat or fart. You digest food and adsorb the monosaccharaides, or it passes through.

High GI Low GI

Much is made of high or GI foods. What the Glycaemic Index of foods is all about is how quickly blood sugar levels rise after eating a particular type of food. You can see from above that this is dependent on how long it takes the starch to be hydrolyzed and absorbed. The GI estimates how much each gram of available carbohydrate (total carbohydrate minus fiber) in a food raises a person's blood glucose level following consumption of the food, relative to consumption of pure glucose. Glucose has a glycaemic index of 100. The blood sugar level is measured over two hours and there are various parameters. Developed for people with diabetes, it is one of those dietary factors that is made much of, but the issue of how much carbohydrate and what is the insulin response is probably more important. Low GI foods (55 or less) include fructose, beans, small seeds, intact grains, most vegetables, and most sweet fruits. Medium GI (56-69) include sucrose, not intact whole wheat, unpeeled potatoes, and some fruits. High GI (70 or above) include glucose, white bread, maltose, and peeled potatoes.

Take-Out Fructose, Take-Out Simple Carbs

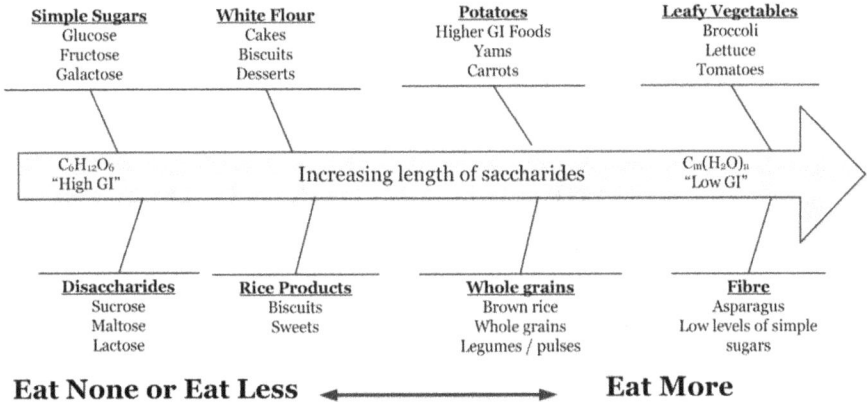

Simple Sugars	White Flour	Potatoes	Leafy Vegetables
Glucose	Cakes	Higher GI Foods	Broccoli
Fructose	Biscuits	Yams	Lettuce
Galactose	Desserts	Carrots	Tomatoes

$C_6H_{12}O_6$
"High GI"   Increasing length of saccharides $C_m(H_2O)_n$ "Low GI"

Disaccharides	Rice Products	Whole grains	Fibre
Sucrose	Biscuits	Brown rice	Asparagus
Maltose	Sweets	Whole grains	Low levels of simple
Lactose		Legumes / pulses	sugars

Eat None or Eat Less ⟵⟶ **Eat More**

Figure 20 Carbohydrates – from Sugar to Leafy Vegetables

Conclusion

I've come to the conclusion that I do not need to eat simple carbohydrates. From a biochemical perspective they are not needed for energy; not essential for nutrients, and simple carbohydrates, especially fructose, have substantial health risks. GI values may be relevant if you are eating 45% to 55% of your diet as carbohydrates, but if you choose a lower carbohydrate diet, ignore GI. The only carbohydrates you will want to eat will be the complex ones. We will see in other chapters that eliminating fructose from your diet, and reducing simple carbohydrates, improves health, helps manage appetite, and is a major contributor to weight reduction.

References

a. Fructose: http://en.wikipedia.org/wiki/Fructose
b. Carbohydrates: http://en.wikipedia.org/wiki/Carbohydrate
c. Bray G. (2007) How bad is fructose?. Am J Clin Nutr October 2007 vol. 86 no. 4 895-896
d. Kretowowicz M, Johnson R, Ishimoto T, Nakagawa T, Manitius J. (2011) The impact of fructose on renal function and Blood Pressure. Int. J Nephrology. http://dx.doi.org/10.4061/2011/315879
e. Cordain L, Eaton SB, Sebastian A, Mann N, Lindeberg S, Watkins B, O'Keefe J, Brand-Miller J. (2005) Origins and evolution of the Western diet: health implications for the 21st century Am J Clin Nutr February vol 81(2)341-354
f. Homer Simpson. Episode 17. http://youtu.be/h5BmrPkgYeA
g. Glycemic Index. http://en.wikipedia.org/wiki/Glycemic_index

CHAPTER 20
LEPTIN AND GHRELIN – HUNGER HORMONES

Get the Facts

➤ Hormonal control of diet through insulin, leptin, ghrelin and another 40 other hormones is extremely complicated.

➤ Dietary control processes such as hormones and the mind are all interconnected.

➤ Working correctly and harmoniously, these hormones provide a finely balanced system.

➤ Working incorrectly, calorie excess causes obesity, and obesity worsens calorie excess.

➤ Fructose interferes with all these critical hormones.

Understand the Science

During the past 15 years, there has been much research published on understanding the control mechanism of the appetite. These studies alter food intake through actions on the vagus nerve, the brainstem, and the hypothalamus. They also influence food preferences and the rewarding properties of food. Response to these signals is not only through direct alteration in food intake, but also through effects on metabolic rate and through nerves vagal stimulation of different internal organs. The vagus nerve or the pneumogastric nerve interfaces with the parasympathetic control of the heart and the digestive tract. It is "involuntary".

Eating is Complicated

The whole process of hunger, satiety, and eating is a very complicated process. We burn energy, and we consume energy. If we consume more than we burn, we store energy. The environment, our lifestyle, our individual wiring affects every process. This next figure shows the overall process and some of the major components. It expands on the 3-legged stool model.

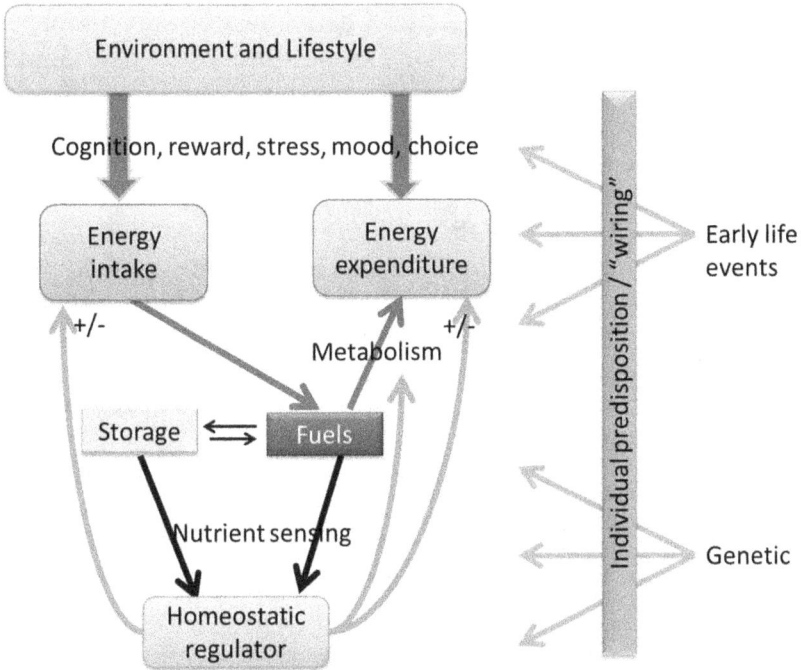

Figure 21 Dietary Control (Lenard and Berthoud)

Here are just some of the factors for hunger and satiety which influence our control processes.

Satiety Factors	Hunger Factors
Stomach and duodenum distension (n. vagus)	Hunger contractions
Heat	Cold
Increase in glucose, amino acids, lipids in blood	decrease in glucose, amino acids, lipids in blood
Catecholamines	Orexins
Serotonin	Endorphins
ACTH	Galanin
Insulin (food in stomach)	Glutamic acid
Leptin	Cortisol
CCK (lipids in duodenum)	Neuropeptide Y
MSH	GABA
Glucagon (also secreted by the pancreas)	Ghrelin
Peptide YY	AMPK

If we take these factors, and put them together, then it is not surprising that the genetic control is far from understood. When people say obesity is simply a matter of eating less or moving more, they fail to recognize that we are very complicate as the next figure shows. The 40 plus hormones that we know about are not shown in the diagram, and we can keep getting more and more detailed. We have not 1, but 2 nervous systems: autonomic and sympathetic. Different parts of the brain. Most organs in the body. It is no wonder there are a large number of diets out there that focus on just one or two concepts. It is not that simple. In this next picture from student lecture notes from Leeds University, Dr Illingworth attempts to show some of the physical and hormonal interactions. Take smell as an example. Bad smells may turn off our hunger. Good smells turn it on. Smells are known to evoke memories, but they also turn on responses such as saliva.

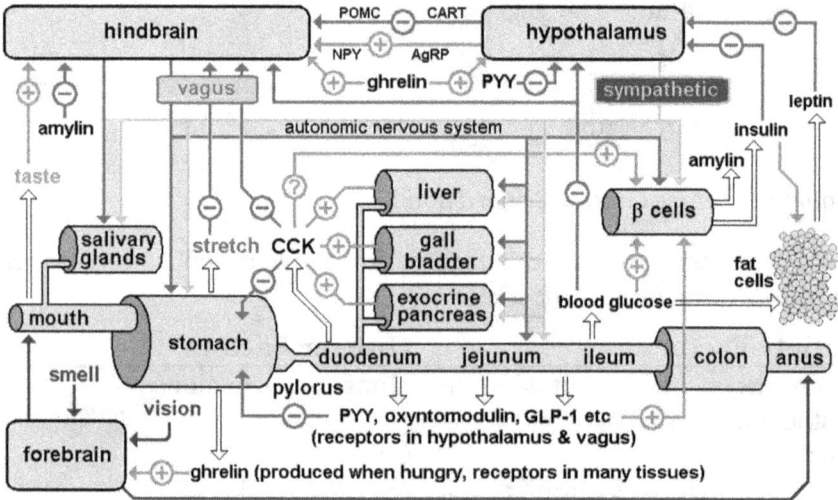

hindbrain   POMC   CART   hypothalamus
NPY   AgRP
vagus   ghrelin   PYY   sympathetic   leptin
amylin   autonomic nervous system   insulin
amylin
taste   liver   β cells
salivary   stretch   CCK   gall
glands   bladder   fat cells
mouth   exocrine   blood glucose
pancreas
smell   stomach   duodenum   jejunum   ileum   colon   anus
pylorus
vision   PYY, oxyntomodulin, GLP-1 etc
(receptors in hypothalamus & vagus)
forebrain
ghrelin (produced when hungry, receptors in many tissues)

Figure 22 Complex Dietary mechanisms.

The model above from Dr Illingworth from Leeds University is too complicated, so we will now look at a simpler model with just 4 of the hormones; leptin, ghrelin, PYY and insulin. The primary area in the brain that focuses on hunger is the hypothalamus, which is centered on a small area in the middle of the brain. A specialized area called the arcuate nucleus is where the signals controlling metabolic rate, hunger, and satiety are located. In the arcuate nucleus are two cell types.

- Hunger Cell type. One cell type is the NPY/AgRP (Neuropeptide Y/Agouti Related Protein) cell. This hunger cell, if stimulated, makes you feel hungry, and your metabolic rate drops.

- Satiety Cell type. Another cell type is the POMC (Proopiomelanocortin) cell. If the satiety cell is stimulated, you feel full, and your metabolic rate increases.

The brain-stem is also involved in this process.

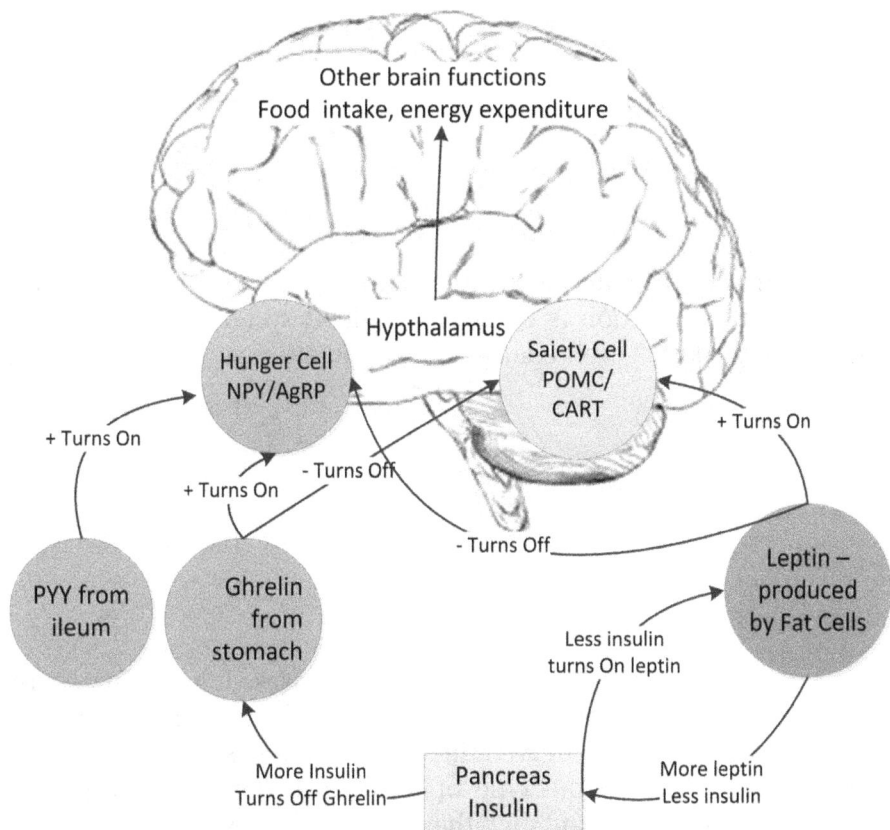

Figure 23 Simplified hormonal control (4 major hormones)

These 4 hormones have different actions.

- Ghrelin is produced by the stomach and travels to the brain where it turns on the hunger cell and turns off the satiety cell. There are two types of ghrelin, acylated and unacylated, and the acylated binds to a growth hormone activating receptor and increases appetite. Unacylated also has a range of metabolic effects.

127

- Leptin is produced by the fat cells of the body, and it travels to the brain where it turns on the satiety cell and turns off the hunger cell.

- Insulin causes a decrease in the release of ghrelin and an increase in the release of leptin. In turn, leptin decreases insulin release.

- PYY (Peptide tyrosine or pancreatic peptide YY3-36) is also part of this complexity. Produced in the ileum and colon, PYY increases after eating, and it decreases by fasting, and works on the hunger cell (NPY receptors).

While the two principle hormones are ghrelin and leptin, all four are interconnected. PYY is less important, but still part of this complicated mechanism. These connections allow the body to recognize and respond to hunger, satiety, and overall nutritional status. Communication is by both the blood system (vascular) and by nerves (vagus). Levels change before and after eating.

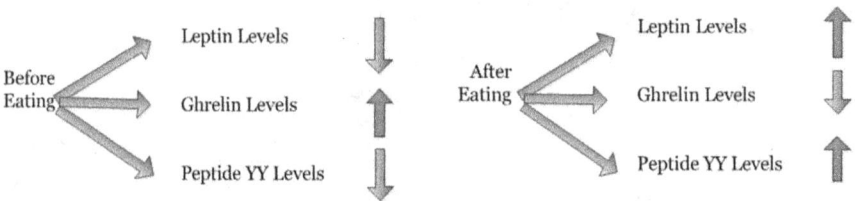

Figure 24 Main hunger hormones

What you eat changes some of these responses. E.g. Eating more protein seems to dampen hormones down and you feel less hungry. One of the changes observed in obese people is they get leptin resistance, similar to the type of resistance that diabetics get to insulin. It also turns out that there is ghrelin resistance in obese people. Obese people don't seem to get the same resistance with PYY as leptin, so there is interest in PYY as an obesity drug. Leptin resistance means you often feel hungry, and no amount of food satisfies that hunger.

Food Shortage – Normal Function

Food shortages mean fewer calories eaten. Insulin levels drop, since insulin is released in response to the intake of calories and the corresponding rise of blood glucose. The lower insulin levels cause a rise in ghrelin, which makes you hungry (i.e. let's go hunting and gathering food). Lower insulin also stimulates the release of stored fatty acids from fat cells. Remember from the chapter on metabolism that in the short term, the liver first metabolizes the glycogen in the liver into glucose, then starts on the fat cells. The fat cells shrink in size and thus produce less leptin. In addition, less insulin has a direct effect on the decreased release of leptin. The lower leptin levels mean that the metabolic rate falls, and you don't burn through the calories as rapidly, again protecting you from the food shortage. This intricate system has kept humans alive through thousands of famines and feasts on the plains of Africa and elsewhere.

Food surpluses – Normal Function

The process above acts in reverse when there is excess food. DNA in mammals mostly controls the processes and animals put on food reserves in times of plenty. Mammals that hibernate may increase fat reserves by 100% to survive during the long winter months when food is not plentiful. Humans have some of this behaviour. But the issue with Western society is not annual or short term body mass increase; it is continual body mass gain.

Normal Function – Other Hormones

We now know it is just not as simple as these 4 hormones. Here are just some of the more than 40. Some hormones produced in the small intestine impact the ghrelin suppression/leptin stimulation pathways and include amylin, oxyntomodulin (OXM), PYY (peptide YY), PP (pancreatic peptide), GLP-1 (glucagon-like peptide 1) and CCK (cholecystokinin). Some, such as PP, amylin, insulin, OXM, GLP-1, GIP, PYY, and CCK are released in response to nutrient ingestion; some such as ghrelin and glucagon in response to fasting. Specifically, OXM responds to protein and carbohydrates in the stomach. PYY and CCK respond to fat and to a lesser degree to protein in the intestines. PP responds to stretching of the stomach. GLP-1 is produced in the panaceas again in response to fat intake.

The type of food eaten changes your response to hunger. Insulin turns ghrelin production off. The fastest way to get insulin levels up is glucose, and glucose is from carbohydrates. Glucose-based carbohydrates and galactose-based carbohydrates (from dairy) are rapidly processed into glucose. Milk satisfies. Fructose based carbohydrates are different. Fructose doesn't stimulate insulin release at all. A fruit juice keeps you hungry! A Swedish study by Nilsson and others showed an evening meal of brown beans, in comparison with white wheat bread lowered blood glucose and insulin both by 15%, increased satiety hormones (PYY 51%) suppressed hunger hormones (ghrelin −14%, and hunger sensations (−15%). Beans also increased GLP-2 concentrations (8.4%), and suppressed inflammatory markers (IL-6 −35%, and IL-18 (−8.3%) at a subsequent standardized breakfast. Not only did the beans change the hormone levels, they changed the microbiome. Beans changed the colonic fermentative activity, with increased breath hydrogen (up 141%), propionate (16%), and isobutyrate (18%).

Ghrelin is also important in many other functions of the body. One of the most important is sleep. In order to efficiently progress though the normal cycles of sleep, you need adequate ghrelin levels. If you don't have them, you will not sleep as efficiently. You will dream less and get less restorative sleep. This will make you more tired the next day, and since dreaming promotes leptin production, you will be hungrier and have a lower metabolic rate.

Food surpluses – Abnormal Function

With chronic calorie excess, there are a number of dysfunctions.

- Insulin levels rise, which turns on the process to move fatty acids into the fat cells. The fat cells become more stretched and release more leptin. Leptin normally acts on the fat cells to increase the production of adiponectin.

- Get more fat cells. Adiponectin is responsible for many things, including making new fat cells.

- Leptin resistance. Over time, the body becomes resistant to leptin, and adiponectin levels fall. The result is that less fat cells are made so existing fat cells get stuffed with fatty acids, creating more and more leptin. Eventually, fatty acids start getting stored in muscle and in the liver.

- Insulin resistance. With the storage of fatty acids in the liver and muscle, these cells become insulin resistant. The process escalates. There is more development of even higher insulin levels, which just drives the whole process more.

- Less use of fatty acids as energy. A consequence of obesity is less movement and a less active lifestyle, and the muscle enzyme "hormone sensitive lipase" starts to fall. This enzyme is responsible for the breakdown of fatty acids for use as energy. With a lower level of this enzyme, fatty acids accumulate even more in the muscle, compounding insulin resistance.

- Ghrelin disruption to hunger cells. Obese people have lots of full fat cells, and leptin levels are generally high. The high leptin levels in combination with high insulin levels turns off the stomach cells that make ghrelin, so ghrelin levels are low. A further complication of high leptin levels is that, over time, it makes the satiety cell insensitive to leptin, and low ghrelin levels make the hunger cell hypersensitive to ghrelin. The result is that even though the leptin levels are high and the ghrelin levels are low, the hunger cells are turned on and the satiety cells are turned off. Ghrelin, when discovered, was hoped to be a simple weight loss pill, but it has not been effective. So the obese person feels famished, and first and foremost is a loss of the conscious signals that tell you when you are full and when you are hungry. A common sign of this is that most obese people don't feel hungry when they get up in the morning. As a result, they often skip breakfast. The brain interprets this as more starvation signals and further shuts down the metabolism. In some studies, the number one risk factor for obesity is skipping breakfast.

- Ghrelin Resistance. There is further complication with these hormones and exercise. Ghrelin has been studied in exercise, as appetite is suppressed after intense exercise. As mentioned, people can get ghrelin resistance as well as leptin resistance. Obese people generally have reduced ghrelin sensitivity and in some studies researchers have found exercise can help in increasing sensitivity.

Simple rule – wait 15 to 20 minutes after you have eaten for some of these other hormones to cut in and provide that satiety and deal with hunger. However, with obese people, this process is often disrupted by insulin, leptin, or ghrelin resistance and / or genetic variation.

In 2013, researchers found more complications. A new circuit in a brain area called the "bed nucleus of the stria terminalis" (BNST) seems to work against, or with, the known area of arcuate nucleus, known to control eating. When the BNST is stimulated, it causes mice to voraciously gorge on food even though they are well fed, and deactivating this circuit keeps starving mice from eating. The findings suggest that a breakdown within this neural network could contribute to unhealthy eating behaviours; it is unknown if the findings are also true of people.

Conclusion

This first leg of the three-legged stool is very complex. Our biochemistry and hormonal control has developed to provide a finely adjusted food intake mechanism to keep us at a stable weight. Hormone levels are changed by what we eat, and when the control mechanisms are disrupted it is not an easy path back to homeostasis. Insulin is a key hormone in this process. Control insulin and that change will cascade to other processes. If you are obese, or have been yo-yo dieting, it's likely you have insulin, ghrelin, and leptin resistance, so any change will be more difficult to overcome. It is not willpower, but chemistry at work. What are some guidelines to make your chemistry work to your advantage?

1. Take-Out fructose from your diet and avoid added sugar. Fructose disrupts the feedback mechanism for feeling full.

2. Take-Out simple carbohydrates because this reduces insulin levels, and increases the feedback mechanism from leptin and helps you eat less.

3. Increase protein levels a little, as that decreases insulin and dampens down hunger.

4. Eat slower and wait for 20 minutes before you go back and fill your plate up again, so the hormone response kicks in and make you feel satisfied without seconds.

5. Eat more complex carbohydrates such as salads and fresh vegetables as this makes the stomach fuller which helps feeling full.

6. Improve your sleep and reduce your hunger.

References

a. Balancing your hunger hormones. http://www.hungerhormones.com/science.html
b. Scott R, Tan T, Bloom S (2013) Vitamins & Hormones Volume 91, 2013, Chapter Seven – Gut Hormones and Obesity: Physiology and Therapies
c. Holst B. (2004) Constitutive ghrelin receptor activity as a signalling set-point in appetite regulation. Trends in Pharmacological Sciences Vol. 25, Issue 3, Pages 113–117 http://www.sciencedirect.com/science/article/pii/S0165614704 000276
d. Berthoud H. (2011) Metabolic and hedonic drives in the neural control of appetite: who is the boss? Current Opinion in

Neurobiology, Vol. 21, Issue 6, Pages 888–896
http://dx.doi.org/10.1016/j.conb.2011.09.004

e. Stocker C. (2008) The influence of leptin on early life programming of obesity Trends in Biotechnology. Vol. 26, Issue 10, Pages 545–551 http://dx.doi.org/10.1016/j.tibtech.2008.06.004

f. Karra E, O'Daly O, Choudhury A, Yousseif A, Millership S, Neary M, Scott W, Chandarana K, Manning S, Hess M, Iwakura H, Akamizu T, Miller Q, Gelegen C, Drew M, Rahman S, Emmanuel J, Williams S, Rüther U, Brüning J, Withers D, Zelaya F, Batterham R. (2013) A link between FTO, ghrelin, and impaired brain food-cue responsivity J Clin Invest. doi:10.1172/JCI44403

g. Circuit That Controls Overeating Found In Brain http://www.huffingtonpost.com/2013/09/27/overeating-brain-circuit-neural-network_n_4002487.html

h. Jennings J, Rizzi G, Stamatakis A, Ung R, Stuber G. (2013) The Inhibitory Circuit Architecture of the Lateral Hypothalamus Orchestrates Feeding. Vol. 341 no. 6153 pp. 1517-1521 DOI: 10.1126/science.1241812

i. King J, Wasse L, Stensel D, Nimmo M. (2013) Exercise and ghrelin. A narrative overview of research. Appetite 68 pp.83-91 doi: 10.1016/j.appet.2013.04.018

j. Nilsson A, Ekström L, Björck I. (2013) Effects of a Brown Beans Evening Meal on Metabolic Risk Markers and Appetite Regulating Hormones at a Subsequent Standardized Breakfast: A Randomized Cross-Over Study PLOS One. DOI: 10.1371/journal.pone.0059985

k. Lenard NR, Berthoud HR. (2008) Central and Peripheral Regulation of Food Intake and Physical Activity: Pathways and Genes. Obesity 16: S11–S22. doi: 10.1038/oby.2008.511

CHAPTER 21
INSULIN AND GLUCOSE

Get the Facts

➤ Insulin is the number one factor in balancing blood sugar levels.

➤ Homeostasis is needed for a healthy, well-functioning body.

➤ Adopt a low carbohydrate diet to minimise glucose spikes and insulin activity.

Understand the Science

When we look at the research on insulin and sugar, it can be pretty daunting to understand the complicated relationship between insulin, glucose, diabetes, obesity, and health. Despite the complexity, and the interaction with hunger, appetite, and food, I will try to keep it simple, yet accurate. There is more information about the role of glucose and insulin in the section on lipogenesis, but let's look at diabetes as a health issue first.

Why are high blood sugar levels bad for you? Glucose is fuel for all the cells in your body when it's present at normal levels, but persistently high sugar levels behave like a slow-acting poison. High sugar levels slowly erode the ability of cells in the pancreas to make insulin. The pancreas overcompensates though and insulin levels remain overly high. Gradually, the pancreas becomes permanently damaged, and it is not just the pancreas that can be damaged. Because blood and the high sugar levels are everywhere throughout the body, the body can be damaged anywhere. Damage to blood vessels, in particular, means no area is safe from too much sugar. High sugar levels and damaged blood vessels cause the multitude of complications that are associated with diabetes:

- Changes that lead to atherosclerosis, a hardening of the blood vessels.

- Kidney disease or kidney failure, requiring dialysis.

- Strokes.

- Heart attacks.

- Vision diminution or blindness.

- Immune system suppression, with increased risk for infections.

- Erectile dysfunction.

- Nerve damage, called neuropathy, causing tingling, pain, or decreased sensation in the feet, legs, and hands.

- Poor circulation to the legs and feet, with poor wound healing.

- In extreme cases, because of the poor wound healing, amputation is required.

Keeping glucose levels closer to normal can prevent many of the complications of diabetes. The American Diabetes Association's goals for glucose control in people with diabetes are glucose levels of 70 to 130 mg/dl before meals, and less than 180 mg/dl after meals, but given that the damage levels are linear, how do you manage your diet to avoid those spikes in glucose and insulin? Why did the Diabetes Association say those levels are ok, whereas they know it's a dose time relationship. Is damage equivalent with a 5 minute exposure to 130 mg/dl compared to a 20 minute exposure to 70 mg/dl? Much research in the past only looked at the peak glucose and insulin levels, but modern techniques can actually measure real time spikes. It turns out that there are large spikes, well over high levels.

Insulin

- Insulin is a simple protein in which two polypeptide chains of amino acids are joined by disulphide linkages. Insulin is produced by the pancreas.

- In the brain and muscle, insulin helps transfer glucose into cells so that they can oxidize the glucose to produce energy.

- In adipose (fat) tissue, insulin facilitates the storage of glucose and its conversion to fatty acids.

- Insulin slows the breakdown of fatty acids.

- In muscle, insulin promotes the uptake of amino acids for making proteins.

- In the liver, insulin helps convert glucose into glycogen.

- Insulin decreases gluconeogenesis, or the formation of glucose, from non-carbohydrate sources.

- The action of insulin is opposed by glucagon, another pancreatic hormone, and by epinephrine.

Glucose Measures and Risk of Disease

There are three primary markers we use to track blood sugar: fasting blood glucose (FBG), oral glucose tolerance test (OGTT), and haemoglobin A1c (A1c). FBG normal level means about 4.2 g (a teaspoon) in our 5 l of blood. If you're interested in health and longevity, instead of just slowing the onset of serious disease by a few years, you might consider shooting for the "normal" targets put out by most diabetes organizations. But remember to interpret the numbers together, and also remember that blood sugar is highly variable. If you wake up one morning and have a fasting blood sugar of 95, but your A1c and post-meal numbers are still normal, that's usually no cause for concern. Likewise, if you see a one-hour post-meal spike of 145 mg/dL, but all of your other numbers are normal, conventional medicine would consider it no cause for concern. Is this lack of concern valid?

Some doctors say that FBG up to 100 is normal. But in one study, patients with FBG of 95 had a 3 times the risk of developing diabetes a decade later, than those under 90. More importantly, FBG is a poor measure for future diabetes.

Marker	Normal	Pre-diabetes	Diabetes
Fasting blood glucose (mg/dL) (FBG)	<99	100-125	>126
Oral Glucose Tolerance Test (OGGT / post-meal, mg/dL after 2 hours)	<140	140-199	>200
Haemoglobin A1c (%)	<6	6-6.4	>6.4

A haemoglobin A1c of 5.1% maps to a blood sugar of about 100mg/dL, but some people measure higher, and some lower. Anything that affects red blood cells will skew the A1c. A1c is a good marker for cardiovascular heart disease. The risk of heart disease in people without diabetes doubles for every percentage point above

4.6%. But, as you can imagine, these tests miss 70 to 94% of individuals with diabetes.

The OGTT test, post meal blood sugars, measures how our blood sugar responds to drinking 75 ml of glucose. As that can be pretty severe the test normally is done post-prandial (post meal), using a glucometer after a meal. The figures in the table are too easy to achieve, as most people can be back down under 120mg/dL within two hours. But if levels stay above 140mg/dL for a period of time, there is irreversible beta cell loss (those cells that produce insulin). Stroke and cardiovascular disease correlate with levels of OGTT above 155gm/dL. Based on this measure, how do you decrease the length of time spent with OGTT levels lower than 140mg/dL? Simple answer: Stop eating.

Conventional recommendations is keep FBG below 100, or A1c below 6. That also is at odds with logic. There are health issues well into the normal range! Increasing glucose levels and macular degeneration (common in diabetics) is linear, so the lower the insulin the less damage. Avoid higher levels, even for short periods or spikes.

Even the Framingham Heart Study has thrown up other data which say that insulin and glucose have some longer term serious consequences. Parekh from Public Health Nutrition at New York University demonstrated links between glucose dysregulation and obesity-related cancers. The team analysed data from the 60-year Framingham Heart Study of 4,615 people; the participants were recruited between 1971 and 1975, and researchers followed them until 2008. Data on diet, exercise, and medical history, were collected from the three generations of people followed in the study. By the end of the study, researchers identified 787 cancers related to obesity with 217 breast cancer cases, 136 colorectal cancer cases, and 219 prostate cancer cases. Researchers found that impaired fasting glucose raised the risk of obesity-related cancer by 27%, after taking into account other factors such as age, alcohol use, smoking, sex, and body mass index. The link between impaired fasting glucose and obesity-related cancer was especially strong among smokers. Obese individuals are more likely to have higher concentrations of both insulin and glucose, an undesirable condition, which may promote cancer cells to grow, multiply, and spread rapidly, as compared to individuals who do not have these abnormalities.

The Core Diabetes Model (Palmer et al) shows that a reduction in HbA$_{1c}$ from 8% to 7% reduced end stage kidney disease by 40%, amputation by 20%, advanced eye disease (Proliferative

Retinopathy) by 42% and myocardial infarction by 15%, over a 5 year modelling period. So it is pretty clear that better glycaemic control in Type 2 diabetes is critical.

Conclusion

If you are a diabetic, increasing glucose levels (and corresponding insulin levels) map strongly to health risks independent of your weight. Do you aim for normal range that the medical industry promotes, or target to have as low a level as possible? Proponents of the low carbohydrate diets and an increasing number of diabetes researchers now suggest the lower the better. And if it is the right advice for a diabetic, or a pre-diabetic, is it correct for the general population as well? Not just for obesity advice, but health. If it reduces the risks of metabolic syndrome, cancer, cardiovascular disease, diabetes, and dementia, then I would suggest it is good advice for everyone, not just diabetics.

If you obese, your risk is at least a 30% increase in risk. Risks for cancer are not as high as for other diseases. Smoking tobacco is the number one cause for lung cancer and the risk of lung cancer from a male heavy smoker ranges from about 17% to 24% compared with a risk of about 2% for a non-smoker. I.e. the risk increases nine times. Look at the chapter on cancer for more detail, but in other chapters we see there are major health risks for consumption of simple carbohydrates.

This data is intriguing because it adds to the theory glucose should be properly viewed as an inflammatory agent. Gary Taubes and others promote the theory that obesity is a reaction to glucose. If you have a table with a sharp edge in the doorway into a room, and every time you walk into that room, you bruise yourself on the edge of the table, what do you do? (A bruise is the body's response to the inflammation from the damage.) Do you treat the bruise repeatedly, or remove the table, thus removing the cause? The Framingham Study for all its faults suggests sugar / glucose is inflammatory, with higher rates of cancer and other diseases. There is work going on in animal studies to look at novel ways to reduce this inflammation.

The practical thing to do is "move the table." Reduce simple carbohydrate consumption, and that reduces glucose spikes. It may or may not result in lower cancer risk, but what is clear is that you have lower risk of diabetes, low risk of diabetes type damage, and that has to be a good thing.

References

a. Niyati Parekh N, Lin Y, Vadiveloo M, Hayes R, Lu-Yao G. (2013) Metabolic Dysregulation of the Insulin–Glucose Axis and Risk of Obesity-Related Cancers in the Framingham Heart Study-Offspring Cohort (1971–2008), 24 Cancer Epidemiol Biomarkers Prev; 22(10); 1–12 doi: 10.1158/1055-9965.EPI-13-0330

b. Insulin Glucose Disruption May Play Role In Obesity-Related Cancers: Study. (2013) http://www.huffingtonpost.com/2013/09/26/obesity-cancer-insulin-glucose-disruption_n_3984441.html

c. Selvin E, Coresh J, Golden S, Brancati F, Folsom A, Steffes M. (2005) Glycemic Control and Coronary Heart Disease Risk in Persons With and Without Diabetes. The Atherosclerosis Risk in Communities Arch Intern Med. 2005;165(16):1910-1916. doi:10.1001/archinte.165.16.1910

d. Kressler C. (2010). Why your normal blood sugar isn't normal. http://chriskresser.com

e. Pan Y; Wang Y; Cai L; Cai Y; Hu J; Yu C; Li J; Feng. Z; Yang S; Li. X; Liang G. (2012) Inhibition of high glucose-induced inflammatory response and macrophage infiltration by a novel curcumin derivative prevents renal injury in diabetic rats. Br J Pharmacol. 2012 166(3):1169-82. doi: 10.1111/j.1476-5381.2012.01854.x

f. Palmer A J, Roze S, Valentine WJ, Spinas GA, Shaw JE, Zimmet PZ. (2004) Intensive lifestyle changes or metformin in patients with impaired glucose tolerance: modeling the long-term health economic implications of the diabetes prevention program in Australia, France, Germany, Switzerland, and the United Kingdom. Clin Ther. 2004 Feb;26(2):304-21. PMID: 15038953

g. Zhang S, Liu H, Chuang C, Li X; Au M; Zhang L; Phillips A; Scott D, Cooper G. (2014) The pathogenic mechanism of diabetes varies with the degree of overexpression and oligomerization of human amylin in the pancreatic islet β cells. FaseB J doi:10.1096/fj.14-251744

CHAPTER 22
EAT GOOD FOOD

Get the Facts

➢ Americans eat 20% of their meals in a car, and eat out 4.8 times a week.

➢ Australians spend 28% of their food budget on eating out.

➢ Fast food on average provides 47% of an adult's daily energy.

➢ It is apparent that diets fail because they fail to take into account the social behaviour and habits that surround eating. If you eat out, you are unlikely to be restricting calories.

➢ Most failed dieters say that the diet was too hard, too restrictive.

➢ Eating out and dieting may be mutually exclusive.

➢ Food is a social activity. Choosing eating strategies that work in your social context.

➢ The 5:2 Diet is built on the premise that you can socialize. It demands less in social behavioural changes.

Understand the Science

Michael Pollan popularized his saying *"Eat food. Not too much. Mostly plants."* His basic premise is that in the Western diet, food has been replaced by nutrients, and common sense, by confusion. As people spend more on eating out, and the average fast food meal provides 47% of an adult's daily energy, it's pretty clear that the consumption of fast food with its higher energy density and glycaemic loads, and excessive portion sizes, is greatly contributing to and escalating obesity. Yet, few are willing to put their head above the "parapet," and take on the food giants with taxes or strategies to reduce this. It is left to you, the reader, to win this battle by not consuming fast food. But it is not just about the food quality. Food is social.

Fifteen years ago, De Castro showed that eating with one other person, increases food intake by 44%, and the bigger the group you eat with, the more you eat. We drink more alcohol and eat more desserts in a social setting. The closer you sit in a restaurant to the dessert bar, the more you eat. The type of company you keep changes what you eat. If you are overweight, you copy what other overweight people eat. So, avoid buffets, and if you must go, sit in the furthest corner to avoid temptation!

Humans are social, and eating out is about enjoyment and experience. Willpower goes. When we eat out we say we want healthier choices 66% of the time, but we eat the treat 71% of the time! With these sorts of issues, the only practicable strategy is to adopt one of two strategies: eat more plants, or find treats that are not loaded with carbohydrates. Eating more unprocessed plants (loaded with fibre) prevents a range of diseases, and the simple rule is fat or fart. If you eat highly soluble food, you will turn it to fat. If you eat roughage, you will have more gas produced by our microbiome. Be anti-social. It is healthier.

USDA figures for the food consumed outside the home is 31% of actual calories. Fast food for adults is over 13% of the calories. What food choices do people make when they eat out? When they eat out, are they eating with other people in a social environment, and eating more than they would when eating at home? In other chapters we discuss some of these issues.

Fast food is the major source of eating-out calories for US Adults and children

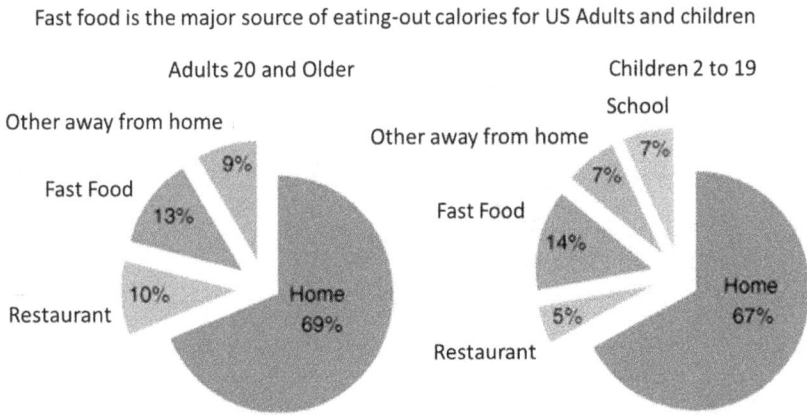

Source: USDA Economic Research Service analysis of 2005-2008 National Health and Nutrition Examination Survey Data

Figure 25 Eating Out in the USA Trends

Food Choices

The sheer novelty and glamor of the Western diet, with its 17,000 new food products every year, and the marketing power of $32 billion a year used to sell those products, has overwhelmed the force of tradition. It has left us relying on science, journalism, government, and marketing to help us decide what to eat. We have changed where we eat. We used to prepare food and eat in our homes. Now we eat out. We eat out a lot. When we go out, we eat fast food, slow food, ethnic food, and so forth, but we rarely eat healthy food when we eat out. We are a mobile society, and are paying for that mobility and freedom with our health.

The NSW Cancer Council found that Australians spend nearly one-third of their weekly household food budget on fast food and eating out. They are spending 50% more on eating out than they did just six years ago. The findings from the Cancer Council are pretty damning against self-regulation by the food industry. They have a voluntary code of conduct; the Australian Quick Service Restaurant Industry (QSRI) Initiative for Responsible Advertising and Marketing to Children.

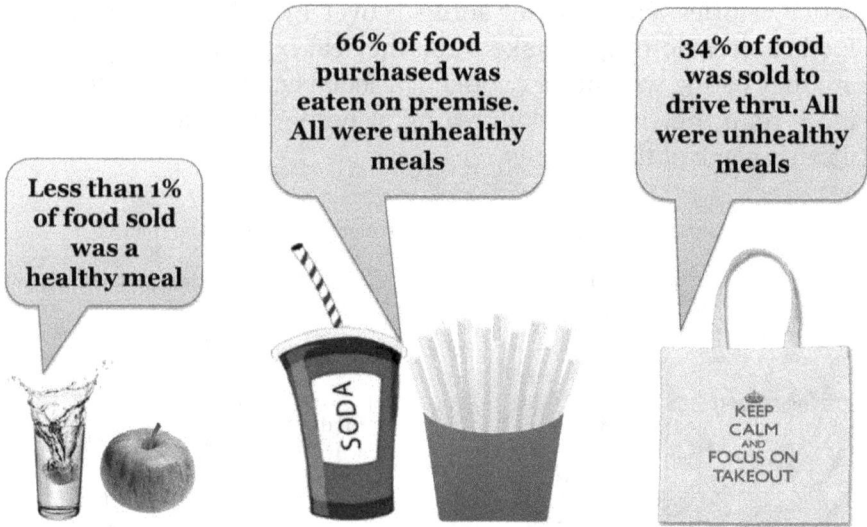

Figure 26 Fast Food Choices are never healthy

Most servings never come close to the 30% of daily requirement guidelines the industry had set themselves. They call it the "healthy options." Some single items exceeded recommended sodium and saturated fat for a whole day. The industry sets itself reasonable goals, but fails to adhere to them. One study looked at what people actually purchased from the food companies. They surveyed exactly what people were purchasing in a global fast food restaurant that promotes "healthy options". In the figure below, only 11 out of 1448 meals (1%) took the "healthy option." None of those healthy meals were sold in the drive-thru. Over 34% of food purchased was drive-thru. All of the customers who purchased and ate food on premise chose unhealthy. Why is this? Why do we eat out more, eat more, and eat worse food that is not as healthy?

The Company We Keep

In 1997, De Castro showed frequency and size of meals are profoundly influenced by the socio-cultural context. Simply eating with one other person increased the amount ingested by 44%, and with more people, the increases were larger. Back in 1992, he said the amount was more like a "power function." In a large group, you will eat up to 75% more than when eating alone. For Christmas dinner, followed by Boxing Day on December 26, a holiday in UK and Australia, you might easily eat around four times your actual calorie requirement. If you restricted calories by 10% per day, it would take you until the end of January to burn off those extra calories!

A Unilever-funded study, "World Menu Report," over ten countries and 5000 diners, confirmed what was evident. Eating out is about the experience and enjoyment of trying new tastes, the atmosphere, a nice break from routine, getting out of the house, catching up with family and friends, enjoying the company, not having to cook or clean up, feeling relaxed and having fun, and no hassles. In other words, eating out means enjoyment! Two-thirds (66%) of the respondents said that they will seek the healthier option on a menu, even if they don't end up choosing it. Next to this, 71% of guests agreed that when eating out they prefer to treat themselves. This highlights the struggle between intention and choice; essentially, what people want to eat, more often than not wins over what they think they should eat. While people have good intentions for eating healthier meals away from home, this does not translate into action.

We also tend to eat what our friends eat. Twenty years ago, Clendenen showed that meals eaten with others are larger than the ones we eat by ourselves. He also showed that females ate more dessert, independent of how long the meal lasted. Twenty years on, Pachucki et al from the Framingham Heart Study, showed that our social networks influence our food choices. Different types of relationships such as spouses, friends, and siblings influenced food choices. The authors classified food into several categories, such as "healthier," "alcohol and snacks," and "meat and soda." A greater share of people (as compared to the overall sample) with higher levels of education, and greater job prestige, consumed food in the "healthier" category. You have more snacks and alcohol if you are more "socially connected." So if you are a part of bigger networks, you probably indulge in more unhealthy food.

We also eat more if we are in the company of other overweight people. Salvy showed that overweight children are more likely to find food more reinforcing than non-overweight youth. Being in the company of overweight peers may give them permission to eat more, or may decrease their inhibitions, this increasing what are seen as the norms of appropriate eating. In a more recent paper, both male and female children consumed less energy from unhealthy snacks, when in the presence of their mothers, than when in the company of their friends. For anyone with teenagers, this is stating the obvious! Conversely, female adolescents consumed less energy from unhealthy snacks and more energy from healthy snacks, when they were with their friends, than when with their mothers. Boys were less concerned than females about healthy food.

It is a double whammy if you are in the lower socio economic bracket, as fruit and vegetables cost more, and junk food is both cheaper and more accessible. It has been suggested that economic policy could help facilitate healthy eating habits among vulnerable groups of young people. (E.g. African and Hispanic Americans.)

Think this is simple? Where you sit in a restaurant changes what and how much you eat. Vanata and others looked at 464 college students' seating location, group size, and gender on their trips to the cafeteria dessert bar in a college dining hall. It is no surprise that the students seated in the section nearest the desserts had the highest number of trips to the dessert bar, while the furthest section from the desserts had the lowest. As the group size increased, trips for desserts increased, with higher proportion of females also getting dessert.

Culture is also a driver. Pollan says he showed the words *chocolate cake* to a group of Americans and recorded their word associations. *Guilt* was the top response. If that strikes you as unexceptional, consider the response of French eaters to the same prompt: *celebration.*

Fast Food

The fast food industry is a $110 billion industry in the USA, with over 160,000 restaurants and over 50 million servings per day. Forty-four percent of Americans eat out once a week, 20% eat out twice a week, 14% eat out three or more times per week, and 6% eat out every day. Only 28% never eat fast food. However, the average

American eats 4.8 meals a week in restaurants, with the most popular meal out, being lunch (2.6 meals), followed by 1.4 sit-down dinners per week, and 0.8 breakfast meals.

In a Spanish study, researchers looked at the impact of fast food in a population with a Mediterranean type diet. The consumption of fast food, more than once per week, increased the risk of overall low diet quality and increased BMI. The risk of being obese increased with the frequency of fast food consumption. Other researchers are less emphatic about junk food and obesity, and in reviews tend to make vague statements such as the following.

> "Consumption of fast foods, which have high energy densities and glycaemic loads, and expose customers to excessive portion sizes, may be greatly contributing to and escalating the rates of overweight and obesity in the USA. Whether an association exists between fast food consumption and weight gain is unclear."

I think these researchers have lost their sense of reality.

Manufactured Food

To quote Pollan again: *"The human animal is adapted to, and apparently can thrive on, an extraordinary range of different diets, but the Western diet, however you define it, does not seem to be one of them."*

And, *"You may not think you eat a lot of corn and soybeans, but you do: 75% of the vegetable oils in your diet come from soy (representing 20% of your daily calories), and more than half of the sweeteners you consume come from corn (representing around 10% of daily calories)."*

The soybean is a notably inauspicious staple food. It contains a whole assortment of "anti-nutrients" or compounds that actually block the body's absorption of vitamins and minerals, interfere with the hormonal system, and prevent the body from breaking down the proteins of the soy itself.

Let's take one example of a manufactured food. David Gillespie, on his blog post provides an example of Goodman Fielder's Praise Creamy Mayonnaise. Mayonnaise used to be egg, beaten with olive oil. The fat free version bears more resemblance to a sugar sweetened beverage (Coke), but with three times less sugar. There is no egg or olive oil. Mayonnaise had 70% water, 26% sugar. Coke has 89% water and 10.6% sugar. There is no caramel in the mayo, but there is many other thickeners, salt, vegetable gums. It should not be called mayonnaise, but called white sugar syrup.

Eat Less Meat

You will see a lot of advice about reducing red meat consumption, or processed meat. But the evidence is far from clear, and comes from epidemiological studies. The documentary headline might read "bacon sandwich raises heart disease and cancer." The advice is eat less red meat, and reduce the level of processed meat.

Researchers at Harvard say a hotdog or two slices of bacon each day is associated with a 20% increase in mortality. Whereas in the EPIC study in Europe, no correlation was found except for those who ate more than 160 g, but that was similar to non-meat eaters. The EPIC study did find more than 40 g per day of processed meat is not good. So if you have a little extra red meat as you deal with the *take-out* of simple carbohydrates, it is probably fine. Switching to high levels of processed meat might not be the best option. Be wary of this research though. That bacon sandwich probably came with all those simple carbohydrates. What is the cause of the health issue? The bacon or the bread? To put these risks into context, Prof David Spiegelhalter from Cambridge, an expert in risk management, says if you eat a bacon sandwich every day, you might live two years less. Smoking 20 cigarettes would take ten years off your life span.

Conclusion

During the past 40 years, society has changed where it eats. Food has become food products. Much is now fast food. Where we eat changes what we eat. So any advice has to take account of our behaviours, or any change will fail.

- Stop buying manufactured, processed food.

- Choose a diet that allows you to eat out, but minimizes the dietary changes that you have to make if you want to lose or maintain weight.

- Adopt a low carbohydrate high fat diet if you socialize a lot.

This may include the following tactics:

- Find some "treats" that are real, whole foods. Do not let the price deter you.

- Enjoy the social events. Devise tactics to avoid manufactured foods.

- Do not try to eat like a mouse when in company. Accept that you will eat more at social events. Just choose wisely.

- The 5:2 Diet allows restricted calories on one or two days a week. It provides the health benefit of intermittent fasting, and does not disrupt the social life.

- Most restaurants will provide food with no added sugar and you can avoid high carbohydrate meals by swapping out the bread, rice and potato with either more protein or more complex carbohydrates. Avoid bread rolls and snacks at the start of a meal. Choose menu items that are whole foods. Make choices that fit within a low carbohydrate style of eating. For example, have an entrée of oysters as a treat instead of a chocolate mousse dessert if that is what you like. Share a desert with others, or make the desert a small cheese platter, or a scoop of CoYo coconut ice-cream with no sugar or dairy. Yum.

References

a. Fast food: exposing the truth. (2013) http://www.cancercouncil.com.au/68208/reduce-risks/diet-exercise/food-labelling-marketing-policy/food-labelling/fast-food-exposing-the-truth-2/
b. Rosenheck R. (2008) Fast food consumption and increased caloric intake: a systematic review of a trajectory towards weight gain and obesity risk. Obes Rev. 2008 Nov;9 (6):535-47. doi: 10.1111/j.1467-789X.2008.00477.x
c. Schröder H, Fito M, Covas M; REGICOR investigators. (2007) Association of fast food consumption with energy intake, diet quality, body mass index and the risk of obesity in a representative Mediterranean population. Br J Nutr. 2007 Dec;98 (6):1274-80. PMID: 17625027.
d. Unilver (2013) World Menu Report http://www.ufs.com/company/media-centre/world-menu-report
e. Pollan, Michael. (2009) In defence of food. Penguin. Pp256 ISBN-13: 978-0143114963
f. Atkins, R. (1998) Dr Atkins' New Diet Revolution Avon Books

g. Saxelberry. (2013) Australians demand more when eating out. http://foodwatch.com.au/blog/in-the-news/item/australians-demand-more-when-dining-out.html

h. Salvy S, Howard M, Read M, Mele E. (2009) The presence of friends increases food intake in youth. Am J Clin Nutr July 2009 ajcn.27658 doi: 10.3945/ajcn.2009.27658

i. Salvy S, Elmo A, Nitecki L, Kluczynski M, Roemmich J. (2011) Influence of parents and friends on children's and adolescents' food intake and food selection Am J Clin Nutr January 2011 vol. 93 no. 1 87-92 doi: 10.3945/ajcn.110.002097

j. Zhylyevskyy O, Jensen H, Garasky SB, Cutrona C, Gibbons F. (2013) Effects of Family, Friends, and Relative Prices on Fruit and Vegetable Consumption by African Americans. Southern Economic Journal, 80 (1): 226 DOI: 10.4284/0038-4038-2011.277

k. De Castro J, Brewer E. (1992) The amount eaten in meals by humans is a power function of the number of people present. Physiol Behav. Vol 51(1):121-5. PMID: 1741437

l. De Castro J.M. (1997) Socio-cultural determinants of meal size and frequency. British Journal of Nutrition Apr;77 Suppl 1:S39-54; discussion S54-5. PMID: 9155493.

m. Vanata D, Hatch A, DePalma G. (2011) Seating Proximity in a Cafeteria Influences Dessert Consumption among College Students International Journal of Humanities and Social Science Vol. 1 No. 4; April 2011

n. Clendenen V, Herman C, Polivy J. (1994). Social facilitation of eating among friends and strangers. Appetite 23 1-13. PMID: 7826053

o. Gillespie D. (2013) http://www.raisin-hell.com/2013/10/you-know-world-has-gone-mad-when-coke.html

p. Spiegelhalter   Risks   (2104) http://www.statslab.cam.ac.uk/Dept/People/Spiegelhalter/davids.html

q. Moseley M. (2014) Documentary: How safe is eating meat? http://www.bbc.com/news/health-28797106

r. USDA (2012) Food and Nutrient Intake Data: Taking a Look at the Nutritional Quality of Foods Eaten at Home and Away From Home http://www.ers.usda.gov/amber-waves/2012-june/data-feature-food-and-nutrient-intake-data.aspx

CHAPTER 23
THE MICROBIOME – OUR GUESTS

Get the Facts

➤ The microbiome is the 100 trillion (and 2 kg) of bacteria, fungi, and archaea that live with us.

➤ They play a role in nutrition, obesity, allergies, autoimmunity, and gender bias.

➤ The existing research creates a new understanding of what we live with.

➤ Don't mess with it. Learn to live with the microbiome, although this is an area of research of which we should expect to see more.

Understand the Science

For more than a century, bacteria (plus fungi and archaea) was seen only as a bane of human existence; the cause of fatal illnesses and gut-cramping food poisoning. In the past decade, bacteria has increasingly come to be seen as benevolent life partners. Most people will carry the same basic set of bacteria over their lifetime. The animal and bacterial kingdoms have co-evolved and co-adapted in response to environmental selective pressures over hundreds of millions of years. There's been some work over time on trying to understand some of this microbiome (sometimes called microbiota, or micro flora), but the research area has recently come into focus.

You are probably familiar with bacteria and fungi. Initially, archaea were viewed as extremophiles that lived in harsh environments, such as hot springs and salt lakes, but they have since been found in a broad range of habitats, including soils, oceans, marshlands, and the human colon and navel. The ones you probably have had a poor experience with are the methanogens in the colon, that aid digestion but create methane.

In 2013, an international team of over 200 scientists from 80 research institutions published the results of the first-ever DNA sequencing of the entire human microbiome. The results of their sequencing of over 242 healthy adults, and with a focus on colonies found on the skin and in the mouth, nose, gut, and vagina are staggering. The human body carries more than 100 trillion bacteria, up to 2 kg (over 4.4lb) of the tiny single-celled organisms. Together, all of the bacteria in the body would be the size of a large liver, and in many ways, scientists say, the microbiome behaves as another organ in the human body. The microbiome is about 1% to 3% of total body mass. Each of our bodies has its own unique microbiome, cultivated from birth, and built from our genes and our diet. It is nurtured by our exposure to a family dog or cat, by how much dirt we ate out of the sandbox, and the antibiotics we've taken for ear infections or strep throat.

Scientists are now expanding on that research, studying the microbiome of infants and of people with particular diseases.

Skin and vaginal sites showed smaller diversity than the mouth and gut. The mouth alone has several hundred species of bacteria. Each tooth is its own ecosystem. Different subspecies (or enterotypes) in the human gut, previously thought to be well-understood, are from a broad spectrum of communities with blurred taxon boundaries. Research shows that the gut microbiome is much less understood than previously thought. More than 1,000 species of bacteria live in the human gut. Many of the bacteria in the digestive tract break down certain nutrients, such as carbohydrates, that humans otherwise could not digest. The majority of these commensal bacteria are anaerobes, meaning they survive in an environment with no oxygen. Generally well behaved, normal flora bacteria can act as opportunistic pathogens at times of lowered immunity.

Escherichia coli (E. coli) is a bacterium that lives in the colon. It is an extensively studied model organism and probably the best-understood bacterium of all. Certain mutated strains of these gut bacteria do cause disease; an example is E. coli O157:H7.

A number of types of bacteria, such as Actinomyces viscosus and A. naeslundii, live in the mouth, where they are part of a sticky substance called plaque. If this is not removed by brushing, it hardens into calculus (also called tartar). The same bacteria also secrete acids that dissolve tooth enamel, causing tooth decay.

One type of calorie may be metabolized differently than another, but the effect of a particular diet depends on a person's genes and bacteria. And that person's bacteria are determined in part by his diet. Metabolism and digestion hinge on an intricate relationship between food, bacteria, and genetics.

Numerous lines of evidence, particularly from rodent models, have suggested that the intestinal microbiota may play a role in the development of obesity. Ridaura et al demonstrate that the microbiota from lean, or obese, humans induces similar phenotypes in mice and, more remarkably, that the microbiota from lean donors can invade and reduce adiposity gain in the obese-recipient mice if the mice are fed an appropriate diet.

Other papers in *Nature*, looked at another way that different bodies metabolize the same diet from Europe. With 300 Danish participants, those with more diverse microbiota in their gut showed fewer signs of metabolic syndrome, including obesity and insulin resistance. Elsewhere, overweight mice were given a high-fiber diet. Those that began with fewer bacterial species saw an increase in bacterial diversity and an improvement in metabolic indicators. This was not the case for those that already had a diverse microbiome, even when fed the same diet. In other studies, bacteria from human stools from identical twins, one twin lean, one twin obese, were transferred to mice, and the mice became obese or lean.

Even the microbiome play a part in gender bias of disease. In a recent science paper, Markle and her colleagues suggested gender bias may be modified and/or reinforced by the microbiome of the person. The microbiome appears to regulate sex hormone levels. It could also affect other autoimmune conditions (inappropriate immune responses that attack self-antigens and destroy host tissue) such as type 1 diabetes mellitus.

Childhood malnutrition is a global health problem that cannot be attributed to food insecurity alone. There is a childhood disease in Africa called *kwashiorkor,* where the child is malnourished, while siblings may not be. The evidence is breast milk composition affects development of the microbiota and immune system.

Probiotic Supplements

One conclusion from the research is that bacteria inside us synthesize hundreds of different types molecules in our mouth, gut, and skin. Drug discovery is one possible long-term benefit from the study of the microbiome, but the more immediate hope is to learn how humans can somehow work with their own bacterial colonies to cure or prevent chronic disease, or just maintain good health.

Over-the-counter probiotics are sold and promoted for bacterial health. Probiotics are, essentially, good bacteria that are mostly associated with improving digestion but they may have other benefits. Many people use probiotics to, in theory, replace some of the healthy bacteria that may be killed by a course of antibiotics.

Study on probiotics is limited, and many microbiologists question whether they're helpful. On the other hand, they're probably not harmful, they say. The same is true for diets thought to promote healthy bacterial colonies.

A recent experiment by Tang at the Muroch Childrens Research Institute in Australia treated children who had severe peanut allergies. Some children received probiotics (Lactobacillus rhamnosus) and peanut oral immunotherapy (OIT), and others placebos or other treatments. Over 18 months, 82% of the children who took the probiotic and peanut OIT were free of peanut allegies.

It also looks like food preservatives are also linked to obesity and gut disease. In Nature in 2015, artificial preservatives used in many processed foods could increase the risk of inflammatory bowel diseases and metabolic disorders. In a study done in mice, chemicals known as emulsifiers were found to alter the make-up of bacteria in the colon — the first time that these additives have been shown to affect health directly.

Artificial sweeteners have also been show to affect the microbiome directly. We have been using non-caloric artificial sweeteners for more than a century. Today the food industry is using them in ever-greater quantities in "diet" foodstuffs and they are recommended for weight loss and for individuals with glucose intolerance and type 2 diabetes mellitus. Elinav and colleagues show that consumption of the three most commonly used non-caloric artificial sweeteners — saccharin, sucralose and aspartame — directly induces a propensity for obesity and glucose intolerance in mice.

Dirtier Prevents Allergies

Bacteria do appear to affect allergies. "*In our study of over 400 children we observed a direct link between the number of different bacteria in their rectums, and the risk of development of allergic disease later in life,*" says Prof Bisgaard, head of the Copenhagen Prospective Studies on Asthma in Childhood. "*Reduced diversity of the intestinal microbiota during infancy was associated with increased risk of allergic disease at school age. But if there was considerable diversity, the risk was reduced, and the greater the variation, the lower the risk. So it makes a difference, if the baby is born vaginally, encountering the first bacteria from its mother's rectum, or by caesarean section, which exposes the newborn to a completely different, reduced variety of bacteria. This may be why far more children born by caesarean section develop allergies."*

Conclusion

Ten years ago, we thought bugs were bad. Now we know they are good (the right ones), most of the time. Stop the antibacterial mouthwash? Reduce the level of cleanliness in our homes and workplaces? Use faecal transplants to treat some gut problems?

How many studies on other things such as nutrients have been confounded with microbiome interactions? Both anecdotal accounts and research trials show us autoimmune diseases can be managed with changes in diet. The exact interactions between microbiome and diet are not clear, but expect more over the next few years. In the meantime, there are really simple things to look after your microbiome. Avoid added sugar and simple carbohydrates. Eat plenty of whole food.

References

a. Human   Microbiome. http://en.wikipedia.org/wiki/Human_microbiome
b. Kostic A, Howitt M, Garrett M. (2013). Exploring host–microbiota interactions in animal models and humans. Genes and Development. 27: 701-718 doi: 10.1101/gad.212522.112
c. Flak M, Neves J, Blumberg R. (2013) Welcome to the Microgenderome Science Vol. 339 no. 6123 pp. 1044-1045 DOI: 10.1126/science.1236226
d. Markle J, Frank DN, Mortin-Toth S, Robertson CE, Feazel L, Rolle-Kampczyk U, von Bergen M, McCoy K, Macpherson A, Danska J. (2103) Sex Differences in the Gut Microbiome Drive Hormone-Dependent Regulation of Autoimmunity. Science 1 March 2013: 1084-1088
e. Gordon J, Dewey K, Mills D, and Medzhitov R. (2012) The Human Gut Microbiota and Undernutrition. Sci Transl Med, Issue 137, p. 137ps12 DOI: 10.1126/scitranslmed.3004347
f. Smith M, Yatsunenko T, Manary M, Trehan I, Mkakosya R, Cheng J, Kau A, Rich S, Concannon P, Mychaleckyj K, Liu J, Houpt E, Li JV, Holmes E, Nicholson J, Knights D, Ursell LK, Knight R, Gordon J. (2013) Gut Microbiomes of Malawian Twin Pairs Discordant for Kwashiorkor (2013) Science 1 February

2013: Vol. 339 no. 6119 pp. 548-554 DOI: 10.1126/science.1229000.

g. Dirt Prevents Allergy, Danish Research Suggests http://www.sciencedaily.com/releases/2011/11/111102125601.htm

h. Ridaura V, Faith J, Rey F, Cheng J, Duncan A, et al. (2013): Gut Microbiota from Twins Discordant for Obesity Modulate Metabolism in Mice Science 6(341) no. 6150 DOI: 10.1126/science.1241214

i. Walker A, Parkhill J. (2013) Fighting Obesity with Bacteria Science 6: 1069-1070 Vol. 341(6150) pp. 1069-1070 DOI: 10.1126/science.1243787

j. Liou A, Paziuk M, Luevano JM, Machineni S, Turnbaugh P, Kaplan L. (2013) Conserved Shifts in the Gut Microbiota Due to Gastric Bypass Reduce Host Weight and Adiposity Sci Transl Med 27 March 2013: 178ra41

k. Flier J, Mekalanos J. (2013) Gut Check: Testing a Role for the Intestinal Microbiome in Human Obesity. Sci Transl Med 11 November 2009: 6ps7.

l. Tang M, Ponsonby A, Orsini F, Tey D, Robinson M, Su E. Licciardi P, Burks W, Donath S (2015) Administration of a probiotic with peanut oral immunotherapy: A randomized trial. The Journal of Allergy and Clinical Immunology. DOI: http://dx.doi.org/10.1016/j.jaci.2014.11.034

m. Chassaing B,Koren O, Goodrich J, Poole A, Srinivasan S,Ley R, Gewirtz A. (2015) Dietary emulsifiers impact the mouse gut microbiota promoting colitis and metabolic syndrome. Nature doi:10.1038/nature14232

n. Artificial sweeteners induce glucose intolerance by altering the gut microbiota (2015) Suez J, Korem T, Zeevi D, Zilberman-Schapira G, Thaiss C, Maza O, Israeli D, Zmora N, Gilad S, Weinberger A, Kuperman Y, Harmelin A, Kolodkin-Gal I, Shapiro H, Halpern Z, Segal E, Elinav E. (2015) Nature 513 ,290 doi:10.1038/513290a

CHAPTER 24
OBESITY BY STEALTH

Get the Facts

➢ At under age 40, most people are overweight and later become obese. Over the age of 40, most slowly but surely become obese at a rate of about 1 lb (0.4 kg) per year!

➢ Less than 30% are in the normal weight range.

➢ Being overweight is caused by what you eat.

➢ Unless you make a change in food intake, you will put on about 1% of your weight each year.

➢ The good news: If you change your food intake, you will lose that weight.

➢ Use a take-out diet. Take-out (or cut out) carbohydrates, starting with added sugar.

Understand the Science

It matters, of course, how many total calories you take in each day, but Lustig says the age-old advice to simply "eat less and exercise more" is naïve. To control weight over the long term, studies show that people benefit more by focusing on "eating right," rather than "eating less." Hu from the Harvard School of Public Health says, "Findings underscore the importance of making wise food choices in preventing weight gain and obesity. The idea that there are no "good" or "bad" foods is a myth that needs to be debunked."

Have you ever wondered why you got the "middle age spread?" Do you wonder how you were svelte and trim in your mid-twenties and by the age of 50, your trousers filled out and made you look like a blimp? Large epidemiological studies (120,000 to 300,000 people) from the USA and Europe / UK show that weight piles on slowly over years.

In the USA, Mozaffarian and his team examined the Nurses' Health Study, the Nurses' Health Study II, and the Health Professionals Follow-up Study. They looked at lifestyle factors and weight gain every four years over 20 years. The review included 120,877 USA women and men who, at the start of the studies, weren't obese and were free of chronic diseases. Other groups have looked at these same groups; Sun and others looked at diabetes and fruit over a four year period. All figures are 4 year intervals.

- Overall : Most gained 1.5 kg (3.35lb) (from -4.1 to 12.4). Only a few (5%) lost weight. Over the 20 years, they increased by 7.7 kg (17.7lb) – a 0.6% increase every year.

- Foods that added weight: Crisps/Chips 0.7 kg (1.69 lb), potatoes 0.6 kg (1.28 lb), sugar-sweetened beverages 0.45 kg (1 lb), unprocessed red meats 0.4 kg (1 lb), processed meats 0.4 (1 lb), desserts and sweets 0.2 kg (0.5 lb), and fruit juice.

- The worst food for weight gain: French fries 1.5 kg (3.35 lb).

- Foods that helped with weight loss: Vegetables 0.1 kg (0.22 lb), whole grains 0.2 kg (0.37 lb), fruits 0.2 kg (0.5 lb), nuts 0.3 kg (0.57 lb), and yogurt 0.3 kg (0.82 lb).

- Diabetes: 6.5% of this group got type 2 diabetes. Replacing fruit juice with blueberries reduced type 2 diabetes by 33%, grapes and raisins (19%), apples and pears (13%), and any combination of whole fruit by 7%.

- If people increased physical activity, they put on less weight 0.8 kg (1.76lb) each year than those who decreased activity.

- One alcoholic drink a day increased weight by 0.2 (0.41 lb) every year.

- Sleeping: Less than 6 hours, or more than 8 hours, a night contributed to weight gain.

- TV: Watching an additional hour of television a day added 1.5 kg (0.31 lb) a year, and encouraged snacking which further increases weight!

- Smoking: New quitters gained 2.3 kg (5.17lb), but repeat quitters 0.06k (0.14 lb).

Note that this review was on non-obese, predominantly white, educated people. Other data shows that the less the education, the more obesity. This study was also based on self-reporting, so participants will have underestimated their eating amounts.

Why were the potatoes, in particular, so fattening? It's not clear. Maybe because they're generally eaten in large quantities. Some previous work has shown that potatoes are the type of food that causes big spikes in blood sugar and insulin, which tends to make people hungrier, and overeat at their next meal.

Other researchers, such as Nestle (NYU) say, "It's not that calories don't count; indeed they do. But it's a lot easier to control calories by eating healthfully and avoiding junk foods and sodas than it is to delude yourself into thinking you can count them accurately." As part of the Take-Out Diet I suggest you do count calories for a period of time to reset your perspective of how many calories are in junk food versus whole food.

Why replace fruit juice with whole fruit? Researchers have said this could be due to high levels of anthocyanins in whole fruit which have been shown to enhance glucose uptake in mice. The same fruits contain naturally-occurring polyphenols which are known to have beneficial effects.

Conclusion

You can see why over years you put on weight. You start out normal weight and 20 years later the average weighs 7 kg (18 lb) heavier. When you consider that you vary in weight 1 kg or more per day, a small change will go undetected. Not only did the study group get heavier, they got sicker. "Wrong" foods appeared to increase weight and increase type 2 diabetes. Remember, though, that epidemiological studies do not show the cause of these responses. These studies do show that there are such things as good and bad foods and good and bad behaviours. Maybe a good way to thing about this is to use a term such as a "take-out" diet. Take-out (remove) some things from your lifestyle such as soft drinks and French fries.

If you look at all diets that give some measure of success, what works best is take-out some things. It can be much easier than trying to stop eating everything in proportion. These people in this study did not appear to over consume. A can of soda a day? Hardly binging. Focusing on one or two items to cut out may have a higher success rate than simply reducing intake. Cutting a can of soda each day is not a huge change. There has been little or no research on this, as the emphasis has been on the biochemistry and hormonal impact and not behaviour. Consider the comparisons of the Atkins Diet versus the restricted low calorie diet. An unrestricted Atkins Diet plan is twice as effective as a low calorie diet. Some of the difference can be explained by the biochemistry, but appetite control is better with a lower carbohydrate diet. The key steps in the Atkins diet is to take-out simple carbohydrates and sugar, and increase consumption of protein and fat. Simple messages are easier to understand than complex ones, and likewise the simple message in the Sugar Free diet is no added sugar. The simple message of the Atkins diet is no carbohydrates. My simple message is take-out some specific foods. All will help avoid obesity sneaking up on you as you age.

References

a. Mozaffarian D, Hao T, Rimm E, Willett W, Huet F. (2011) Changes in Diet and Lifestyle and Long-Term Weight Gain in Women and Men. J Med 2011; 364:2392-2404. http://www.nejm.org/doi/full/10.1056/NEJMoa1014296
b. Malik VS, Popkin BM, Bray GA, Després JP, Hu FB. (2011) Sugar-sweetened beverages, obesity, type 2 diabetes mellitus, and cardiovascular disease risk. Circulation. 23 ;121(11):1356-64.
c. Ostrow N. (2011) Potato Chips Cited as Culprit in U.S. Weight Gain. http://www.bloomberg.com/news/2011-06-22/potato-chips-add-pounds-while-yogurt-slims-harvard-study-finds.html
d. Muraki I. (2013) Fruit consumption and risk of type 2 diabetes: results from three prospective longitudinal cohort studies BMJ 2013; 347 doi: http://dx.doi.org/10.1136/bmj.f5001

CHAPTER 25
ORGANIC IS GOOD FOR YOU

Get the Facts

➤ Organic food is not necessarily nutritionally better for you. It is not worse either.

➤ Organic food may be "cleaner" food, which may diminish putting things into your body that you do not want.

➤ If you have a choice, and the income to justify the spending, organic food may have lower levels of pesticide, but it is unlikely to be of any consequence.

➤ Eating organic is not equivalent to eating well.

Understand the Science

What is organic? To meet organic standards, organic crops must be produced without the use of conventional pesticides (including herbicides), synthetic fertilizers, sewage sludge, bioengineering, or ionizing radiation. Organically raised animals must be given organic feed and kept free of growth hormones and antibiotics. Organic farm animals must have access to the outdoors, including pastureland for grazing. The USDA label says that 95% of the food product has to come from certified organic sources. There is a range of accepted certification systems; and there are substantial differences between organic and conventional fruits and vegetables. They differ with respect to production method, labelling, marketing, and price. Do these changes make any difference to food quality?

Smith-Spangler and team from Stanford University, raised serious questions about the often-touted, nutritional advantage of organic food in a meta-study of 237 peer-reviewed studies with 17 studies in humans and 220 comparing organic and conventional foods and diets. They concluded that *"the published literature lacks strong evidence that organic foods are significantly more nutritious than conventional foods."* Understandably, this drew a great deal of attention and organic advocate defence. Stanford is certainly no ag-school promoting the status quo. Instead, it enjoys a very strong reputation for research excellence. It isn't easy to dismiss these findings. Many commentators, confronted with the highly credible de-mystification of the nutritional advantage of organic, jumped to the paper's slight evidence which supported a 30% reduction in exposure to pesticide residues, as a way to justify paying extra for organic produce.

There was some increase in phosphate levels, but not significant in organic food. Two studies showed slightly lower pesticide levels in school children's urine; slightly higher levels of antibiotic resistance in non-organic chickens' urine, but there was little else, and most things such as bacterial contamination and nutrient levels were similar. Given that pesticide residues in conventional foods is already miniscule – is this reduction of any consequence?

Here is what Steve Savage commented on pesticide levels from a USDA food sampling program.

> *"When most people hear the word "pesticide" they imagine something quite dangerous. What they don't know is that over the last several decades, the old chemicals have been steadily replaced by much less hazardous ones that have emerged from a multi-billion dollar discovery effort. That is why 36.6% of the residues detected in 2010 were for chemicals that are less toxic to mammals than things like salt, vinegar, or the citric acid in your lemons. Seventy-three percent of the detections were for pesticides that are less toxic than the vanilla that is in your ice cream. Over 90% of the pesticides detected were less toxic per gram than the ibuprofen that is in the Advil / Nurofen tablets that tens of millions of people take on a regular basis.*
>
> *Ninety-five point four percent of the detected residues were from chemicals that are less toxic than the caffeine that is in your coffee each morning. "Pesticide" does not equal "danger". The reason that the USDA can look at their data and make strong statements about safety is that the residues they find are virtually all below the tolerances, mostly far below. Only 7.8% of the residues detected in 2010 were even within the range of 0.1 to 1 times the tolerance. More than half were less than 1% of the tolerance."*

Conclusion

Should you eat only organic food? There are few demonstrated science studies on the topic, but emotions run high. So should you be concerned about pesticides in existing food products? Certainly not if the food product is produced under the strict USA, Australian,

NZ, or European regulations. I have concerns about food produced in some of China, Asia, and India; they have a more varied level of regulation; there is continued use of pesticides no longer accepted in the more regulated countries, and there may be high usage of hormones. Conversely, most of the intensive farming practices used in modern agriculture give us food (size, colour, seedless, etc.) that our ancestors would simply not recognize. There are issues in intensive aquaculture or feedlot production systems that have ongoing question marks about the food produced and food produced is not the same as wild seafood or range farmed animals. Does it make any difference to our health? Possibly. Can I change it? Probably not. Most certainly not without a substantial change in my lifestyle, and besides it's unclear whether that would be detrimental or beneficial.

References

a. Smith-Spangler C, Brandeau M, Hunter G, Bavinger C, Pearson M, Eschbach, Sundaram P, Liu H, Schirmer P, Stave C, Olkin I, Bravata D. (2012) Are Organic Foods Safer or Healthier Than Conventional Alternatives?: A Systematic Review Ann Intern Med.   157(5):348-366.   doi:10.7326/0003-4819-157-5-201209040-00007
b. Savage S. (2012) Do You Really Need to Buy Organic Foods To Avoid   Pesticide   Residues? http://appliedmythology.blogspot.com/2012/09/to-you-really-need-to-buy-organic-foods.html

CHAPTER 26
EIGHT GLASSES OF WATER

Get the Facts

➢ Your body needs some water. Drink water.
➢ Do you need eight x 8oz (1.9l) per day? No. Include tea and coffee in your consumption figures.
➢ Do not drink sweetened sugar beverages (SSB). That means avoid gin and tonic, rum and Coke, or any alcohol with SSBs. Change your drink. Just enjoy it on the rocks.

Understand the Science

Dr Karl from the Australian ABC Network affiliate says:

"You see them everywhere. Those ubiquitous bottles of water, it seems, are an absolutely essential part of many people's lives. Presumably, without this life-giving bottled water, people wither up, die, and turn into a pile of dust waiting to be blown away by the next breeze. You come across the exhortation to "drink at least eight glasses of water a day" everywhere. This advice has been in a health column in the New York Times, and published by many writers in the popular press. It even appears in a pamphlet from the University of California Los Angeles, which advises the students to carry a water bottle with you. Drink often while sitting in class"

Another part of the "eight glasses of water per day" mantra is that we are all chronically dehydrated, and yet our bodies are not sensitive enough to correct this by making us thirsty. From a physiological point of view, this is rubbish.

The conventional advice is that the average individual needs at least 1ml of fluid for every calorie burned. That's approximately eight, 8-oz glasses per day for a 2000-calorie diet. This equation is based on panel advice, but there is little science to back this up. You are likely to have to go to the toilet regularly and may possibly deplete minerals with constant urinating. While adequate hydration is essential for maintaining blood volume, kidney function, and for preventing constipation, also consider that you get lots of water from green leafy vegetables and fruits. If you eat processed foods, your requirement for water may be higher. Furthermore, the admonition not to count coffee, tea, or beer, as water replacement, is also wrong.

Conclusion

Does drinking water have some benefits? Yes, of course, but it's important that you don't substitute sugar sweetened beverages (SSBs) for water. Water has no calories or additives, is widely available, inexpensive, and generally safe. It is a good beverage choice! Epidemiological studies show that energy intake is significantly lower (9%, or 194 kcal/d) in water drinkers compared to non-water drinkers. German schoolchildren, in just one year of drinking water rather than SSBs, reduced the risk of being overweight by 31%. Another benefit of water is it has no calories. Consuming water before or with a meal reduces feelings of hunger and increases satiety, in contrast to both diet and regular soft drinks. It's also thought that the intense sweet flavour of SSBs may stimulate appetite. Coffee and tea are reasonable alternatives to water provided that caloric sweeteners and creamers are avoided or used sparingly.

References

a. Panel on Dietary Reference Intakes for Electrolytes and Water. 2005
b. Jequier E, Constant F. (2009) Water as an essential nutrient: the physiological basis of hydration. Eur J Clin Nutr. 2;
c. Valtin H. (2002) "Drink at least eight glasses of water a day." Really? Is there scientific evidence for "8 x 8"? Am J Physiol Regul Integr Comp Physiol. 283(5):R993-1004 PMID: 12376390
d. Popkin BM, Barclay DV, Nielsen SJ. Water and food consumption patterns of U.S. adults from 1999 to 2001. Obes Res. 2005;13:2146–2152
e. Muckelbauer R, Libuda L, Clausen K, Toschke AM, Reinehr T, Kersting M. Promotion and provision of drinking water in schools for overweight prevention: randomized, controlled cluster trial. Pediatrics. 2009;123:e661–667
f. Stookey JD, Constant F, Gardner CD, Popkin BM. Replacing sweetened caloric beverages with drinking water is associated with lower energy intake. Obesity (Silver Spring) 2007;15:3013–3022.

g. Dennis EA, Dengo AL, Comber DL, Flack KD, Savla J, Davy KP, Davy BM. Water Consumption Increases Weight Loss During a Hypocaloric Diet Intervention in Middle-aged and Older Adults. Obesity (Silver Spring) 2009 Aug 6

h. Black RM, Leiter LA, Anderson GH. Consuming aspartame with and without taste: differential effects on appetite and food intake of young adult males. Physiol Behav. 1993;53:459–466.

i. Almiron-Roig E, Drewnowski A. Hunger, thirst, and energy intakes following consumption of caloric beverages. Physiol Behav. 2003;79:767–773.

CHAPTER 27
INTERMITTENT FASTING AND THE 5:2 DIET

Get the Facts

➤ Animals and humans do not eat the same amount of food every day, yet long term, they maintain a normal weight range by adjusting their consumption.

➤ The only mammals that become obese are humans and animals fed by humans (such as house pets).

➤ Restricted calories on some days is normal, and can be beneficial for maintaining a good weight.

➤ Animals with restricted calories live longer and healthier lives, but this is unproven in humans.

➤ Eating five meals a day, or "grazing," could be dangerous to your health.

➤ The 5:2 Diet is a good diet for weight loss as it creates a weekly calorie deficit in the two days of reduced food intake.

➤ The 5:2 Diet appears to have benefits for blood pressure, sugar response, and hormones implicated in longevity.

➤ Intermittent dietary regimes appear to reduce cognitive diseases such as Alzheimer's.

Understand the Science

Periods of feast and famine are the norm for most animals except humans. We eat three meals a day and snack in between meals. We graze – a cafe latte here, cookies, chips, smoothies, sports drinks, etc. there. Eating throughout the day has become the norm, and to do the absolute opposite meets with some medical opposition, whereas in many cultures, some form of fasting is intricately legislated even within their religion. The concept of eating little and often as a good thing, has been driven by the snack manufacturers and fad diet programs, and subsequently became medical dogmas. We now know that eating often causes you to end up eating more. Humans are eating 120 calories per day on average more today than 20 years ago.

On a day-to-day basis, humans do not eat the same amount of calories each day, unless they are very strict and conscientious. I decided to use a calorie counter from myFitnesspal to understand exactly what I ate, and to calibrate my eating. I wanted to understand where my soft spots were and why for three years, in spite of exercise and diet, my weight had stayed the same, my cholesterol was still considered to be high, and my pants were still XL.

A "normal" female eats about 1,800 calories per day. A "normal" male eats about 2080 calories per day (8700 kj). As you age, your metabolism slows down and you need to eat fewer calories (200 less from 20 to 60 years of age), and when you do not, you can gain more weight. Importantly, it is very difficult to eat the same each day, so, to try to do so in a diet, is likely to lead to behavioural issues. For many people, work and schedules vary and create variables in what is eaten. We also like to eat different foods each day rather than the same thing every day. Rats in research trials are often forced to eat the same food and the same amount every day.

My calorie counter suggested that to lose 0.5 kg per week, I would need to eat (net of exercise) about 1800 calories initially, and then get down to 1600 calories per day as I got closer to my goal weight. This is actually what I consumed over a six-month period from the beginning of my measuring.

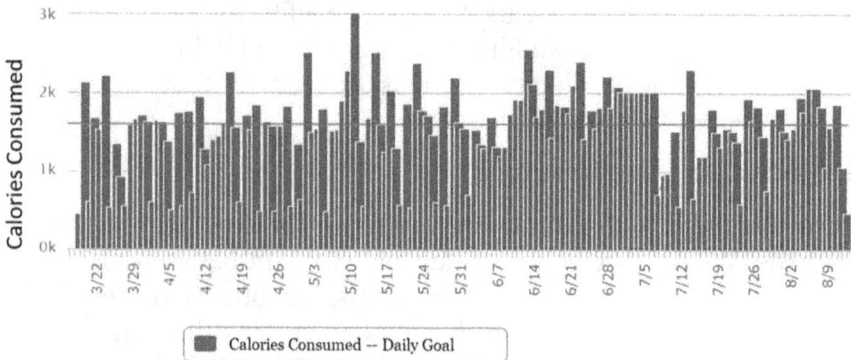

Figure 27 Variable Calorie Intake of Author

The software accounts for exercise, so if you show the net calories which takes away the exercise, some of the peaks are even less, or on fasting days, shows very few calories. The fasting days (25% of normal calories, or 600 calories) show up as the down days. For me, June was four weeks on holidays in Europe, and travel is very disruptive for normal diets. A spike on May 10th was a birthday party. If you eat 3,000 calories in a day, then it would take ten days, at a 30% reduction in normal caloric intake, to make up for extra calories on that day. Have you ever wondered why you put on weight over a Thanksgiving or Christmas period? Dieting fails (see section on why diets fail) and one of the features of intermittent fasting programs is that you don't have to count calories every day. Counting calories is difficult and most people do not want to be bothered with counting calories in every food they eat. That's why Weight Watchers came up with a simplified form of calorie counting – points. To lose weight you have to consume fewer calories over a period of time (weeks or month) and consume fewer calories than you expend.

I suggest as part of the *Take-Out* diet that you do use a calorie counting app for a short period of at least 2 weeks. Continuing to use it for 12 weeks over the *Take-Out* first period to reinforce the change management. Performance measures should be part of any change management process. Calorie counting does 3 things.

- Helps recalibrate what daily caloric intake should be, and what portion size is reasonable.

- Helps define what 500 or 600 calories looks like on a 5:2 diet.

- Helps in the decision-making about food products.

Calorie counters should not be used to make food choices. Calorie counters are great to understand what is going on in your diet, but poor for making decisions about food and health. While I have maintained a daily counter for over 2 years, it is for research only. I don't advise others to do so. Instead of counting calories, consume the right kind of food.

Eat, Fast, Live

In August, 2012, a documentary by Michael Mosley, a BBC Horizon science reporter and director, was shown during the London Olympics. The producers thought that showing it at that time might have a reduced audience, but it was the converse, and was one of the most watched documentaries on BBC. Mosley had gone to a number of science groups in the USA and UK who were researching diets, fasting, and longevity. If you want longevity, you want to be healthy for the duration. Quality of life is important. Part of his story is about hormesis or "when a little poison is good for you". Hormesis is a biological response but is a little controversial. Body building is an example. You do a little exercise which damages muscle, and it grows stronger. Some researchers say fasting is a hormesis response, but the scientific evidence is not there yet.

The first group Mosley visited was one with over 50,000 adherents called Calorie Restriction with Optimal Nutrition (CRONies). That lifestyle is similar to the Calorie Restricted Diet, Longevity Diet, and Anti-Aging Plan. The nutrient-rich, very low calorie diet was developed by Roy and Lisa Walford and Brian Delaney out of research in the mid-1980s that showed that mice lived up to 50% longer with increasing calorie restriction. The lifestyle is based on a 20% calorie restriction (i.e. males consume about 1800 Calories per day), and it also attempts to provide the recommended daily amounts of various nutrients. Mosley looked at the requirements and discipline, but decided he could not adhere to the very detailed planning. When he was compared with some of the "CRONies" it was said his risk of illness (Cardio vascular / cancer) was 10%. Cronies are reportedly at less than 1% risk. So while calorie restriction has substantial health benefits, it is not clear what the benefits are from. Are they from reduced calories, the type of diet, or other factors from adopting a "healthy" lifestyle?

Why does "calorie restriction" significantly lengthen the lifespan of many non-primate species, everything from worms to fleas to mice? A trial by Partridge at University College London, UK, tested if the effect was merely due to a reduction of total calories or of particular nutrients in the diet of fruit flies. Fruit flies have simple and well understood DNA and simple life processes. The flies on the calorie restricted diet lived the longest, at about 82% longer compared to those on "standard" food for fruit flies. Lowering the amount of protein and fat in the flies' diet helped increase lifespan by nearly 65%, and accounted for nearly all of the effect. It was not just calories. Eating less sugar increased longevity only by about 9%. The question is how relevant is this to other species? We are left with a number of questions about the CRON lifestyle.

What about full fasting? Mosley then met Valter Longo, Director of the USC -Longevity Institute. Longo's research goes into why we age, particularly age-related diseases such as cancer and diabetes. Longo explains, "There is lots of evidence that temporary periodic fasting can induce long-lasting changes that are beneficial against aging and diseases." He further says, "The effects can be much more effective than a cocktail of drugs."

Mosley did a prolonged four-day fast under medical supervision. A hormone called Insulin Growth Factor-1 Hormone (IGF-1) halved, his blood glucose levels fell, and he lost 1.5 kg fat. IGF-1 is a good marker for cancer risk and is thought important in longevity. High levels of protein keep IGF-1 high. But Mosley would not or could not do this every month, which is what he would need to do in order to maintain this improvement in biological markers in the longer term.

Mosley then looked at intermittent fasting, and in particular, at Dr Krista Varady's work at the University of Illinois at Chicago. Varady asked obese women to restrict calories to 25% of a daily diet (all at lunch) on one day, and then were asked to eat 125% of a normal diet on the alternate days for eight weeks. Half the group were on a low fat diet: low-fat cheeses, lean meats, and lots of fruit and vegetables. The other group ate high fat food such as pizzas, high fat lasagnes (typical Americans with 35 to 45% fat in their diets). To Varady's surprise, those on the high fat plan lost more weight than the low fat (5.6 vs 4.2 kg) dieters; both lost 7 cm on their waist, had significant falls in LDL cholesterol, and their blood pressure was down. Furthermore, they only ate about 110% on the "feast days", and they did not lose muscle tissue. More and longer studies on the comparison of low-fat and high-fat diets are underway. (This is a common theme with diets: high protein, high fat diets are more successful than low fat diets.)

Mosley included animal studies in the BBC documentary but made no mention that this research is not necessarily reproducible in humans, but that's documentaries! The Salt Institute for Biological Studies took mice and fed them a high fat diet. Half could eat whenever they wanted to eat. The others, with the same amount of food, only had an eight-hour feeding period. After 100 days, the mice that could eat whenever and whatever had high cholesterol, high blood glucose, and liver damage. The "involuntary fasting" mice weighed 28% less and had lower chronic inflammation, despite eating the same food. The researchers assume the results are due to the snacking mice having constant elevated insulin levels.

Mosley didn't like the alternate day diet. He felt they are socially inconvenient and emotionally demanding. He was not obese, nor concerned about losing too much weight. He decided to try the 25% diet, but only two days per week and to do it for one month. This became the basis of the 5:2 Diet, or Fast Diet book and hundreds of thousands of people have taken this up. This type of diet has been researched elsewhere, such as the Genesis Breast Cancer Prevention Centre at Manchester, UK, where Harvie looked at a two-day fast for intervention on breast cancer risk for over six years. Cutting calories for two days a week gave the same benefits, or more, than a normal calorie-reduced diet. Benefits were reduced obesity and lowered insulin resistance levels. These and many other studies show intermittent-fasting diets are a safe and effective alternative to daily dieting. As we know, daily dieting fails. A research question remains: are there some metabolic effects from intermittent fasting? Or is it just a lifestyle that is achievable over a longer period?

Lastly, Mosley was really excited about the evidence that shows fasting protects the brain, regenerates neurons, stops dementia, and increases cognitive responses. It is the memory function improvement which is most exciting. Much science has shown that walking and aerobic exercise are effective at reversing hippocampal volume loss in late adulthood, and contribute to improved memory function. Erikson found this could be from one to two years additional life, and this can be very important for older people with limited life expectancy. Two years staying out of a nursing home has high economic and social value. Take home message if you are older: keep walking.

Mark Mattson, Professor of Neuroscience at the National Institute of Aging, is studying dementia, a disease afflicting over 26m people globally. His "dementia sensitive" mice research is pretty clear. Eating junk food (high fat / high fructose) makes the mice fat and stupid, and they die young with diseases.

Intermittent energy restricted mice, on the other hand, do not develop detectable dementia. In human terms, instead of developing dementia at age 50, it might not happen until age 80.

Mice on the restricted diet get increased brain-derived neurotropic factor (BDNF), and researchers see development of new brain cells and neurons.

Aging can be reversed!

Increased BDNF also improves mood. The effects are the same as anti-depressants, but occur within three days. Over 17% of humans get depression at some point in their lives, so is this a contributor to the rise of obesity?

As is much of the popular science research, science can appear more certain that it actually is. The Mosley documentary linked animal research with human research, and viewers came away thinking the intermittent fasting is a sure-fire solution. The reality is that is work in progress. Many viewers took on board the comments from Prof

Mark Mattson from the USA National Institute of Aging and took up the diet just for this reason alone.

> *"The age-related cognitive declines in Alzheimer's disease ... are occurring very early, maybe decades before the subject starts to have learning and memory problems. That's why it's critical to start dietary regimes early on, when people are young or middle-aged so that they can slow down these aging processes, and live to 90 with their brain functioning perfectly well."*

Personally, I found it easy to cut calories for two days per week instead of trying to restrict calories every day. It doesn't cause disruption socially, is flexible, and is not mentally demanding. Does it increase yo-yo diet syndrome or add to the eating disorders in society? It does seem to for some according to various internet forums, but there may be other factors involved. I suspect that some of this yo-yo dieting is caused by consumption of simple carbohydrates (especially fructose, simple sugars, and carbohydrates) on the "normal" days. We know from other research that simple carbohydrates increase what you eat the next meal, and the "Last Supper" effect is real, so these effects may be important for some 5:2 dieters. Lowering body mass is important for health (research is indisputable), but are there other long term health benefits from CRON, or intermittent fasting? It may be that the 5:2 diet enables a form of intermittent fasting with three-fold benefits: better metabolic indicators, reduction in weight, and reversing of aging. The 5:2 Diet is now a fad diet, and diets have well-deserved bad reputations. Many fail to recognize that diet is merely one part of a health regime; including eating appropriate food, exercise, sleep, community, and a sense of well-being.

Conclusion

The 5:2 Diet is an excellent diet. It helps with all 3 legs of the *Take-Out* Diet: biochemical, behavioural and social aspects, and importantly addresses the causes diet failure.

- Biochemical and hormonal: On the fast day, you have to cut out simple carbohydrates. Otherwise that low level of calories make you feel hungry. If you only have 500 calories to eat, most will choose to eat moderate amounts of protein, and many complex carbohydrates. E.g. 100 g of chicken or fish, an egg, and as many complex vegetables as fits on the plate. Sugar and simple carbohydrates have to go as most 5:2ers want more food bulk than just six chocolate cookies! When you review some of the dozens of 5:2 recipe books now

171

available, the striking thing is they look like low carbohydrate diet books.

- Internal behaviour: The 5:2 Diet removes the whole issue of "guilt" and "bad foods" associated with dieting. You have to count calories on the fasting days, but for the rest of the time there are no "bad" foods. The dieter learns new portion sizes. You cannot graze or snack. Restricting calories on the two days appears to reduce food intake on the normal (or feast) days. Is it because they are on a "diet" or way of eating? (WOE). I suggest it is a combination of less snacking, learning better portion size, changing the type of food eaten, less sugar and simple carbohydrates eaten, and eating more protein to reduce appetite. They get good weight loss so they feel better about the diet and grow in confidence. Lastly, willpower is only for one day at a time and most can cope with just a single day. Just like alcoholism recovery programs, it's one day at a time, and then, only 2 days out of 7. If you fail to diet for one week or a month, the diet program says that is acceptable, and just get back on the program again.

- Social compliance: One of the major causes of people abandoning diets is the social inconvenience of dieting. With 37% or more of food eaten out, any diet will be a difficult social inhibitor. (Molly and Jeff are coming for dinner. She / he is on that weird diet and can't eat eggs/ meat / pasta / carbohydrates / red foods / vegan / vegetarian / grain / etc. Most people have 2 days a week they don't socialize, so those more solitary days can easily become the fasting days.

For these various reasons and from my own experience, I suggest the 5:2 is a good candidate as a short-term diet to lose weight. If combined with the Take-Out sugar and Take-Out simple carbohydrates actions then the weight loss can be 1 kg per week. Most importantly, it has the least conscious change management needed.

References

a. Mair W, Piper MDW, Partridge L (2005) Calories Do Not Explain Extension of Life Span by Dietary Restriction in Drosophila. PLoS Biol 3(7): e223. doi:10.1371/journal.pbio.0030223
b. CRON-diet. http://en.wikipedia.org/wiki/CRON-diet

c. Spindler S. (2010). "Biological Effects of Calorie Restriction: Implications for Modification of Human Aging". The Future of Aging. pp. 367–438. doi:10.1007/978-90-481-3999-6_12. ISBN 978-90-481-3998-9.

d. Dr Michael Mosley and Mimi Spencer. (2013) The Fast Diet: The Secret of Intermittent Fasting - Lose Weight, Stay Healthy, Live Longer. Short Books. PP256 ISBN-13: 978-1780721675

e. Erickson K.   Voss M, Prakash RS, Basak C, Szabo A, et al. (2011) Exercise training increases size of hippocampus and improves memory PNAS doi: 10.1073/pnas.1015950108

f. Shirayamn Y et.al. (2002) Brain-Derived Neurotrophic Factor Produces Antidepressant. Effects in Behavioral Models of Depression   J.   Neuroscience,   22(8):3251–3261 http://www.jneurosci.org/content/22/8/3251.full.pdf

g. Hormesis. http://en.wikipedia.org/wiki/Hormesis

h. Rattan, S. (2008). "Hormesis in aging". Ageing Research Reviews 7 (1): 63–78. doi:10.1016/j.arr.2007.03.002

i. Gems D, Partideg L. (2008). "Stress-Response Hormesis and Aging: "That which Does Not Kill Us Makes Us Stronger". Cell Metabolism 7 (3): 200–3. doi:10.1016/j.cmet.2008.01.001

CHAPTER 28
BIOCHEMISTRY OF FATS AND OILS

Get the Facts

➤ Fats and oils chemistry is complex, but understandable. It's worth the read and research to understand!

➤ Fats and oils are used for energy, for cell structure and as precursors for many hormones.

➤ Science is still very uncertain about many health aspects of omega-3 or omega-6 families of fatty acids, so do not believe all the myths about Omega fatty acids.

➤ You probably consume adequate essential fatty acids without any supplements.

Understand the Science

To understand the complexity of fats and oils, we have to understand some biochemistry. Don't groan at the word "biochemistry"! I have put all the information in clear, easy-to-understand form in this chapter. Read on with confidence. It is important to grasp the concepts. These are important as fats are our very life. Without fat we wouldn't have cells, or life. We would be nothing. Fats are important sources of fuel because, when metabolized, they yield large quantities of energy in usable form. They act as building blocks for all sorts of essential compounds particularly the endocrinology systems, and lastly, they are integral to our brain and cell walls. Like much of biochemistry and the organic world, the exact chemical structure makes a world of difference. Two molecules can differ by a single molecule, or 1 bond, yet the compounds may have completely different biological activity. There are less than five concepts needed to understand this biochemistry: oils and fats, fatty acids, triglycerides, saturation, and bonds.

- Fats and oils mean the same. Fats are sometimes confused with the hard fat and oils, but essentially they are all fat, or all oils! We tend to say that oils are liquid and fats are hard, but in reality they are all fats. Organic fats are more complex than inorganic fats, such as motor oil. We can't use mineral oil, although some specialized bacteria can, but engines can use organic fats as energy.

- Don't confuse fats (trigylcerides) and fatty acids. Fats (triglycerides) are made up of fatty acids (FA) and glycerol (a glucose-like compound). Think of the letter E. Un-kinked, the vertical "I" is the glycerol, and each of the three horizontal "—"s are a fatty acid. (The chapter on Lipogenesis has a diagram explaining this.) The triglyceride is named from the type of fatty acid that it is made from, the degree of hydrogenation (saturation), and the chemical bond type. Cholesterol is a particular type of fatty acid.

- A fatty acid is a carboxylic acid with a long aliphatic tail (chain), which is either saturated or unsaturated. Omega-3 fatty acid, and Omega-6 fatty acid refer to particular fatty acids. Most naturally occurring fatty acids have a chain of an even number of carbon atoms, from four to 28. Fatty acids are usually bound up in triglycerides or phospholipids. When they are not attached to other molecules, they are known as "free" fatty acids. Particular fatty acids might include ALA (Alpha-linolenic acid), EPA (Eicosapentaenoic acid), and DHA (Docosahexaenoic acid). Fatty acids have complicated names and the length of the fatty acid, the saturation and the bond type provides a common name for the fatty acid. E.g. myristic saturated is C14, palmitic saturated is C16, and some of the C18 fatty acids include stearic saturated C18, oleic monounsaturated cis-bond C18, linoleic polyunsaturated C18, vaccenic monounsaturated trans-fat C18 and elaidic monounsaturated trans-fat C18.

- Saturation. Fatty acids can be further categorized by the level of saturation. On the fatty acid molecule there are open spaces, like parking spots. When all the available spots, or parking spaces, on the carbon atom are filled (i.e., saturated) with hydrogen atoms, the fatty acid is said to be saturated. If one or more places on the carbon are not filled with hydrogen, the fatty acid is called unsaturated. A fat molecule with one empty space is called a monounsaturated fat. If two or more spots on the atom are empty, the fat is known as a polyunsaturated fat.

o   Saturated fats contain no double bonds. E.g. lard, coconut oil.

o   Monounsaturated fats contain one double bond. E.g. olive oil, canola, nut oils.

o   Polyunsaturated fats contain two or more double bonds. E.g. vegetable oils, seafood.

- Bonds. The type of chemical bond is the last of the concepts to grasp. The term Cis or Trans refers to the geometric arrangement of the carbon double bonds. Cis-fats are common in nature, and trans-fats uncommon. Trans-fats are created in manufacturing processes and present in partially hydrogenated vegetable oils. The manufacturing processes now avoid creating them by keeping the manufacturing temperatures down.

Fats for Energy

Fats are used as an energy store. Tri-glycerides / fat are broken down in the body to release glycerol and free fatty acids. The glycerol can be converted to glucose, and thus used as a source of energy. There is more of this in the Chapter on energy usage and Lipogenesis. The fatty acids are used in heart and skeletal muscle, as those muscles prefer fatty acids. Despite long-standing assertions to the contrary, the brain can use fatty acids as a source of fuel in addition to glucose and ketone bodies.

Fats for Structures

Fats / triglycerides are insoluble in water, so they do not exist in the blood as fats. They are combined with proteins and then travel around in the blood and are called lipoproteins. If you imagine the lipoprotein as a cargo ship, and the triglycerides as cargo, you can begin to understand why geometric shape (bonds) and the chemical structure is very important.

In the 1940's Danielli-Davson proposed a rigid model of cell membranes, and this was modified by Singer and Nicholas to the "Fluid Mosaic Model" membrane in 1972. The lining layer on both inside and outside of the cell is a protein layer (phospholipids). The middle of the cell member is often drawn like springs and are neatly arranged between the two layers of phospholipids. Scattered in the membrane are various structures. Integral proteins and protein channels go right through from top to bottom and help move compounds such as carbohydrates and proteins in and out of the cell. Some structures go partway through such as surface proteins, globular proteins, peripheral proteins and cholesterol. Lipids are integral to life and research is continuing on how they operate so well, and what happens when they stop working as well.

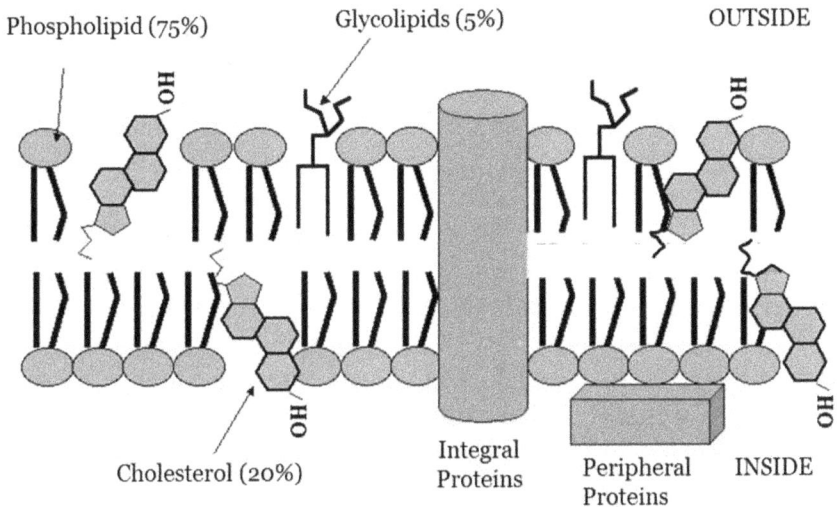

Figure 28 Cell Wall Membrane Simple Schematic Diagram

Most people never understand how important fat is in our life. Fat is generally thought of as "bad", but you can see from above that fat should be thought of good. Damage cell walls and health suffers.

Cholesterol

Cholesterol, a particular type of triglyceride, acts as both a precursor for hormones and as a part of cellular membranes. Its chemical structure is ($C_{27}H_{46}O$). It is important for the production of oestrogen in women, testosterone in men and processing vitamin D. Cholesterol helps keep a cell fluid and functioning. The human body produces 2 g of cholesterol per day, making up about 85 percent of blood cholesterol levels. The other 15 percent comes from a person's diet. We will talk some more about cholesterol in the Chapter on Statins.

Fatty Acids

All fatty acids are synthesized by humans except for 2 notable ones, which you will have heard of. Humans and other animals *must* ingest these 2 because the body requires them for good health, but cannot synthesize them. The term "essential fatty acid" (EFA) refers to fatty acids required for biological processes, but does not include the fats that only act as fuel. The two are alpha-linoleic acid (ALA), an Omega-3 fatty acid, and linoleic acid (an Omega-6 fatty acid). Even now, there is doubt about linoleic acid "essentiality" and some of the previous science may be in error.

The Omega-3 fatty acid group, also known as n-3 fatty acids are polyunsaturated fatty acids with a double bond at the 3rd carbon atom. Omega-3s include ALA, found in some vegetable oils, such as soybean, rapeseed or canola, flaxseed, walnuts, and green vegetables such as Brussels sprouts, kale, spinach, and salad greens. Others in this family include EPA (Eicosapentaenoic acid), and DHA (Docosahexaenoic acid), both found in marine oils. Some of the shorter Omega-3s, such as ALA, can be used to build the longer EPA and DHA, but the process can be inefficient. We don't know whether the vegetable or the fish oil type of Omega-3 is more important, even though there is a widespread practice of taking fish oil tablets with higher levels of EPA and DHA. We only need a small amount of Omega-3 – a handful of walnuts, or a tablespoon of flax seed oil. Omega-3 are converted to Eicosanoids.

Omega-6 fatty acid group (n-6 fatty acids) is a family of polyunsaturated fatty acids that have that have in common a double bond in the 6th carbon atom. Linoleic acid is the shortest of the Omega-6 group. The fatty acids are converted to Omega-6 Eicosanoids with major sources from crops of palm, soybean, rapeseed, and sunflower. Global production is over 32mT of Omega-6 and 4mT of Omega-3 ALA. Omega-6 fatty acids lower LDL cholesterol (the "bad" cholesterol) and reduce inflammation, and they are protective against heart disease. Groups such as the Harvard School of Health still maintain that the ratio is immaterial with little evidence to show the ratio is important. Don't tell that to other researchers who disagree vehemently, or to dieting proponents such as the Paleo dieters or other groups.

Conjugated Linoleic Acids (CLAs) are an area of research within this whole Omega-6 arena. The "conjugated" part is the bond arrangements within linoleic acids and there are 28 different forms of CLA. They occur naturally in animal fat, especially grass fed ruminants (cows, sheep, goats), but much of what we eat is from manufactured plant CLA. Supposedly CLA can help you lose weight, but there are also concerns about side effects including fatty liver disease and diabetes.

Food / Plant	Omega -3 (%)	Omega -6 (%)	Omega -9 (%)	6 to 3 ratio	Saturated fat (%)
Avocado Oil	-	18	65	18:1	17
Borage Oil	-	60	26	No n-3	14
Canola Oil	10	24	54	2.4:1	8
Corn Oil	-	59	27	59:1	13
Coconut Oil	-	1	8	No n-3	91
Cottonseed Oil	-	56	18	56:1	26
Flaxseed Oil	57	16	19	0.3:1	6-9
Leafy vegetables (broccoli)	1.3				
Macadamia Nut Oil	-	2	84	1:1	12
Almond Oil	-	28	65	28:1	7
Walnut Oil	5	58	28	7:1	9
Oily fish	75	-	-		25
Olive Oil	-	12	72	12:1	14
Palm Oil	-	10	39	10:1	51
Palm Kernel Oil	-	2	14	2:1	84
Peanut Oil	-	34	48	43:1	17
Primrose Oil	-	81	9	No n-3	10
Pumpkin Seed Oil	-	60	20	20:1	17
Rice Bran Oil	-	27	46	27:1	26
Safflower Oil	-	56	24	78:1	8
Sesame	-	45	40	45:1	15
Soybean Oil	5	56	24	11:1	15
Sunflower Oil (high Oleic)	-	11	81	7:1	19
Butter	1	1	32	1:1	65
Lard or Pork Fat	-	12	48	12:1	40
Beef Tallow	-	5	40	5:1	55
Goose fat	-	13	52	13:1	35

CLA is involved with insulin regulation and work is continuing. Stay tuned. The table shows which oils are from different plant sources, and some of the concerns are the Omega 6 to 3 ratio. Many of these oils are "seed oil" produced from seeds of plants and only available with modern technology in the past 40 years. Many scientists and authors focus on these as a concern for health. This is discussed in other chapters. Omega-9 fatty acids are common components of animal fat and vegetable oil, and include oleic acid (main component of olive oil, macadamia oils) and erucic acids, which are found in rapeseed, wallflower, and mustard seed. If you look at this table you can see that levels of different Omega fatty acids vary substantially. Some fats have no omega-3, some no omega-6, and some are such as coconut oil and animal fats are mostly omega-9s or saturated fats. Plants rich in Omega-3 Fatty acids include green leafy vegetables (lettuce, broccoli, spinach, kale), legume seeds (mungo, kidney navy, or pinto beans, peas), citrus fruits, melons, cherries and ground flaxseed.

Fats for Hormones - Eicosanoids

Fatty acids are often the precursor (or building blocks) for other important compounds too. As in most biological processes, the more you know, the more complexity you find. Fatty acids are precursors for other compounds. Eicosanoids (or icosanoids) are signalling molecules made from either Omega-3 or Omega-6 fatty acids. They exert complex control over many bodily systems, mainly in inflammation or immunity, and work as messengers in the central nervous system. The networks of controls that depend upon Eicosanoids are among the most complex in the human body. Normal diets will provide all the Omega-3 or Omega-6 required but the amounts and balance of these fats in a person's diet may affect the body's Eicosanoids-controlled functions. We need Omega-3 fatty acids for numerous normal body functions, such as controlling blood clotting and building cell membranes in the brain. Omega-3 fatty acids are also associated with many health benefits, including protection against heart disease and possibly stroke. New studies are identifying potential benefits for a wide range of conditions including cancer, inflammatory bowel disease, autoimmune diseases such as lupus and rheumatoid arthritis. The role of omega acids and eicosanoids is also studied in mental processes including bi-polar, depression, intelligence, and dementia. Anti-inflammatory drugs such as aspirin and other non-steroidal anti-inflammatory drugs (NSAID) act by down-regulating eicosanoid synthesis.

Trans-Fats

Trans-fats cause cardiovascular disease, obesity, cancer, and diabetes, and even back in 1997 it was estimated over 30,000 deaths in the USA were attributable to trans-fats. One cause was that they raised LDL cholesterol levels and lowered HDL cholesterol levels, but this did not explain all of the increase shown in the Framingham Nurses Study. In the 1990s, it was quite likely that the so-called positive effects of polyunsaturated fatty acids was completely negated by the levels of trans-fats in other food products. Even today, who is to say if the hydrogenation process has zero levels of co-production of trans-fats? What is a safe level? Food companies have changed the fats so that now palm oil makes up 50% of fats used in food products. Trans-fats are usually found on store shelves in breads, cookies, and lots of other baked goods and snacks. Look for food packaging that states "no trans-fats." As we discuss in the section on margarine, food labelling is such that the level of trans-fats do not need to be specified if they are below the minimum criteria. Given their role in disease, are minute amounts of trans-fats important or not?

Conclusion

In conclusion, we can't get away from fats; they are integral in our lives. They are used for energy, for building blocks for other compounds, and in every cell in our bodies. What difference has a change in consumption made? We do know that the modern human diet has much more Omega-6 and polyunsaturated oils than it used to have, and this change may, or may not, have had profound changes to human health. Is this change a cause of increasing ill health? Exactly what change is unclear. I think there is enough evidence to be prudent about consumption of seed oils. Studies using animal models say polyunsaturated fats can be toxic. Together, with the dearth of evidence that saturated fats are harmful, I have chosen to *Take-Out* seed oils from my diet. I have substituted, and use in preference, animal fats, coconut, and olive oil. My guess is I eat enough leafy green vegetables and fish to get adequate levels of these essential fatty acids. More of this in the next chapter.

References

a. Wikipedia. Fat http://en.wikipedia.org/wiki/Fat
b. Wikipedia. Essential fatty acids. http://en.wikipedia.org/wiki/Essential_fatty_acids
c. Wikipedia. Omega-3 fatty acids http://en.wikipedia.org/wiki/Omega-3_fatty_acid
d. Wikipedia. Omega-6 fatty acids http://en.wikipedia.org/wiki/Omega-6_fatty_acid
e. Wikipedia. Omega-9 fatty acids. http://en.wikipedia.org/wiki/Omega-9_fatty_acid
f. Wikipedia. Cell membranes and transport. http://en.wikibooks.org/wiki/A-level_Biology/Biology_Foundation/cell_membranes_and_transport
g. Wikipedia. Eicosanoid. http://en.wikipedia.org/wiki/Eicosanoid
h. Sacks, F. (2014) Ask the Expert: Omega-3 Fatty Acids http://www.hsph.harvard.edu/nutritionsource/omega-3/

i.   Ascherio A, Willett W. (1997) Health effects of trans fatty acids. Am J Clin Nutr vol. 66(4) 1006S-1010S

j.   Mensink R, Katan M. (1990) Effect of Dietary trans Fatty Acids on High-Density and Low-Density Lipoprotein Cholesterol Levels in Healthy Subjects. N Engl J Med 323:439-44 DOI: 10.1056/NEJM199008163230703

k.   Lopez-Garcia E, Schulze M, Meigs J, Manson J, Rifai N, Stampfer M, Willett M, Hu F. (2005) Consumption of Trans Fatty Acids Is Related to Plasma Biomarkers of Inflammation and Endothelial Dysfunction J. Nutr. vol. 135(3) 562-566

l.   Whigham L, Watras A, Schoeller D. (2007) Efficacy of conjugated linoleic acid for reducing fat mass: a meta-analysis in humans Am J Clin Nutr 85(5) 1203-1211

m.   Castro-Webb N, Ruiz-Narváez E, Campos H. (2012) Cross-sectional study of conjugated linoleic acid in adipose tissue and risk of diabetes Am J Clin Nutr. 96(1)175-181 doi: 10.3945/ajcn.111.011858

n.   Pescatore F. (2005) The Science of Fats, Fatty Acids and Edible Oils Choosing the Right Oils and Fat. http://www.diabetesincontrol.com/component/content/article/64-feature-writer-article/2385&Itemid=8

CHAPTER 29
STOP CONSUMING VEGETABLE OILS

Get the Facts

➤ Oils ain't oils, as Castrol Motor Oil Company once promoted.
➤ Consumption of vegetable oils is a contentious scientific area of research and polarizes nutritionists / medical researchers / health practitioners / and industry.
➤ Many diets recommend cutting out seed oils (polyunsaturated oils such as soybean, cottonseed, safflower, sunflower, peanut, sesame, rapeseed, and rice bran).
➤ Avoid all margarines and fake butters.
➤ Use butter, olive oil, or coconut oil.
➤ Palm oil has substituted for margarine from the 1990s, which replaced lard in the 1950s, as the preferred oil in food products.
➤ Avoid over consumption of oils – they are calorie dense and can undo the best of diets.

Understand the Science

The consumption of processed seed and vegetable oils has increased dramatically in the past century. These were not available to humans until the twentieth century, because we simply didn't have the technology to extract them. Extraction of oil can involve bleaching, deodorizing, and use of the solvent hexane. Due to their low price and manufacturing stability, these oils have made their way into most processed foods, including "healthy" salad dressings, butter replicates, mayonnaise, cookies, and bread. Books such as *Toxic Oils* by David Gillespie say research evidence is unequivocal. Short but concise articles including a review by Chris Gunner, at Authority Nutrition, is an excellent evidence-based argument against Omega-6 over-consumption.

We are dealing with a 30-year scientific theory that says saturated fats are bad, and polyunsaturated oils are good. The conspirators view the multi-billion dollar investment and profits from seed oils as the reason for continuing this theory. So the arguments about oil are scientific, political (entrenched views), and financially driven. When considering the value of study results, it's a good idea to look at who sponsored the research. If industry sponsored, view with suspicion.

Past research has often been confounded or compromised. Few epidemiological studies looked at the type of oil that people were consuming, and researchers only looked at short term studies. Animal studies are dismissed by the "industry" as not relevant. Disease is generally a long term process and many diseases may take twenty-years between exposure and disease. Because oils or fats are found in most things we eat, it is almost impossible to do proper experiments. Any experiment changing the ratio of what oils are in a diet will be confounded by the baseline consumption.

In the previous section we looked at different types of fatty acids and three in particular; Omega-3, Omega-6 and Omega-9, and in foods they are found. One measure is the ratio of Omega-3 to Omega-6. A primary concern is that certain types of polyunsaturated oil cause inflammation in animals and humans, and may be the cause of metabolic syndrome. Of particular concern is the level of Omega-6 polyunsaturated fatty acids compared with Omega-3 in our diet. We need some Omega-3 and Omega-6 essential fatty acids because the body can't produce them.

Inflammation

There has been a great deal of research on the saturated fats and the impact on increased serum cholesterol and consequential cardiovascular disease. The link between higher consumption of saturated fats and obesity or chronic illness is now pretty much disproved, even though it is still part of the current medical advice. That may only change slowly. It's not known if there is inflammation from saturated fats, and like most fats we eat, we burn for energy. There are those that think that the saturated fat in coconut oil is beneficial in diets, rather than just neutral.

The primary concern throughout this discussion on saturated, monounsaturated, and polyunsaturated fatty acids, including Omega-3 / 6 / 9, is the chemical activity and the inflammation from these compounds. The essential fatty acids (Omega-3, Omega-6) are very active compounds, both in themselves, their Eicosanoids derivatives, and inclusion of these compounds into cell membranes throughout the body. Inflammationis an underlying factor in some of the most common diseases including cardiovascular disease, cancer, diabetes, and arthritis. The concern is that unsaturated fats get incorporated in cell structures, the unsaturated fat oxidises, and the cell structure is damaged. The extent appears unknown.

Seed Oils

Throughout evolution, humans got Omega-3 to Omega-6 in a ratio of about 1:1 up to 1:3 in our food. That's changed during the past century of food industrialization. The ratio is now about 1:16. Polyunsaturated fatty acids in seed oils (usually labelled as vegetable oils) are now in most processed food and it is exceedingly difficult to avoid Omega-6. Many argue that consumption of these oils has increased at the expense of other healthy fats like butter. They were labelled as "heart-healthy" and governments all around the world encouraged us to eat more of them. Figure 28 shows how consumption of polyunsaturated fats, mainly Omega-6, has increased in the USA to levels previously never known to humans.

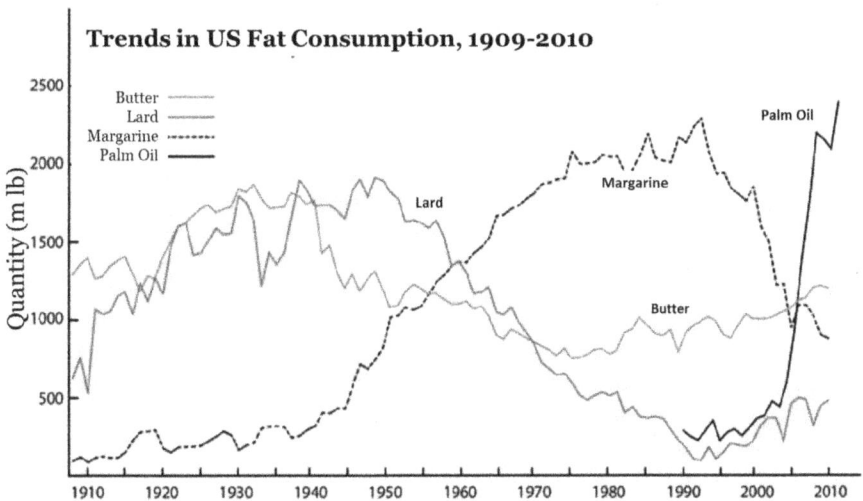

Figure 29 USA Trends in fat consumption 1909 to 2010 (Bonner)

The popularity of butter and lard declined in the 1940s and 1950s, giving way to margarine. Butter has had a resurgence, possibly due to the popularity of Atkins / Paleo / Low carbohydrate diets, and changing food habits. The increase to margarine was driven by the mistaken belief that vascular health could be improved by switching from saturated animal fats to unsaturated plant oils. The consumption of margarine fell from 1990, when it was discovered that plant-oil solidification produces metabolically harmful trans-fat. The physical-chemical properties of lard make it ideal for baking, and palm oil is an effective substitute because its chemical composition is almost identical with 49% saturated fatty acid

185

(palmitic), 37% monounsaturated (oleic), and only 9% polyunsaturated (linoleic). (Lard is 43:47:10). Much of the objection to palm oil comes from the association with deforestation of rain forests and associated animal habitat loss. It has no cholesterol. There is some controversy about the health effects of palm oil with several studies linking palm oil and cardiovascular disease and others with health benefits increasing good cholesterol.

What is interesting is Figure 29 from Guyenet, who reviewed all the papers he could find on Omega-6 content in our body fat stores.

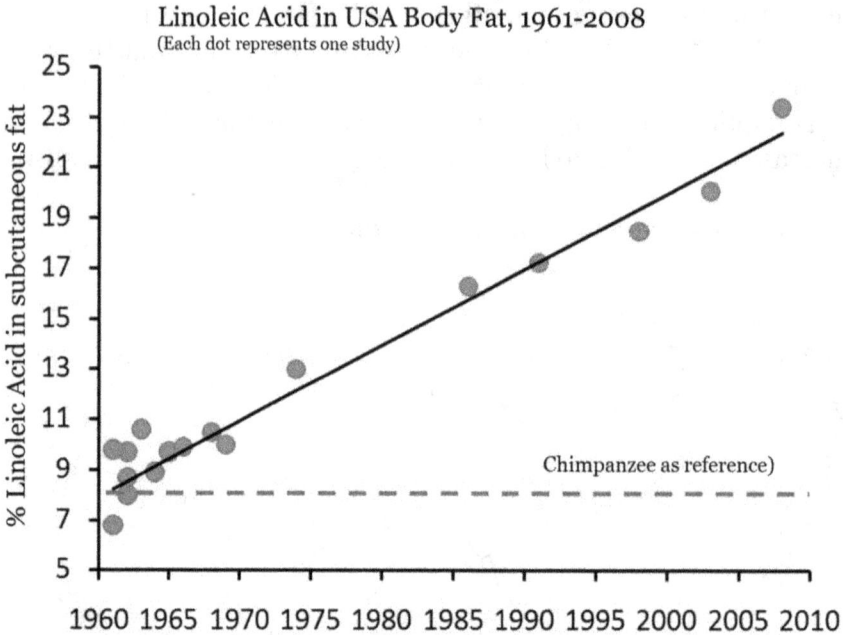

Figure 30 Linoleic Acid in USA Body Fat (Guyenet)

These 7 papers surprised him – the level of Omega-6 was linear and increased 300% over the last 40 years. Some Omega-6 will be burned for energy like most other fats, but it also accumulates in tissue. These oils (that are very sensitive to chemical reactions) are stored and incorporated into cells with physiological changes. In the previous section we looked at the bonds in these fatty acids, and the problem with polyunsaturated fats is that all these double bonds make them susceptible to oxidation. Oxidation is where the fatty acids react with oxygen, and this damages them. That is why margarine can go rancid when the polyunsaturated fats oxidize. It suggests that if we have a lot of these fatty acids in our bodies our cell membranes are more sensitive to oxidation.

It's important to note that not all plant oils are bad. For example, coconut oil and olive oil are both excellent. Most critics of omega-6 high oils suggest do not eat seed oils, avoiding their high Omega-6 content. Oils include Canola, Corn, Cottonseed, Peanut, Safflower, Soybean, Sesame, Sunflower, and Rice Bran.

Furthermore, the jury is out on additional Omega-3 supplements. We will discuss in the Omega-3 Chapter. There's some evidence Omega-3 fats contribute to cancer. However, this doesn't mean we should refrain from eating them. Cardiovascular disease causes more deaths than cancer, and Omega-3 fats are protective against CVD.

- Eat enough oily marine fish to achieve Omega-6 and Omega-3 balance.

- Minimize Omega-6 intake so that balance is achieved at the lowest possible intake of polyunsaturated fats.

- All nutrients can be eaten in excess, even Omega-3 fats. The right amount of oily fish is probably about one to two meals per week.

Mainstream View

There is a much discussion about this complex issue. Research is at best ambivalent, and you can choose a range of studies to confirm the hypothesis you want proven. A 2012 systematic review by Johnson & Fritsche of randomized controlled trials (considered one of the highest forms of evidence) found there is no data in *"healthy human beings to show that the addition of linoleic acid (an omega-6 fatty acid) to diets increase markers of inflammation"*. I.e. dietary omega-6 does not contribute to inflammation.

The American Heart Association's scientific advice is similar. *"Aggregate data from randomized trials, case-control and cohort studies, and long-term animal feeding experiments indicate that the consumption of at least 5% to 10% of energy from omega-6 polyunsaturated fatty acids reduces the risk of CVD relative to lower intakes. To reduce omega-6 intakes from their current levels would be more likely to increase than to decrease risk for CVD."*

Many nutrition professionals, medical associations and their members, and some alternative health practitioners, still consider seed oils as health foods, or promote additional Omega-3 oils. Bodies include the Australian Heart Foundation.

Coconut Oil

Coconut oil is extracted from the "meat" inside the hard-shelled fruit of the coconut palm (*Cocos nucifera*). Like lard, it is solid at room temperature, is stable at high temperature, and has a long shelf life of up to 2 years, which makes it attractive for many kinds of food processing and baking. For years it had a bad reputation because it is very high in saturated fat, the kind found mostly in animal products. In the 1980s a media campaign demonized coconut and other tropical oils and blamed them for heart attacks because of their saturated fat content, and the health establishment quickly jumped on board. As a result, food companies stopped using tropical oils, replacing them largely with partially hydrogenated oils. Most health organisations continue to advise against consumption of high amounts of coconut oil due to its high level of saturated fats.

Coconut oil is unusual because it contains a high percentage of lauric acid (often claimed to be a medium-chain triglyceride or MCT) compared with other saturated fats. Most oils consist of long-chain triglycerides (LCTs). The difference matters because our bodies metabolise MCTs differently from LCTs. MCTs are transported directly from the intestinal tract to the liver where they're likely to be burned off as fuel. That means they are less likely to be deposited in fat tissues – and this is what gives rise to the weight-loss claim by coconut oil supporters.

In the past few years with the rise of the Paleo diet and the realisation that trans-fats were produced in hydrogenation of polyunsaturated seed oils, coconut has gained its own cult status. It's fine to use coconut oil, but I don't go out of my way to consume it, and I don't see much evidence for the claimed benefits to heart health. What I read is people who promote and consume coconut oil also recommend decreasing consumption of sugars and simple carbohydrates, and increasing eating whole foods.

Conclusion

Some things are really clear: if you want to reduce the risk for allergies to your children by 50%, stop feeding them margarine and seed oils. If you don't want glaucoma, stop eating seed oils. If you want lower cardiovascular disease or cancer, avoid any products with trans-fats. Animal studies are even more alarming. Yet other studies show mixed benefits or few detrimental effects. So what are we supposed to do? These are long term, complex issues, with complex biochemistry, and no-one seems to have absolute clarity – except the zealots.

For me the simple thing is to minimize or reduce those dietary changes and risks. Don't be a food zealot. If you do, it makes food choices very difficult, as the social implications are very severe. Do you need to remove 100% of seed oils from your diet? How would you eat out socially if you decided to completely avoid seed oils? If you *take-out* simple carbohydrates from your diet, then most seed oils will also be gone. I have removed 95% of the canola and seed oils from my diet. I have changed to using olive oil for salad dressings and fry less food or grill to avoid the risk of producing trans-fats during cooking. I've taken-out from my diet most food products, and eat more whole food. Other simple steps to further reduce seed oil consumption include:

- Eliminate margarine from the diet and use butter sparingly.

- Use olive oil, coconut oil, butter or lard. Get rid of seed oils from your pantry.

- Avoid foods cooked with high levels of polyunsaturated oils.

- Limit consumption of both Omega-3 and Omega-6.

- Eat green leafy vegetables and a couple of fish meals a week to make sure you have enough essential fatty acids.

While others propose radical changes, it makes sense to reduce these long term risks by taking an 80/20 approach. Do I have fried fish and chips with friends down at the beach on a Friday night, given what I know now? My choice is yes. The social benefits outweigh going without / different food choices, or being a food zealot. It's a choice that you will have to make to suit you. My tactics? Reduce the chips. Add a few fresh prawns. It is a tough change with eliminating most food products and is an extra challenge because of the size and reach of global food businesses that control our food supply.

I have no doubt this area of oils will continue to be a vigorous area of research and commentary.

References

a. Gillespie, David. (2012) Toxic Oil. Why Vegetable Oil will kill you & How to Save Yourself ISBN 978-1-7425-3582-1
b. Gunnars, K (2013) Are Vegetable and Seed Oils Bad For Your Health? A Critical Look http://authoritynutrition.com/are-vegetable-and-seed-oils-bad/
c. A.P. Simopoulos (2006) Evolutionary aspects of diet, the omega-6/omega-3 ratio and genetic variation: nutritional implications

for chronic diseases. Biomedicine & Pharmacotherapy 60(9) Pages 502–507 DOI: 10.1016/j.biopha.2006.07.080

d. Guyenet S. (2011) Seed Oils and Body Fatness: A Problematic Revisit http://wholehealthsource.blogspot.com/2011/08/seed-oils-and-body-fatness-problematic.html

e. Jaminet, Paul. (2013) Omega-3 Fats and Cancer http://perfecthealthdiet.com/category/nutrients/omega-3-and-omega-6-fats/

f. Johnson GH, Fritsche K. (2012) Effect of dietary linoleic acid on markers of inflammation in healthy person: a systematic review of randomised controlled trials. J Acad Nutr Diet. 2012 Jul;112(7):1029-41, 1041.e1-15. doi: 10.1016/j.jand.2012.03.029.

g. Australian Heart Foundation. (2009)Summary of evidence. Dietary fats and dietary cholesterol for cardiovascular health (2009) http://www.heartfoundation.org.au/.../Dietary-fats...

h. Australian Heart Foundation (2009) Position statement. Dietary fats and dietary sterols for cardiovascular health (2009) http://www.heartfoundation.org.au/.../Dietary-fats.

i. Wu et al (2014) Circulating Omega-6 Polyunsaturated Fatty Acids and Total and Cause-Specific Mortality: The Cardiovascular Health Study http://circ.ahajournals.org/.../CIRCULATIONAHA.114.011590.

j. The Cochrane Database of Systematic Reviews (Hooper et al), 2012, Reduced or modified dietary fat for preventing cardiovascular disease. http://www.ncbi.nlm.nih.gov/pubmed/22592684

k. The World Health Organization: Fats and fatty acids in human nutrition: Report of an expert consultation (2010) http://www.who.int/.../fatsandfattyacids.../en/index.html

l. Mozaffarian D, Micha R, Wallace S (2010) Effects on Coronary Heart Disease of Increasing Polyunsaturated Fat in Place of Saturated Fat: A Systematic Review and Meta-Analysis of Randomized Controlled Trials. Ploa Medicine 7 (3) DOI: 10.1371/journal.pmed.1000252.

m. Jakobsen MU, O'Reilly EJ, Heitmann BL, Pereira MA, Bälter K, Fraser GE, Goldbourt U, Hallmans G, Knekt P, Liu S, Pietinen P, Spiegelman D, Stevens J, Virtamo J, Willett WC, Ascherio A. (2009) Major types of dietary fat and risk of coronary heart disease: a pooled analysis of 11 cohort studies. Am J Clin Nutr. 89(5):1425-32. doi: 10.3945/ajcn.2008.27124.

n. Bonner, J (2013) From pork lard to palm oil and back. NATURE 492 (41) doi:10.1038/492041b

o. Coconut Oil. (2015). Consumer New Zealand. https://www.consumer.org.nz/articles/coconut-oil

p. Is Coconut oil a Miracle Food? (2014) Berkley Wellness. http://www.berkeleywellness.com/healthy-eating/diet-weight-loss/food/nutrition/article/coconut-oil-all-its-cracked-be

CHAPTER 30
BUTTER VS MARGARINE

Get the Facts

➢ Butter got "bad press" as the message was out to reduce fat intake and reduce polyunsaturated fats.

➢ Butter is a healthy fat and consumption has begun to increase from years of decrease.

➢ Polyunsaturated fats from vegetable oils increase allergies and present other health problems.

➢ Avoid margarine during pregnancy, and up to at least the first three years of the child's life.

Understand the Science

Margarine was first developed in the nineteenth century as an inexpensive alternative to butter. Early on, it was a popular butter substitute for people who could not afford butter, or where butter was not available, including soldiers on the battlefield. Margarine can be made from animal fats and/or vegetable oils. The bulk of the industry today is comprised of vegetable oil based margarines.

This increase in consumption of margarine was partly attributable to the relationship between a diet high in saturated fat, in animal fat, and the risk of heart disease. Plant oils tend to have less saturated fatty acids and do not contain cholesterol. More specifically, plant oils have much lower amounts of three types of saturated fatty acids (i.e.16:0, 14:0, and 12:0), which are the saturated fatty acids that seemed to be most associated with raising blood cholesterol levels.

Margarine is made by adding hydrogen to unsaturated fatty acids in plant oils. This "hydrogenation" is a process where oils are heated up in a container and hydrogen gas is applied. The degree of change depends upon how much hydrogenation is allowed to take place. The more the hydrogenation, the more solid the oil. For instance, margarines that come in block form are typically more hydrogenated than softer tub margarine. The hydrogenation chemistry process means that some polyunsaturated fatty acids are converted to monounsaturated fatty acids and some of the monounsaturated fatty acids are converted to saturated fatty acids. This converts the liquid oil to semisolid, or to solid fat. The most popular plant oils used for hydrogenation are soybean or canola oil. Because of their relatively high content of mono and poly unsaturated fatty acids, margarines made from soybean, canola, sunflower, safflower, olive, palm and cottonseed oils are perceived to be healthier than butter.

There is a problem with this process and it involves the type of chemical bonds between the molecules. There are both "cis" type bonds and "trans" type bonds. (Check out the Biochemistry of Oils Chapter.) Trans-fats are a known health risk. When heat is applied to plant oils during hydrogenation, a small number of the cis-double bonds can be converted to trans-double bonds, which helps solidify the oil. In fact, conventional margarines have a higher trans-fatty acid content than butter, and typically, the harder the margarine, the higher the trans-fat acid level. Food companies have been working successfully over the past decade to alter their process for forming margarine and to lower and supposedly eliminate the trans-fat content which is reflected on the food labels. How bad is this? While trans-fats are naturally occurring, research pretty much says avoid trans-fats. Trans-fat is considered by many doctors to be the worst type of fat you can eat.

Margarine and Allergies

Children who consume more margarine have double the rate of medically diagnosed eczema, hay fever, allergies, and asthma. This has been seen in Finnish children and German two-year olds. Early childhood, especially up to 3 years old, is important as it is when these allergies develop.

These allergies are turned on if their mother ate margarine or vegetable oils during the last four weeks of pregnancy. In that case, children have at least a 50% greater chance of having eczema, hay fever, or allergies for life. There is a very direct relationship between the level of polyunsaturated fat in the placental cord blood supply and the risk of allergy disease. Not only that, the relationship is clearly dose-dependent.

Want to give someone allergies, eczema, hay fever, or asthma for life? Just increase the polyunsaturated fats in their diet. Want to decrease the risk? Just decrease the polyunsaturated fats.

The mechanism is understood. Long-chain polyunsaturated fatty acids reduce T-cell activation and dampen inflammation. They counteract the neonatal immune activation and hamper normal tolerance development to harmless environmental antigens.

So what does a margarine ingredient label says are the ingredients? Water, vegetable mono and diglycerides, salt, rice starch, gelatin, natural and artificial flavours, lactose, colour including yellow 5 and yellow 6, vegetable datem, potassium sorbate, lactic acid, and calcium disodium EDTA added as preservatives, Soy Lecithin, Vitamin A (Palmitate) added.

What is butter made from? Milk, cream. Sometimes salt. Enough said.

References

a. Barman M, Johansson S, Hesselmar B, Wold AE, Sandberg A-S, et al. (2013) High Levels of Both n-3 and n-6 Long-Chain Polyunsaturated Fatty Acids in Cord Serum Phospholipids Predict Allergy Development. PLoS ONE 8(7): e67920. doi:10.1371/journal.pone.0067920

b. Sausenthaler S, Koletzko S, Schaaf B, Lehmann I, Borte M, Herbarth O, von Berg A, Wichmann HE, Heinrich J. (2007) Maternal diet during pregnancy in relation to eczema and allergic sensitization in the offspring at 2 y of age. (2007) Am J Clin Nutr February 2007 vol. 85 no. 2 530-537

c. von Mutius E, Weiland SK, Fritzsch C, Duhme H, Keil U. (1998) Increasing prevalence of hay fever and atopy among children in Leipzig, East Germany. Lancet. 1998 Mar 21;351(9106):862-6.

d. Dunder T, Kuikka L, Turtinen J, Räsänen L, Uhari M. (2001) Diet, serum fatty acids, and atopic diseases in childhood Allergy Vol 56(5)p 425–428 DOI: 10.1034/j.1398-9995.2001.056005425.x

e. Sausenthaler S, Kompauer I, Borte M, Herbarth O, Schaaf B, von Berg A, Zutavern A, Heinrich J (2006) Margarine and butter consumption, eczema and allergic sensitization in children. The LISA birth cohort study. (2006) Pediatric Allergy and Immunology, Vol 17 (2), p 85–93, DOI: 10.1111/j.1399-3038.2005.00366.x

f. David Gillespie (2013) Want kids with allergies and asthma? Feed them margarine. http://www.raisin-hell.com/2013/09/want-kids-with-allergies-and-asthma.html

Chapter 31
Exercise Benefits and Weight Loss

Get the Facts

➢ Medical advice has not caught up with science when it comes to exercise.

➢ Exercise does not reduce weight long term.

➢ If you are exercising for weight loss, stop it.

➢ It is unclear whether you eat more to compensate for hunger created by exercise, or that exercise makes people hungry.

➢ If you are overweight or obese, change your diet first to lose that weight.

➢ Focus on weight loss as that provides most of the health benefits first. Exercise is easier when you have lost weight.

➢ Exercise for health. It is good for mobility, increasing basal metabolism, reducing risk of depression, promoting better sleep, and helping with some mobility issues.

➢ Exercise may reduce cardiovascular disease and dementia.

➢ Move slowly most of the time

➢ Avoid sitting for more than 30 minutes at a time.

➢ Move fast occasionally.

➢ Continue to move as you get older. When the elderly stop moving about 500m (1/3 mile) a day, they become very frail, and are likely to die within a few months.

Understand the Science

Medical advice has not caught up with the science regarding exercise. Health professionals continue to mislead the public because they do not understand or else they confound the facts of exercise science. Exercise for weight loss is so ineffective it is a waste of time. In a second or two we can easily eat hundreds of calories and it would take hours to burn those calories by exercising. A Starbucks Grande Frap is 450 calories, a fast food chain meal is over 1500. Thirty minutes a day of exercise will not create any weight loss. It should make you feel good, make you healthier, may assist in diseases such as osteoporosis, but it is ineffective for weight loss. Furthermore, because you exercise, you will eat more to compensate for the hunger you feel after exercising. Or you will reward yourself. In just a few minutes, the latte, an "energy" drink, or that "healthy" oat bar at the coffee shop will replace those calories burned with exercise. People who exercise to lose weight also tend to pay less attention to their diet, which makes it even more difficult for them to lose weight. Exercise for weight loss is a serious long-term health risk because of the added load on the body's organs. Thin people need to exercise more than those who are overweight to achieve similar improvements for health.

Back in 1996, a very detailed look at identical twins put them under a 650 calorie deficit – in a controlled environment, and what they discovered is that genetics plays a very large part of our response to exercise.

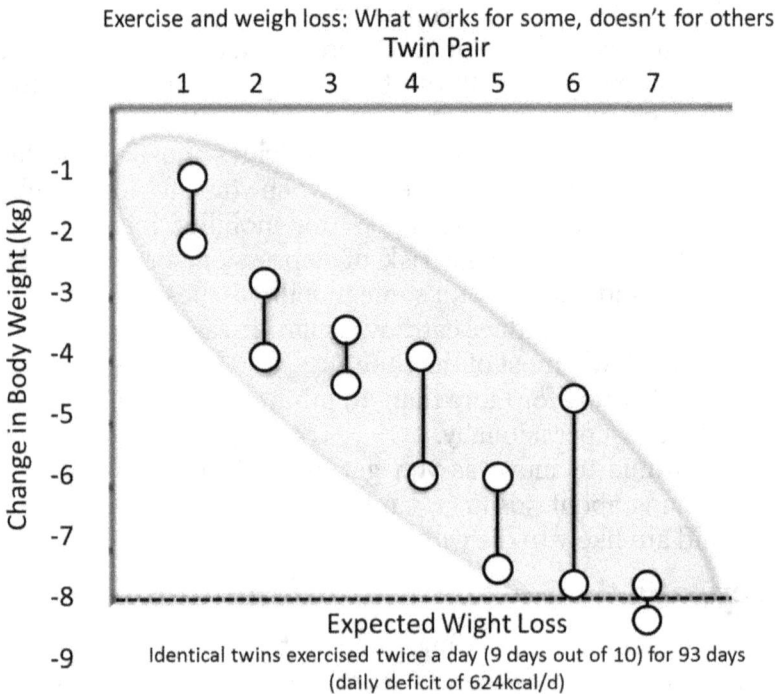

Figure 31 Exercise Sensitivity from Twinning Studies (Bouchard)

Twin studies are excellent because each set of twins (twin pair) have the same genetics and therefore the researchers can focus on the treatments. In this study, the expected weight loss from the exercise regime was 8 kg, but the outcome was surprising. The seven pairs of twins lost between nothing and 8 kg over three months. I.e. weight loss from exercise depends on your DNA. For twin pair 1, they only lost about 1 kg, whereas Twin pair 7 lost the expected 8 kg. While each of the twin pairs lost slightly amount of weight, the biggest difference is from their genes. We know genes are particularly strong for the changes in body mass, body composition, subcutaneous fat distribution and abdominal visceral fat. Bouchard says they don't know the genetic basis for this difference.

Humans are designed to be very efficient walking / running machines and it has been said that the human is the most efficient mammal alive. A cheetah can run faster, a horse can walk further, but, a human can jog for hundreds of kilometers. A 155 lb (70 kg) person uses about 560 calories an hour at 8 kph (5 mph). Depending on speed and the weight of the individual, a marathon runner will burn 2600 to 3400 calories at a 10 kph (6 min per mile) pace. If you walked 7 hours, every day, for a week, you would lose just 1 kg. Even worse, if your genes are like Twin Pair 1, and not Twin Pair 7, you could lose no weight. Some individuals are not "responsive" to exercise. That's distressing news for those who hit the gym, pound the pavement, or encourage others to go to the gym. Yet the medical community continues to push the line. In the USA, exercise is a huge priority, and yet, a large part of the population is overweight and unhealthy.

Exercise is touted as a health fix, but the whole picture isn't always presented. Susan Anderson, National Director of Healthy Weight at the Heart Foundation, says it's careless to suggest that exercise for weight loss is useless. *"It's irresponsible because movement is fundamental to health and therefore necessary for an individual to achieve and maintain an ideal healthy weight......All overweight people, and adults who are starting or re-starting physical activity and exercise regimes, should consult their doctor before beginning an exercise routine and gradually increase the intensity and duration of their activity. There is abundant evidence that adopting a healthy eating pattern and being physically active can control weight."* Perhaps she has some evidence that is not in the literature?

Julie Gilbert, a spokeswoman for the Dietitians Association of Australia, says weight loss comes from a combination of diet and exercise. *"We know that 70 percent of weight loss comes from cutting your portion size down and 30 percent comes from exercise,"* she says. *"Exercise plays the biggest role, not so much in terms of weight loss, but in terms of helping people to maintain their weight."* The Australian National Health and Medical Research Council guidelines for the management of people who are overweight and obese, suggest a modest weight loss with physical activity alone of only 1.8 kilograms over a year doing three to five hours of moderate or vigorous exercise each week. But that exercise is combined with a cut in kilojoule intake; the weight loss can be as high as 7.5 kilograms in just 12 weeks. Which is easier? A take-out of some of the food you consume which takes zero time, or 9-15 hours of exercise? My son said, *"Drop the fork, forget the walk."*

Physical Health Benefits from Exercise

While exercise is not effective for weight loss, it is important with respect to health. Reportedly, physical inactivity accounts for 6% of global deaths. Dana King found that baby boomers born after World War II are less healthy than those born in the previous generation. King's team analysed data from two USA National Health and Nutrition Examination Surveys, focusing on 6000 people who were around the age of 54 between 1988 and 1994, or 2007 and 2010. Key differences were 50% of the baby boomer group didn't exercise at all, compared with 17% of their forebears, and obesity rose from 29% to 39%. "People who grew up in the 30s, 40s and 50s did a lot more running around, and had fewer labour-saving devices, whereas baby boomers grew up in a time of rapid change, with a decline in walking to school and less activity," says King. Hypertension, diabetes, hypercholesterolemia were all higher. It is this type of research that has linked the weight and exercise dogma and results mirror the increase on weight. The question remains: Do people move less now because they are more obese, or are they obese because they move less? It is a correlation; not the primary cause. Society has changed behaviours; lifestyle and work are different. Whereas most jobs used to require physical labour, now, many do not. Today, more jobs require sitting, or standing in one place, for hours per day.

The conclusion from a meta-study by Vissers looked specifically at the effect of exercise on visceral adipose tissue (VAT), without diet changes. He came to the conclusion you could reduce VAT. Moderate to vigorous aerobic exercise does reduce VAT, but weight training was of little value. As with most trials on diets, exercise is similar: people stop exercising and put the VAT back on. An evidence-based view is that exercise is a complete waste of time in the effort to lose weight. Sure, there is good solid science-based evidence that exercise has a range of metabolic benefits and so forget weight loss, but focus on the associated health benefits. The Paleo

Diet / lifestyle strategies are defined as "move slowly most of the time, lift heavy things and move fast occasionally" and as it turns out, that is pretty much the best advice on what we now know to be evidence based.

Recent results from the European EPIC involved researchers assessing exercise levels and waist lines of 334,161 Europeans over 12 years, recording every death. The risk of death was reduced from avoiding inactivity by 7.35 per cent, while having a BMI under the level of obesity only lowered mortality by an estimated 3.66 per cent. This was consistent in normal weight, overweight and obese people. If you look at the results a little closer, you can reduce your risk of mortality by 20% to 30% if you are moderately active, and up to 41% if you are active and lean.

Physiological Benefits of Exercise:

- Walking has been shown to increase the size of the hippocampus, and will delay the onset of dementia by two years.

- Increased muscle mass with its associated increased mitochondrial activity leads to higher basal metabolism.

- Reduced fat in cells.

- Posture improves with better core stability, body shape and less muscular / skeletal problems.

- Cardiovascular fitness increases.

Mental Health Benefits from Exercise

These benefits are listed in Sustrans, a UK charity that works with communities, policy makers, and partner organizations.

- Twenty percent will experience some kind of mental health problem in the course of a year, and 45% will experience a mental health problem at some point in their lives. The UK figures are that each year more than 250,000 people are admitted to psychiatric hospitals.

- Regular physical activity improves mood, helps relieve depression, and increases feelings of well-being.

- Physical activity is effective in the treatment of clinical depression and can be as successful as psychotherapy or medication, particularly in the longer term.

- Physical activity can be used for its therapeutic effects on mental illness, and also for its impact on mental health in the general population.

- Physical activity can help reduce physiological reactions to stress, improve sleep, and reduce anxiety.

- Rhythmic aerobic forms of exercise, including brisk walking and cycling, appear to be most consistently effective.

- Regular physical activity reduces the risk of depression and has positive benefits for mental health, including reduced anxiety, and enhanced mood and self-esteem.

In another study (self-reported survey data of 3500 people in UK), time spent sitting when not at work, such as watching TV, using a computer, driving, was negatively associated with mental health for women. Men got off comparatively easy. Only sitting time at the computer negatively impacted their mental well-being.

Sitting is Another New Tobacco

This is the one piece of bad news about exercise. Sitting for hours on end, every day, is bad for your health. Sitting at work is bad for you. Sitting after work is bad for you. Sitting is the new smoking, except that the furniture lobby probably isn't as powerful as the tobacco lobby!

We love our office chairs, La-Z Boys, couches, and cushions, and it is all bad news. Even a healthy amount of exercise can't save you from the negative effects of too much sitting. If you work in an office setting, sitting is hard to avoid, unless you're an early adopter of the treadmill desk. You might laze around the house on your days off, but McCrady and Levine (in a study of 21 people, aged about 40, BMI around 28) found that people spend more time sitting and do less standing or walking on work days compared to their leisure days. The subjects burned about 527 calories on work days, and 586 on leisure days.

Reduced Life Expectancy

By reducing "excessive sitting" to less than three hours a day, the USA life expectancy could increase by two years, according to a July 2012 study in BMJ Open. Reducing TV time to less than two hours a day would bump it up by 1.4 years. (By comparison, smoking knocks off 2.5 years of life expectancy for men and 1.8 years for women.) The study estimated that the average adult spends 55% of his or her day doing something sedentary, but also notes that even high levels of self-reported sitting could be conservative. It's not easy to remember all the time you've spent sitting during the day, since it's not necessarily a domain-specific behaviour, like watching TV.

Kidney Disease

A self-reported survey of 6,379 people (ages 40 to 75), found that even accounting for physical activity and BMI, those who sat less had lower risk of chronic kidney disease. When women cut down their sitting time from a full workday to only three hours, their risk fell by more than 30%, double that of men at 15% decrease.

Chronic Disease and Metabolic Syndrome

Research consistently shows the more time spent sitting, the more likely you are to have a chronic disease, regardless of body mass index or how much exercise you do. Those who sat at least 6 hours per day were significantly more likely to have diabetes. Obese individuals sit 2.5 more hours a day than lean individuals, according to a 2009 obesity study. In turn, sitting more is associated with Metabolic Syndrome, a combination of factors such as abdominal obesity, low levels of good cholesterol, high blood pressure, high triglyceride levels or hyperglycaemia, which together, put you at a higher risk for serious medical issues like heart disease, stroke, and diabetes. People who spent more time being sedentary were 73% more likely to have metabolic syndrome. In 2005, a group of researchers theorized that reducing TV and computer use to less than 1 hr per day outside of work could reduce the prevalence of adult metabolic syndrome in the USA by 30 to 35%.

Colorectal Cancer

Even if you've been diagnosed with cancer, sitting could still be what kills you. More leisure time spent sitting down meant a higher risk of death. The study tracked the self-reported habits of more than 2000 patients with colorectal cancer, for up to 16 years after their diagnosis. The most physically active had a 28% lower chance of dying than those who exercised less. Those who spent at least six leisure hours a day sitting had a 36% greater risk of dying than those who sat less than three hours a day.

The Sitting Death Trap

An Australian study of 200,000 individuals 45 years and older found that regardless of sex, age, and body mass, sitting puts you at a higher risk for mortality from all causes. People who sat more than 11 hours a day had a 40% higher risk of dying within three years. The risk of death was much lower for people who exercised five hours a week or more, but it didn't negate the sitting death-trap.

Conclusion

So it is pretty clear. There is no value to exercise for weight loss but there huge value for health. You have to move to maintain or improve health, but more importantly, you have to stop sitting. The best recommendation I could work out is to not sit for more than 20 minutes at a time. This is why it becomes one of the Take-Out actions. Take-out sitting down. As part of Change Management, it should be easier than deciding to go to the gym, or going for long walks or some other activity to take up, especially if you are overweight and it is hard to move. If you have a desk job, stand up and walk every 20 minutes.

Most people in the western world do not exercise enough. It is estimated 80% of Americans do not meet the recommended 2.5 hours of exercise per week, and even in sports mad Australia only 1 in 3 play sport or exercise twice a week or more. Are you one of those 60% who don't exercise? Change management principles says this is a big change to make. So instead of doing more exercise, put down this book. Stop sitting for 5 minutes? Do that every 20 to 30 minutes.

References

a. King D, Matheson E, Chirina S, Shankar A, Broman-Fulks J. (2013) The Status of Baby Boomers' Health in the United States: The Healthiest Generation? JAMA Intern Med. 2013; 173(5):385-386. doi: 10.1001/jamainternmed.2013.2006
b. World Health Organization. Global Health Risks: Mortality and Burden of Disease Attributable to Selected Major Risks. Geneva, Switzerland: WHO Press; 2009
c. McCrady S, Levine JA (2102) Sedentariness at Work: How Much Do We Really Sit? Obesity. Vol 17(11) 2103-2105 DOI: 10.1038/oby.2009.117

d. George E, Rosenkranz R, Kol G. (2013) Chronic disease and sitting time in middle-aged Australian males: findings from the 45 and Up Study International Journal of Behavioral Nutrition and Physical Activity 2013, 10:20 doi:10.1186/1479-5868-10-20

e. Katzmarzyk P, Lee IM. (2012) Sedentary behaviour and life expectancy in the USA: a cause-deleted life table analysis. BMJ Open 2(4) doi:10.1136/bmjopen-2012-000828

f. Bharakhada N, Yates T, Davies MJ, Wilmot EG, Edwardson C, Henson J, Webb D, Khunti, K. (2012) Association of sitting time and physical activity with CKD: a cross-sectional study in family practices. Am J Kidney Dis. 2012 Oct;60(4):583-90. doi: 10.1053/j.ajkd.2012.04.024

g. Edwardson CL, Gorely T, Davies MJ, Gray LJ, Khunti K, et al. (2012) Association of Sedentary Behaviour with Metabolic Syndrome: A Meta-Analysis. PLoS ONE 7(4): e34916. doi:10.1371/journal.pone.0034916

h. Campbell P, Patel A, Newton C, Jacobs E, Gapstur S. (2013) Associations of Recreational Physical Activity and Leisure Time Spent Sitting With Colorectal Cancer Survival, J of Clinical Oncology. doi: 10.1200/ JCO.2012.45.9735

i. van der Ploeg H, Chey T, Korda R, Banks E, Bauman A. (2012) Sitting Time and All-Cause Mortality Risk in 222 497 Australian Adults Arch Intern Med. 2012;172(6):494-500. doi:10.1001/archinternmed.2011.2174

j. Shaunacy Ferro (2013) 7 Ways Sitting Will Kill You- Let's count the ways. http://www.popsci.com/science/article/2013-02/many-reasons-chair-killing-you

k. Exercise may not be helping you lose weight. Body and Soul. http://www.bodyandsoul.com.au/weight+loss/diets/exercise+may+not+be+helping+you+lose+weight,6739

l. Michael Mosley (2012) The Truth about Exercise. BBC Horizon documentary. www.bbc.co.uk/news/health-17177251

m. SANE. Facts and figures about mental illnesses. http://www.sane.org/information/factsheets-podcasts/204-facts-and-figures

n. UK Chief Medical Officer. (2004) At least five a week: Evidence on the impact of physical activity and its relationship to health http://webarchive.nationalarchives.gov.uk/20130107105354/http://www.dh.gov.uk/en/Publicationsandstatistics/Publications/PublicationsPolicyAndGuidance/DH_4080994

o. Bouchard C, Tremblay A, Després JP, Thériault G, Nadeau A, Lupien PJ, Moorjani S, Prudhomme D, Fournier G. (1994) The response to exercise with constant energy intake in identical twins. Obes Res. Sep;2(5):400-10 PMID: 16358397.

p. Bouchard C, Tremblay A. (1997) Genetic Influences on the Response of Body Fat and Fat Distribution to Positive and Negative Energy Balances in Human Identical Twins J. Nutr. 127 (5) 943S-947S

q. Volek J. (2013) The Many Facets of Keto-Adaptation: Health Performance and Beyond http://youtu.be/GC1vMBRFiwE.

r. Vissers D, Hens W, Taeymans J, Baeyens JP, Poortmans J, Van Gaal L. (2013) The Effect of Exercise on Visceral Adipose Tissue in Overweight Adults: A Systematic Review and Meta-Analysis. PLoS ONE 8(2): e56415. doi:10.1371/journal.pone.0056415

s. Ekelund U, Ward H, Norat T, Luan J, et al (2015) Physical activity and all-cause mortality across levels of overall and abdominal adiposity in European men and women: the European Prospective Investigation into Cancer and Nutrition Study (EPIC)Am J Clin Nutr March 2015 ajcn.100065

CHAPTER 32
HIGH INTENSITY WORKOUTS

Get the Facts

➤ Optimal vascular function is critical for health, and endurance training (ET) has been shown to be an effective method of improving this.

➤ ET is 3 to 5 hours per week of running or some form of exercise (walking, normal gym, exercise).

➤ The medical benefits of exercise include decreasing arterial stiffness, increasing skeletal muscle capillarization and improving the basic energy processes deep within our cells in the mitochondria.

➤ High Intensity Training (HIT) and sprint interval training (SIT) are both as effective as ET for most medical benefits.

➤ Both training modes improve skeletal muscle microvascular and macro vascular function, with SIT being a time efficient alternative.

Understand the Science

Instead of long stints in the gym and miles of running in the cold, the same results could be achieved in less than a third of the time according to Wagenmakers from Liverpool John Moores University. This was documented in a BBC Horizon Documentary with Dr Michael Mosley.

The current recommendation of the World Health Organization (WHO) and health departments in most countries is that people of all ages should do 3 to 5 hours of endurance training (ET) per week to increase health and fitness and prevent chronic diseases and premature mortality. Most people find it difficult to set aside this much time in their busy lives. If you are a gym junkie or road warrior, it is no big deal, but for the 70% plus people in the world, it is a huge deal. In Australia, 29% play a sport or exercise twice a week or more. Insufficient time due to work or "study" was the most common reason (22%) for not participating. The activities were walking (25%), aerobics (13%), swimming (9%), and cycling (6%).

The USA rates are half that of Australians (16%). They also spend five times more time watching TV than exercising. The UK has 40% of men, and 28% of women, exercising once a week or more.

HIT is 15 to 60 second bursts of high intensity cycling interspersed with 2 to 4 minute intervals of low intensity cycling. HIT can be delivered on simple spinning bikes that are present in commercial gyms and are affordable for use at home or in the workplace. HIT is suitable for any individual. SIT is 4 to 6 repeated 30 second "all out" sprints on special laboratory bikes interspersed with 4 to 5 minutes of very low intensity cycling (30 minutes, three times a week). Due to the very high workload of the sprints, this method is more suited to young and healthy individuals. Both HIT and SIT can make a massive difference to our health and aerobic fitness. Three sessions of SIT, taking just 90 minutes of time per week, are as effective as 5 sessions of traditional ET, taking 5 hours per week, in increasing whole body insulin sensitivity.

There are two independent mechanisms thought causing this increased sensitivity. One mechanism involves improved delivery of insulin and glucose to the skeletal muscle, and the other involves improved burning of the fat stored in skeletal muscle fibers. Additionally, there is reduced stiffness of large arteries, important in reducing the risk of vascular disease. These results are not "one off." Professor Wagenmakers expects that HIT and SIT will turn out to be unique alternative exercise modes suitable to prevent blood vessel disease, hypertension, diabetes, and most of the other ageing and obesity related chronic diseases. Celebrities such as Dame Helen Mirren are advocates.

You can see the obvious value. Based on a pilot study currently ongoing in the Sports Centre at the University of Birmingham the researchers said, "Previously sedentary individuals in the age-range of 25 to 60 also find HIT on spinning bikes much more enjoyable and attractive than endurance training and it has a more positive effect on mood and feelings of well-being. This could imply that HIT is more suitable for achieving sustainable changes in exercise behaviour." HIT, therefore, seems to provide the ideal alternative to outdoor running, dangerous cycling trips, and long, boring endurance cycling sessions in health and fitness gyms. That is why the researchers believe that there will be a great future for HIT for obese and elderly individuals, and potentially also for patients with hypertension, diabetes, and cardiovascular disease.

Conclusion

I personally don't see that it will do much to change the 70% of people who don't exercise. It comes back to change management and personal motivation. I was highly motivated while I was writing this book, and I heard myself say on numerous occasions "I can't be bothered to go to the gym." I've tried SIT. It is not easy. Sure it takes less time than other exercise, but you can't get away from the reality that to be effective, it is still hard work, no matter how it is sold. I cannot see people doing this unless there is some motivating factor to drive changes in behaviour. Those who play some sport generally do so for other reasons than fitness such as social interaction, giving relief to competitive urges or it is just good fun. SIT or HIT may assist gyms in marketing and promoting that you get more for less (more fit, less time). Lastly, neither are HIT or SIT a replacement for weights based exercises which provides improved muscle mass, improvement in bone density, and improvement in cognitive skills.

References

a. Getting Fit Fast: Inactive People Can Achieve Major Health and Fitness Gains in a Fraction of the Time http://www.sciencedaily.com/releases/2013/02/130201090405.htm
b. Cocks M, Shaw CS, Shepherd SO, Fisher J, Ranasinghe A, Barker T, Tipton K, Wagenmakers A. (2013) Sprint interval and endurance training are equally effective in increasing muscle microvascular density and eNOS content in sedentary males. The Journal of Physiology, 591, 641-656 doi: 10.1113/jphysiol.2012.239566
c. Michael Mosley (2012) The Truth about Exercise. BBC Horizon documentary. www.bbc.co.uk/news/health-17177251
d. ABS 4177.0 - Participation in Sports and Physical Recreation, Australia, 2005-06
e. Bureau of labour Statistics. http://www.bls.gov/spotlight/2008/sports/
f. Sustrans. Physical activity and health – facts and figures http://www.sustrans.org.uk/policy-evidence/related-academic-research/physical-activity-and-health-facts-and-figures

CHAPTER 33
MAINTAIN AND LIVE THE HEALTHY LIFESTYLE

Get the Facts

➤ Why are diets so spectacularly unsuccessful?

➤ Is it easier to take weight off, or to maintain a good weight?

➤ Is there a "set point" or natural weight or hormesis.

➤ Some say it is harder to maintain as the body wants to go back to the weight that it was before the diet. Other research says that the set point depends on the behaviour of the individual.

➤ Obesity leads to lifetime changes. If you have been obese, you may need to continue to eat 200 calories less per day because of lower leptin production.

➤ As you age, your energy requirement falls.

Understand the Science

Maintenance of a healthy lifestyle seems to take ongoing effort. Many who are overweight, and lose weight on a diet, seem to return to the same weight. Many revert to an increased weight, but this might be age related (Chapter on obesity by stealth). Why do less than 20% maintain the loss for a year, and only 8% after 7 years? Do people have a "set point?" Or is this increase back to their starting weight, or higher, due to no basic change to lifestyle and making the same food choices that got them overweight in the first place? Is it biochemical or behavioural, or a mix of each? The set point theory is that the body maintains its normal weight and body fat level with internal regulatory controls that dictate how much fat one has. Some individuals have a high setting, meaning they tend to have a naturally higher weight as a set point, and others have a low set point, and therefore a naturally lower body weight. Some refer to the set point theory as an internal "thermostat" that regulates body fat. It's a convenient theory, but even back in 1990 Harris said it was unlikely and was instead due to multiple factors, and that is consistent with the 3-legged stool model in this book.

We know that DNA and genetics that humans vary in size. We use terms and cliches such as "can't fatten a thoroughbred," or call people gazelles or elephants. We know from identical twin studies that genes determine much of our size. Recent endocrinology research suggests that part of the set point may be hormonal. Leibel and Rosenbaum from Columbia Medical Center say that the complex processes including slower metabolism, combined with changes in hunger, contribute to 20% excess calories consumed with overweight people. This 20% accounts for most of any weight gain. People do have different Total Daily Requirements (TDRs), but even after two years of diet change, the TDR remained the same. In other words, the body has a mind of its own. What controls the appetite?

The research was complex, and they compared two similar people (both female, same height). One dieted and lost 20% of her body mass, and the other remained the same. Should the TDR be 20% less for the dieter? While there are some minor metabolic changes, the dieter will need to eat less to remain at the lower weight. In closed system experiments where everything is monitored, the dieter actually continued to eat the same as the non-dieter.

The conclusion, unfortunately, is that appetite signalling does not catch up with the change in body mass. Subjects continued to eat at pre-diet levels and returned to the same weight. When Roseberg provided leptin to the levels it was before they lost weight, he discovered that thyroid normalizes, metabolic changes reverse, and the brain thinks you are back to normal, and your appetite adjusts to the new lower weight. The conclusion from this then that the set point is actually an indication of appetite, and that is determined by hormonal levels.

Losing weight quickly is better than losing it slowly. Nackers reported on groups drawn from participants in the TOURS trial, which included a sample of middle-aged (average 59.3 years) obese women (avg BMI = 36.8) who received a six-month lifestyle intervention, followed by a one-year extended care program. Participants were encouraged to reduce caloric intake to achieve weight losses of 1 lb/week (0.45 kg). Some lost weight faster, some slower. The dropout rate was 48%. Fast losers (11 kg in six months) were 5 times more likely than slow losers (4 kg) to achieve a 10% weight loss at 18 months. So if you need to lose weight, try to lose it quickly.

Very low calorie diets (VLCDs) reached the height of popularity in the USA when Oprah Winfrey announced to her TV audience in 1988 she had lost 67 lb (30 kg). Interest waned somewhat 2 years later after she had regained it all and said she would never diet again! VLCDs are just as effective as LCDs, and the drop-out rate is no better or worse than low calorie diets. Drop-out rate is generally about 20% in trials compared with 80% in the real world. When you look at weight loss trials, remember that these subjects usually are volunteers, they have researchers interested in them, and sometimes have all their food paid for. It is not surprising that the drop-out rate is less than 20%. For the real world, more than 80% will drop-out after 18 months, and as few as 8% will keep that weight off. When you review dieting studies, keep this in mind.

Conclusion

If you are obese and go on a weight loss program, lose weight quickly. You will lose more, and keep more off. The reasons for this are not clear. If there is a "set point" it may be that hormonal changes needed to adjust to the new body mass happen quicker. Alternatively, it may be behavioural where people who lose weight actually change their eating behaviours. Smokers who quit cold turkey are more successful at quitting than those who try to give up slowly. In change management, the principles are to change as fast as possible in order to avoid long transition periods. Any effective weight loss is always described as a "life style change." In the Take-Out Diet, I recommend as fast a weight loss as practical in as short a time as possible to minimize the pain of change, to make people feel really good about themselves, and to reset the hormonal regulation to get used to the new weight. The best diet is one that you continue for longer than 2 years.

References

a. Nackers L, Ross K,Perri M. (2010) The Association Between Rate of Initial Weight Loss and Long-Term Success in Obesity Treatment: Does Slow and Steady Win the Race? Int J Behav Med.   2010   September;   17(3):   161–167 http://www.ncbi.nlm.nih.gov/pmc/articles/PMC3780395/ doi: 10.1007/s12529-010-9092

b. Ryttig KR, Flaten H, Rössner S (1997) Long-term effects of a very low calorie diet (Nutrilett) in obesity treatment. A prospective, randomized, comparison between VLCD and a hypocaloric diet+behavior modification and their combination. Obes   Relat   Metab   Disord.   1997   Jul;21(7):574-9. www.ncbi.nlm.nih.gov/pubmed/9226488

c. The Quest to Understand the Biology of Weight Loss (HBO: The Weight of the Nation) http://www.youtube.com/watch?v=2i_cmltmQ6A

d. Tsai AG, Wadden TA. (2012) The Evolution of Very-Low-Calorie Diets: An Update and Meta-analysis Obesity 14(8) 1283-1293 DOI: 10.1038/oby.2006.146

e. Harris R. (1990) FASEB J. Role of set-point theory in regulation of body weight. 4(15):3310-8 PMID: 2253845.

Chapter 34
80/20 Rule

Get the Facts

➢ The 80/20 rule or the Pareto Principle applies to lifestyle and health as well as business.

➢ Identify one or two changes in your lifestyle that will make the most difference (the 20%).

➢ Adopt a "take-out" approach. Take something out, rather than putting something extra back into your health program.

➢ Stop consuming added sugar. If you smoke tobacco or drink more than recommended, stop these two first.

➢ When you have achieved reduced sugar consumption, look to the next most valuable health change of reducing simple carbohydrate consumption.

Understand the Science

Business-management consultant Joseph Juran suggested the 80/20 principle and named it after the Italian economist Vilfredo Pareto, who observed in 1906, that 80% of the land in Italy was owned by 20% of the population. He developed the principle by observing that 20% of the pea pods in his garden contained 80% of the peas. To Pareto's surprise, other countries also had 80% of the wealth owned by 20%. The Pareto Principle is also known as the 80-20 rule; the law of the vital few; and the principle of factor scarcity. The rule states that, for many events, roughly 80% of the effects come from 20% of the causes.

Mathematically, the 80-20 rule is roughly followed by a power law distribution (also known as a Pareto distribution) for a particular set of parameters, and many natural phenomena have been shown to exhibit such a distribution. As an example, a common rule of thumb in business is that 80% of your sales come from 20% of your clients. In customer relationship management, it seems that if you try to focus on every customer your business is less likely to succeed than if you focus on the top 20% of clients.

Why do airlines have frequent flyer programs? It is to target those 20% of customers who travel frequently with them, and provide 80% of the airline's profits. These frequent flyers are loyal customers with short booking lead times, who are prepared to pay higher cost fares, and who are value and not price driven.

Conclusion

The 80/20 rule appears applicable to health and diet. No-one has looked closely at this so far. In the added sugar debate, many advocates find that they can eliminate one food and get 80% of the benefits. The Standard American Western Diet (SAD) has 15% of calories coming from added sugar. If you eliminate that added sugar, it explains why many people who go on a no-sugar diet get 80% of the weight loss they want.

Many see the whole health and diet subject as having been overly complicated. Obesity is blamed on gluttony and slothfulness, and obese people are told to simply eat less and move more. But it is clear that this approach requires a high level of self-control, discipline, motivation, and long term commitment. Where people have focused on eliminating sugar or go on a simplified diet such as the 5:2 *Eat, Fast, Live Diet*, compliance rates increase. Why? Most likely the 80/20 rule applies. The 5:2 is close to 80/20. You only diet 30% of the time!Focus on the 20% and achieve 80% of the benefit.

Most people do not have absolute self-control. They have some self-control, but not in every aspect of their life. Dieting gets too hard. There are too many temptations. So don't focus on a big change. Focus on a small change that will provide a big result.

References

a. http://en.wikipedia.org/wiki/Pareto_principle

CHAPTER 35
OBESITY AND DISEASE

Get the Facts

➢   People are fat and getting fatter.
➢   Is it true that some people can eat like a horse and stay lean while others get as big as a horse?
➢   Increased obesity in children is bringing a rising tide of health issues.
➢   Metabolic Syndrome, which is the precursor to a range of diseases has increased. Obesity is an indicator and/or cause of Metabolic Syndrome
➢   Some normal-weight people also have metabolic syndrome, so it is not just obesity that is increasing the rates of metabolic syndrome.
➢   We know enough about obesity and its causes to know we must change our diet to prevent even more severe rates of obesity.

Understand the Science

In the chapter on BMI measures, overweight means a BMI of over 25 kg/m^2 and obese is over 30 kg/m^2. The headline reads, "In every region of the world, obesity doubled between 1980 and 2008," says Dr Ties Boerma, Director of the Department of Health Statistics and Information Systems at WHO. "Today, half a billion people (12% of the world's population) are considered obese." By any measure, the obesity rates are alarming. Health budgets, drained by treating obese people, is greater than the national GDP of most nations. The numbers on obesity are staggering.

• There are over 1.0b overweight and 0.5b (560m) obese.

• Global obesity has doubled in 30 years, going from 7.9% of women in 1980 to 13.8% in 2008, and for men from 4.8% to 9.8%.

- As people age, they become more obese, especially after 40 years old.

- Males are more obese than females.

- 65% of people live in countries where you are more likely to die from complications from obesity than from malnutrition.

- Obesity accounts for 1-3% of total health expenditures in most OECD countries.

- Obesity is 5-10% of the health expenditure in USA, and exceed $300b in the USA and Canada.

- Obese people have 25% higher health costs.

- Obese people earn up to 18% less than non-obese.

Here are the numbers from the OECD nations, with Korea or Japan at 3% and the USA at 34% obese. If you take the median, rates were 9% in 1990, 13% in 2000, and 17% in 2009.

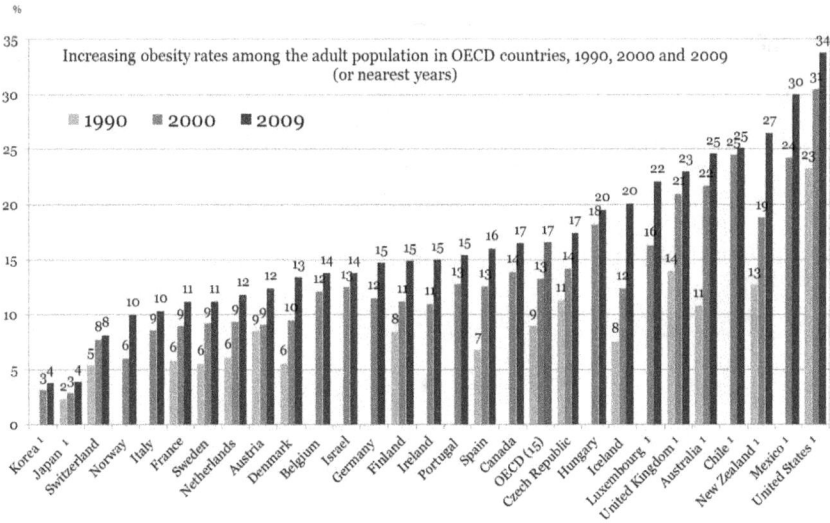

Figure 32 Global Obesity data from OECD

Australia is in the global race to be the fattest nation. (Perhaps the crowds at the football matches should chant "oink, oink oink", rather than "ozzie, ozzie, ozzie, oi, oi, oi."). As in sport they may have to beat New Zealanders who are leading the charge, probably due the higher number of Pacific Island descendants. Mexico was reported in 2013 to be the fattest at 32.8%. Every country has their own figures, and in Australia they are as alarming as anywhere.

- Out of 23 m total population, 14m are overweight or obese, with more than 5m obese.

- More disconcerting is that 25% of children are overweight or obese, with over 0.6m children obese.

- Obesity has doubled in the last 20 years.

- Obesity has overtaken smoking as the leading cause of premature death and illness.

- Aboriginal and Torres Strait Islander people are 1.9 times as likely as non-indigenous Australians to be obese.

- If weight gain continues at current levels, by 2025, close to 80% of all Australian adults and a third of all children will be overweight or obese.

- The estimated health costs is over $35b a year.

- If you get to hospital, direct costs are more than $4b. One is every 6 days spent in hospital is related to overweight and obesity issues among the over 45's.

Rank	Country	% Overweight
1	Naura	94.5%
2	Micronesia	91.1%
3	Cook Islands	90.9%
4	Tonga	90.8%
5	Niue	81.7%
6	Samoa	80.4%
7	Palau	78.4%
8	Kuwait	74.2%
9	USA	74.1%
10	Kiribati	73.6%

A group of Pacific Islands nations holds 8 out of the top 10 of the most overweight citizens. Most nations are still getting more obese. USA leads the way from Mexico, New Zealand but not by much.

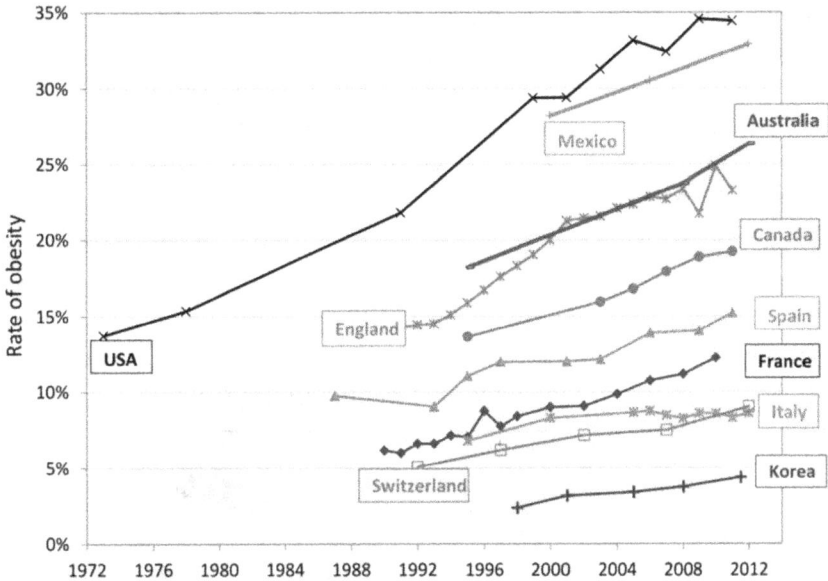

Figure 33 Global Obesity Rates

These OECD figures shows every country has increasing rates of obesity during the past 40 years. In the past three years, the OECD have said the rate has stabilized in a number of countries. However the rate of obese and overweight children continues to rise.

You Are What You Eat

We have already discussed genetics as a factor. You are what you eat, maybe. One of the intriguing notions is that the same diet may be treated differently by different people. Majzoub, of Boston Children's Hospital, deleted a gene called Mrap2 in mice and showed that this helps to control appetite. Surprisingly, however, even when the *mutant mice* ate the same as normal mice, they still gained more weight. Why that is remains unclear, but it may be through Mrap2's effect on another gene, called Mc4r, which is known to be involved in weight gain. Microbiome plays a role as discussed. Understanding this mechanism will be an important break-through in understanding weight gain and weight loss. While the scientists slowly move to better understanding of these processes, there are some very simple steps to halt the obesity epidemic right now. A magic pill will not be enough.

What Is The Linkage to Disease?

Throughout this book, the linkages are not always clear. Some researchers like to use different words to describe the outcomes and it is the health outcomes that I am interested in. Remember that the outcomes are usually risk factors for diseases, not the disease itself. If the risk factor for prostate cancer is 10%, then it means 1 in 10 men will get the cancer. You might be that one, or you might be one of the 9 men who does not get cancer. If you increase your risk by 50%, you now have a 1.5 in 10 chance of cancer, not that 50% of men will get prostate cancer.

One view of obesity is shown below. Which comes first? Obesity or the complication? Is obesity a complication of poor diet? Obesity certainly causes physical stress, and that leads to some of the other outcomes. However, does obesity reduce self-esteem? Or does low self-esteem result in poor diet which results in obesity?

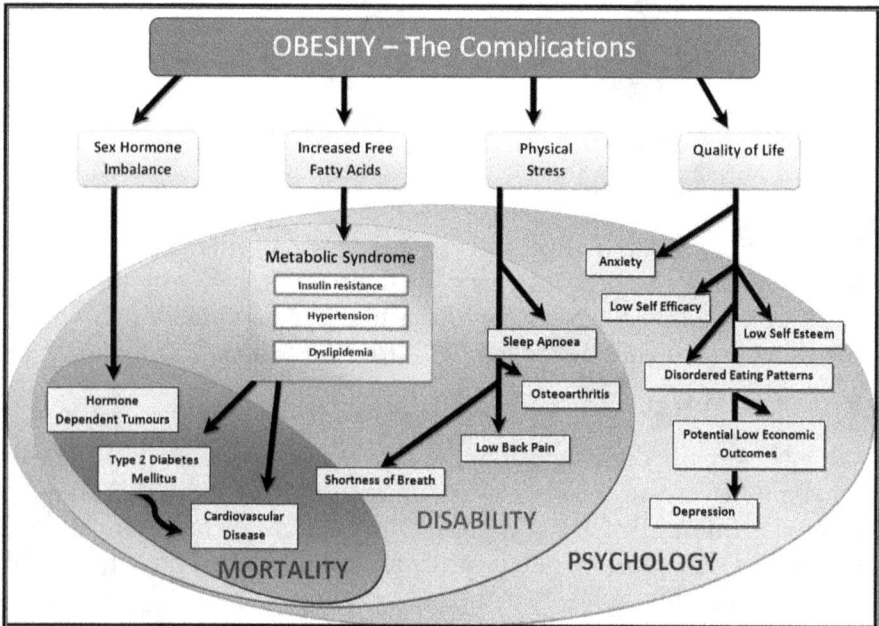

Figure 34 Complications from Obesity

We know that depression causes poor food choices and subsequently obesity, although it is also true that people with obesity may get depression. While this diagram is useful to understand the various issues, we are still left with poor understanding of why people become obese.

The next figure puts this in the context of a person organs. Obesity is also a key component in a range of autoimmune diseases.

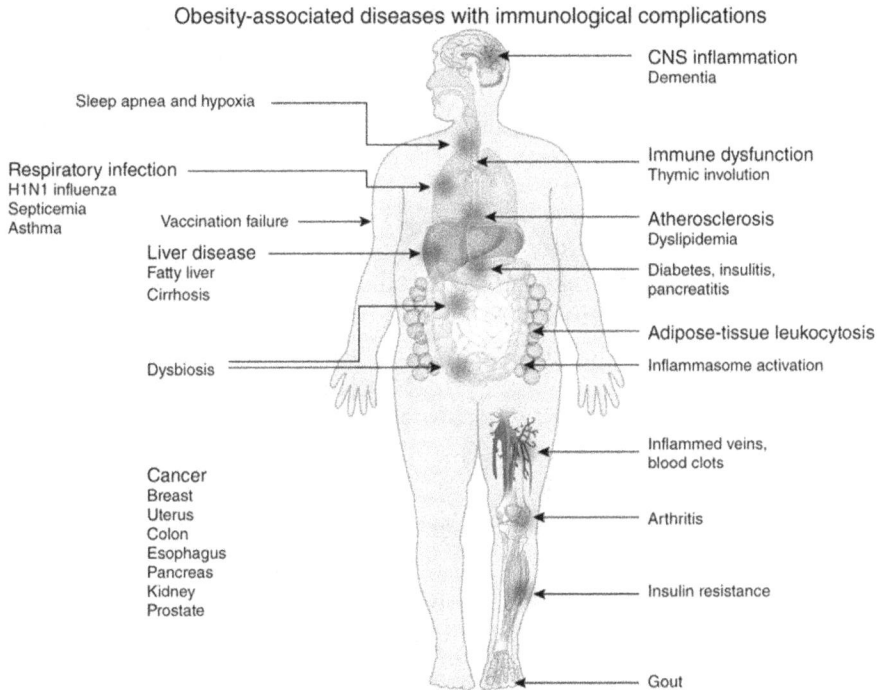

Obesity-associated diseases with immunological complications

- CNS inflammation
  Dementia
- Sleep apnea and hypoxia
- Respiratory infection
  H1N1 influenza
  Septicemia
  Asthma
- Vaccination failure
- Liver disease
  Fatty liver
  Cirrhosis
- Dysbiosis
- Cancer
  Breast
  Uterus
  Colon
  Esophagus
  Pancreas
  Kidney
  Prostate
- Immune dysfunction
  Thymic involution
- Atherosclerosis
  Dyslipidemia
- Diabetes, insulitis,
  pancreatitis
- Adipose-tissue leukocytosis
- Inflammasome activation
- Inflammed veins,
  blood clots
- Arthritis
- Insulin resistance
- Gout

Figure 35 Obesity autoimmune diseases (Kanneganti)

Metabolic syndrome (MetS) leads to a range of other complications.

Metabolic Syndrome (MetS), also referred to as "syndrome X," or "insulin-resistance syndrome" is defined as a grouping of several related risk factors, including abdominal fat, dyslipidaemia, hyperglycaemia, and hypertension. These are risk factors for a large range of diseases including cardiovascular disease, stroke, kidney disease, type 2 diabetes mellitus, fatty liver disease, cholesterol gallstones, gout, depression, or polycystic ovarian syndrome. Mechanical stress is a direct result of obesity.

Obesity and physical inactivity are important contributors to metabolic syndrome, as are genetic and racial composition, aging, and the presence of other endocrine disorders. MetS prevalence has increased over time, reflecting the obesity epidemic and predictions of a greater incidence of diabetes. An analysis of the 2003 to 2006 National Health and Nutrition Examination Survey revealed that, based on a waist circumference threshold of greater than 102 cm for men and 88 cm for women, the age-adjusted prevalence of metabolic syndrome in American adults was 34.3% (36.1% for men; 32.4% for women). This percentage increased to 38.5% for all adults when racial- or ethnic-specific criteria were used (41.9% for men;

35.0% for women). The prevalence increases with age, peaking in the 60 to 69 years group, which parallels a correlation with weight gain with increasing age. One question is why don't all overweight or obese people have MetS? And why do normal, or slightly overweight, also have MetS?

It is worthwhile to look at the paper by St-Onge back in 2004, as the conclusion is that the "normal" body mass index (BMI) recommendations need to be revisited. St-Onge used the data from that same National Health Survey, but instead of looking at the overweight people, they focused on the normal weight people. What was found was that over 20% had MetS in the normal BMI range, and 17% to 22% in the overweight BMI class. Women had greater incidence of MetS; and white Americans more than black. The ATP III criteria for BMI include a waist measurement. People with a BMI in the range of 23 to 25 kg/m^2 (i.e. normal range) have twice the odds ratio for MetS than a 21 to 22 range. If you move up to a 25 to 27 range, your odds ratio is 3 times higher. If you exclude waist measurement, you still look at doubling of risk.

> The message is pretty clear. The "beer belly" has to go.
>
> If you want to be healthy, aim for a BMI of <22 kg/m^2. Don't figure that just being "a little overweight" is ok. Women are less at risk than men.

There is conflicting evidence in other studies. These are correlation studies, not experiments and we know other things are likely to be going on. We will discuss some possible dietary causes for this increased risk of MetS in normal weight people elsewhere.

Only recently has a direct link between obesity and disease been proven. It was always assumed. Cowley and his team from Monash showed obese people generally have elevated blood pressure and elevated blood pressure increases risk of heart diseases. Was this correlation, or causation - a specific pathway? Leptin has always been implicated in this process, but Cowley showed leptin directly affects blood pressure, through both the production of leptin, and the receptors for leptin. Leptin acts through the dorsomedial hypothalamus to increase blood pressure. When the leptin signalling was blocked, it reduced blood pressure in obese mice. Humans with defects in leptin signalling are protected from obesity caused hypertension. This then suggests it is not obesity per se that causes the high blood pressure. The high blood pressure comes from the leptin signalling process, and losing weight improves health.

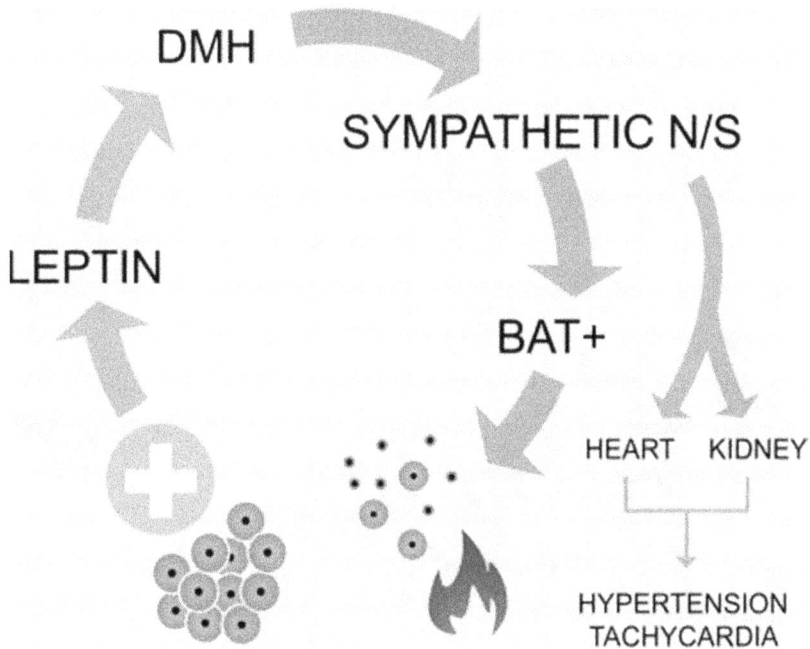

Figure 36 Leptin pathways for hypertension (Cowley)

Childhood Obesity

Children are slowly getting more obese. Children who are overweight or obese, are at greater risk of poor health in adolescence, as well as in adulthood. Among young overweight people there are orthopaedic problems and psychosocial problems such as low self-image, depression and impaired quality of life.

Excess weight problems in childhood are associated with an increased risk of being an obese adult. We know increased MetS gives poorer health outcomes such as more cardiovascular disease, diabetes, certain forms of cancer, osteoarthritis, a reduced quality of life, and premature death.

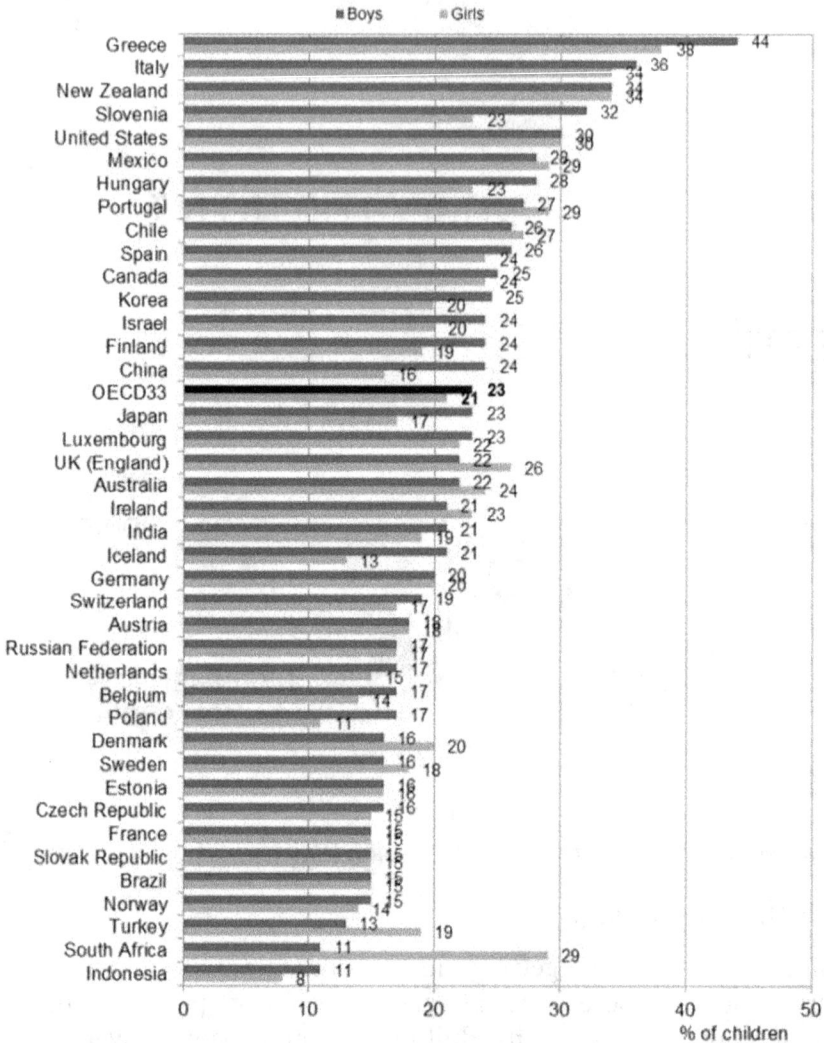

Figure 37 Overweight Children aged 5-17, 2010 (OECD)

Figure 37 looks at measured childhood obesity, with some surprising results. Thirty four percent of Chinese boys are overweight or obese, 22% of Australia children, and 34% of New Zealanders who are higher than USA. Why are Greek children most overweight with 44% of boys overweight or obese?

Measures can vary between studies. Australian data in 2009 showed that 17% of boys, and 14% of girls, aged two to three years were overweight or obese with 4% of them obese. By age 4 to 8 years, 13% of boys and 15% girls were overweight (5% and 6% obese). There have been changes in the last decade, and between 1995 and 2007 overweight two to three year old boys increased by 2.4% while overweight girls decreased by 2.5%. The prevalence of obesity in two to three year old boys increased by 2.0% between 1995 and 2007, and decreased for girls by 2.1%. Obesity generally increased by 2%.

Prevalence of overweight and obesity in Australian Children aged 2-3 years 1995 (left) and 2007 (right)

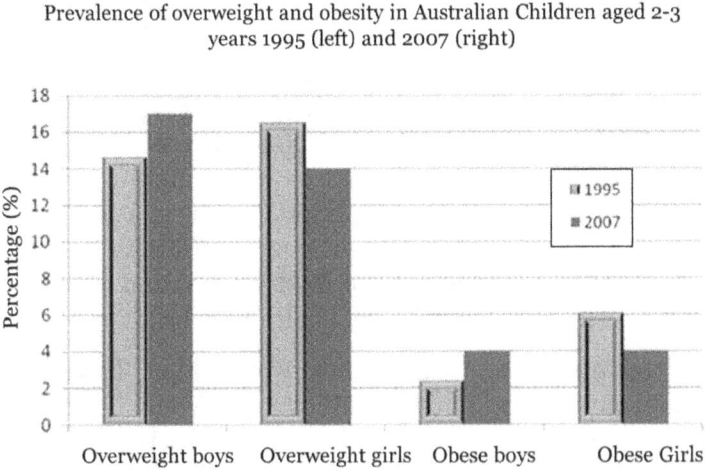

Figure 38 Australian childhood obesity 2-3 year olds

Prevalence of overweight and obesity in Australian Children aged 4-8 years 1995 and 2007

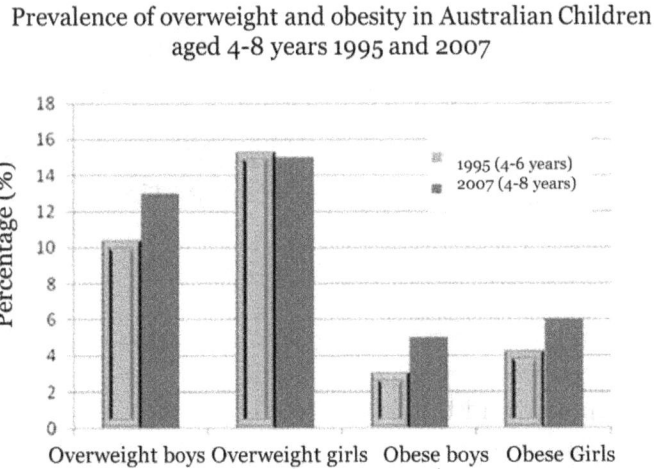

Figure 39 Australian childhood Obesity 4-8 year olds

It appears there may be a slowdown in the rate of obesity increase in the 2 to 3 year olds, but 4 to 8 year olds are still getting bigger. Older children also became more overweight or obese.

Conclusion

The increase in global obesity, or a pandemic as some describe it, is shaping up to be the most costly health issue society has faced. Hospitals are already dealing with complications of heavier equipment, much more complex surgery due to patient obesity, and ever-increasing incidences of MetS and associated chronic diseases.

The puzzle is that if you are obese, you would expect everyone to have a high risk of MetS, but not all do. Furthermore, if you are normal weight, up to 20% may have MetS. So is it obesity that is causing these outcomes? It is clearly not with the normal weight people. Others argue that obesity is simply a marker. It may be that the saccharine disease, as Cleave proposed in the 1960s, is the cause, and obesity a consequence. If you want to be healthy and reduce your risk of illness, you have to target a middle of the range BMI and not be complacent if you are "a little bit overweight". As we see in other chapters, health is also about the food we eat, and is not just weight. Even if obesity is not your issue, health may be.

This research prompted me to lose more weight than I originally targeted, and to get to the middle BMI range. When I started, I thought getting to a BMI of 24 would be good and I would be at a weight of about 78 kg (170 lb). Reviewing this data prompted me to continue to lose weight down to low 70's and a BMI of 22.

References

a. OECD (2011), "OECD 50th Anniversary", in Health at a Glance 2011: OECD Indicators, OECD Publishing. http://dx.doi.org/10.1787/888932523196
b. OECD (2014) More efforts needed to tackle rising obesity, says http://www.oecd.org/els/health-systems/Obesity-Update-2014.pdf
c. Obesity: Mexico Overtakes United States As World's Fattest Country (2013) http://www.huffingtonpost.co.uk/2013/07/10/obesity-mexico-united-states-fattest-country_n_3571988.html
d. OECD (2010) Obesity and the Economics of Prevention: Fit not Fat. www.oecd.org/health/fitnotfat ISBN: 978-92-64084865
e. OECD (2013), Health at a Glance 2013: OECD Indicators, OECD Publishing. http://dx.doi.org/10.1787/health_glance-2013-1-en
f. OECD (2012) Obesity Update. http://www.oecd.org/health/49716427.pdf
g. WHO. New data highlights increases in hypertension, diabetes incidence. (2012) http://www.who.int/mediacentre/news/releases/2012/world_health_statistics_20120516/en/
h. AJMC The Controversial Question of Metabolic Syndrome (2013) http://www.ajmc.com/publications/evidence-based-

diabetes-management/2013/2013-1-vol19-sp2/the-controversial-question-of-metabolic-syndrome

i. St-Onge M. Janssen I, Heymsfield S. (2004) Metabolic Syndrome in Normal-Weight Americans. New definition of the metabolically obese, normal-weight individual Diabetes Care September 27 (9) 2222-2228 doi: 10.2337/diacare.27.9.2222

j. Australian Government Departments of Health and Ageing, Agriculture, Fisheries and Forestry, and the Australian Food and Grocery Council, "Children's Nutrition and Physical Activity Survey: Main Findings", prepared by the Commonwealth Scientific Industrial Research Organisation (CSIRO) Preventive Health National Research Flagship, and the University of South Australia, Canberra, 2007, viewed 21 April 2009, http://www.health.gov.au/internet/main/publishing.nsf/Content/health-pubhlth-strateg-food-monitoring.htm#07survey.

k. Matarese G, Procaccini C, De Rosa V. (2012). At the crossroad of T cells, adipose tissue, and diabetes. Immunological reviews, 249(1), 116–34. doi:10.1111/j.1600-065X.2012.01154.x

l. Simonds S, Pryor J, Ravussin E, Greenway F, Dileone R, Allen A, Bassi J, Elmquist J, Keogh J, Henning E, Myers M, Licinio J, Brown R, Enriori P, O'Rahilly S, Sternson S, Grove K, Spanswick D, Farooqiemail I, Cowley M. (2014) Leptin Mediates the Increase in Blood Pressure Associated with Obesity DOI: J Cell. http://dx.doi.org/10.1016/j.cell.2014.10.058

m. Kanneganti T, Dixit V. (2012) Immunological complications of obesity. Nature Immunology 13, 707–712 doi:10.1038/ni.2343

n. Cole TJ, Lobstein T. (2012), Extended international (IOTF) body mass index cut-offs for thinness, overweight and obesity. Pediatric obesity 7(4) p 284-94 2010; PMID: 22715120

o. OECD/European Union (2014), Health at a Glance: Europe 2014, OECD Publishing. DOI: 10.1787/health_glance_eur-2014-en

p. Korda R. (2014) Obesity is sending over-45s to hospital http://www.abc.net.au/worldtoday/content/2014/s4118877.htm

q. Joshy G, Korda R, Attia J, Liu B, Bauman A, Banks E. (2014) Body mass index and incident hospitalisation for cardiovascular disease in 158 546 participants from the 45 and Up Study. International Journal of Obesity 38(6):848-56. doi: 10.1038/ijo.2013.192

CHAPTER 36
THE CURSE OF SUGAR SWEETENED BEVERAGES

Get the Facts

➤ Sugar consumption in sugar sweetened beverages (SSBs) is driving Metabolic Syndrome (MetS).

➤ Increased MetS risks increases diseases such as cardiovascular disease and cancer. The high dietary glycaemic load (GL) leads to inflammation, insulin resistance, and impaired ß-cell function and death.

➤ Why is there little political will to control sugar sweetened beverages? The conclusions from over 13 meta-studies globally say SSBs lead to MetS and the diseases associated with MetS.

➤ Drink no more than one sugary beverage per month. No ifs, no buts, no maybes. The bad news: fruit juices are as bad if not worse.

➤ When you can, take-out diet drinks as well. Think of diet drinks like nicotine patches.

Understand the Science

Recently, a comprehensive meta-review was published by Vasanti Malik and authors, from the Harvard School of Public Health. This builds on their previous work on sugar sweetened beverages (SSB). SSBs are always part of large-scale obesity prevention efforts, by many countries across the globe although SSB manufacturers try to downplay the association between obesity and SSBs. Malik's conclusions about SSBs are:

• SSB intake increase tracks with rising rate of obesity. The more sugar consumed, the fatter you are.

• The SSB effect is under-reported. They say the studies adopt cautious conclusions.

• SSBs are the greatest contributor to added sugar intake in the USA.

- Their intake is a significant contributor to weight-gain.

- They have little nutritional value.

- Weight gain is primarily due to incomplete compensation for the calories in the SSB liquids at subsequent meals.

- They increase type 2 diabetes and cardiovascular risk independent of obesity.

- They are a contributor to a high dietary glycaemic loading.

- The increased fructose metabolism leads to inflammation, insulin resistance, impaired beta-cell function, and high blood pressure, as well as accumulation of visceral adiposity/ectopic fat, and increased blood concentrations of LDL cholesterol (bad cholesterol).

Intake of SSBs should be limited and replaced by healthy alternatives such as water or tea (herbal or regular) with no sugar. Why did the American Heart Association release a scientific statement recommending reductions in added sugar to 100-150 Calories per day or 35 g sugar? A can of Coca Cola is 142 Cal. Epidemiological studies show a can of soda (SSB) adds 0.5 kg to your weight every year. Consuming SSBs means you eat more at the next meal. SSB calories consumed are worse than empty calories because they have calories and then you eat more!

Why was the statement released? Because the Heart Foundation still believe in "moderation?" I would say there is overwhelming evidence to minimize consumption of SSBs. There is overwhelming evidence that people do not practice moderation. Diets fail.

There are occasional studies, such as one from Australia that says obesity does not track sugar consumption and there is no link. There are questions about the data and the analytical method, but the overriding reasons for trying to dis-associate obesity from SSBs and say it is only a matter of moderation is the influence of the sugar producers and manufacturers. I discuss this more about this in the politics of fat wars and globalization of food chapters.

SSB Global Pattern

The history of SSBs traces back to the 1760s when carbonated processes were developed to mimic naturally carbonated mineral waters. In the late 1860s, J. S. Pemberton, an Atlanta pharmacist, combined kola, a caffeinated nut from Africa, with cocoa, a stimulant from South America, to create Coca-Cola. He marketed it as a tonic. In 1904, Asa Candler purchased the rights, and he started the first mass production factory. During World War II, Coca-Cola supplied USA Army GIs with free Coke, and worked with the army post war to create Coke manufacturing plants in European countries with the support of the government. Coke is synonymous with SSBs, and the SSB market has expanded to include fruit drinks, energy and vitamin waters, sports drinks, and "health" drinks. Consumption of SSBs rose three fold in 30 years; 3.9% of calories in the late 1970s to 9.2% in 2001. Per capita, consumption has increased in most countries around the world.

Interestingly look at how consumer beverage consumption has changed, firstly from 1965 to 1990, and then from 1990 to 2012.

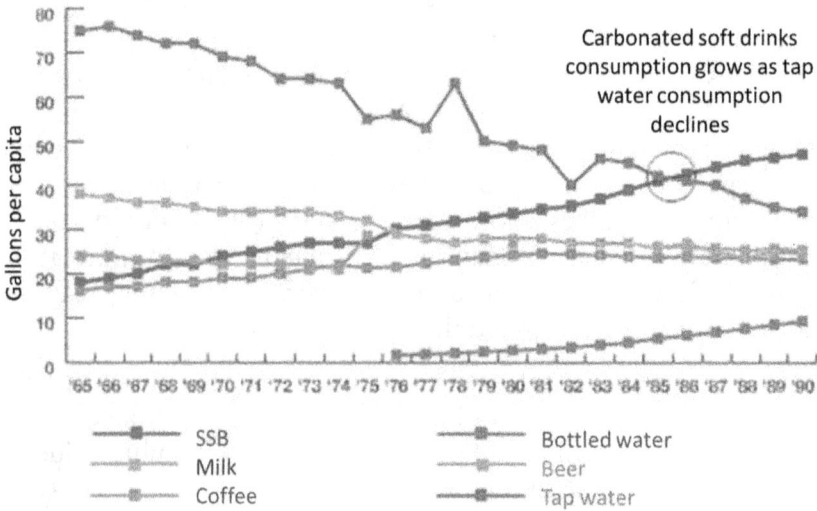

Source: John C Maxwell Beverage Industry 1992

Figure 40 USA Consumption of Beverages 1965-1990

These figures do not include the fruit juices and "healthy" drinks which have increased as SSBs have levelled off or declined. Bottled water has become the growth product for the major beverage corporations. Just how much of this "bottled water" contains sugar is not stated.

USA Consumption 1991-2012

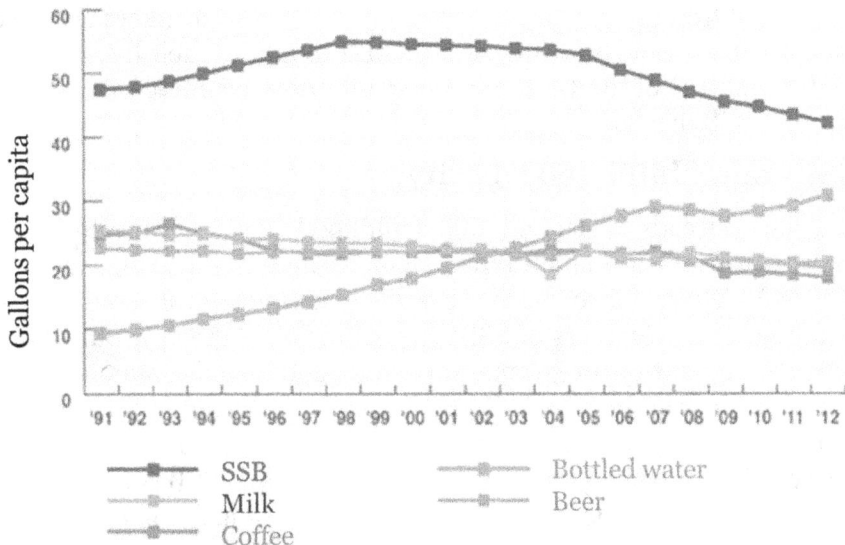

Source: Beverage Marketing Corporation 2012

Figure 41 Consumption of Beverages since 1990 (from Nestle)

What is particularly distressing from a health perspective is the increase in consumption of SSBs by children. The graph below shows consumption within age groups – Mexico on the left, USA on the right.

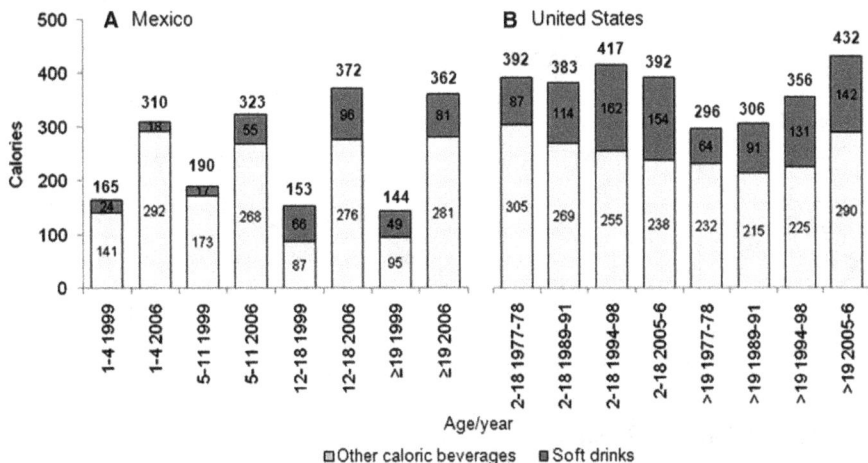

Figure 42 Beverage Consumption in Mexico and USA (Malik)

Children aged 1 to 4 years old had 165 Calories per day in 1999 from drinks, doubling within seven years. Billions of dollars are spent to entice children to drink a particular brand, as SSB drinkers are very loyal to their brand and stay with them throughout their lives. In the mature market of the USA, adult consumption has increased mostly in other SSB drinks.

SSBs and Childhood Obesity

We have already discussed that childhood obesity leads to adult obesity, with the attendant type 2 diabetes and CVD (cardio vascular disease). There have been several epidemiological studies on children. The promoters of SSBs say education is the key. But where school intervention programs have been conducted, data show the benefits are only short term. Intervention (e.g. cut out SSBs from the school canteen) works to decrease the number of overweight and obese children. When followed up after two years, SSB consumption was back to the previous level, and so was overweight and obesity.

SSB Consumption and Weight Gain in Adults

Johnson in 2007 plotted sugar consumption against obesity prevalence from data from 1700 to 2000. Remember this is simply correlation.

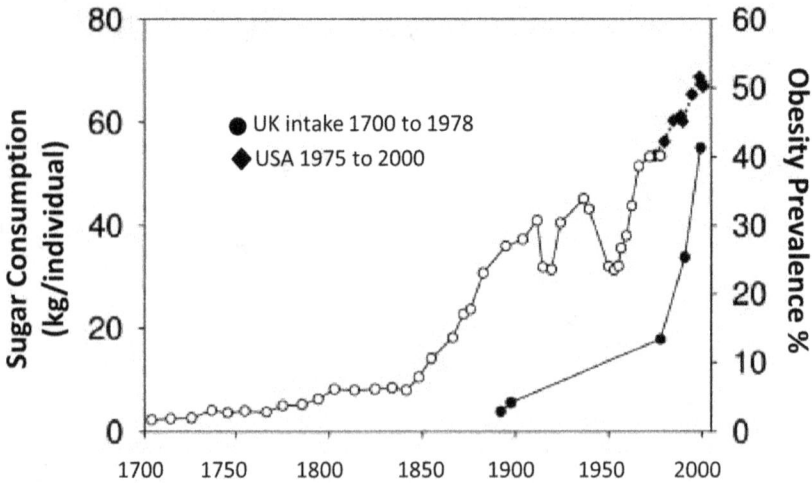

Figure 43 UK and USA sugar vs obesity (Johnson)

Inconsistencies in trial design, methodologies, and data quality have made it difficult to observe consistent effects, so you need to treat most studies with caution. The most reliable are large studies that have a long duration.

One of the results from the Nurses Cohort Studies (over 20 years tracking 120,000 nurses) by Schultz, showed women who increased their SSB consumption from 1991 to 1995, and maintained a high level of intake, gained on average 8.0 kg over the two periods, while women who decreased SSB intake between 1991 and 1995, and maintained a low level of intake, gained on average 2.8 kg over the two periods. The graph below shows those 4 different groups. The 2 kg difference between the two groups in 1991 may be because the more overweight people were trying to diet and were drinking less SSBs. The high group were those who drank 1 can per day; the low group less than 1 can per week.

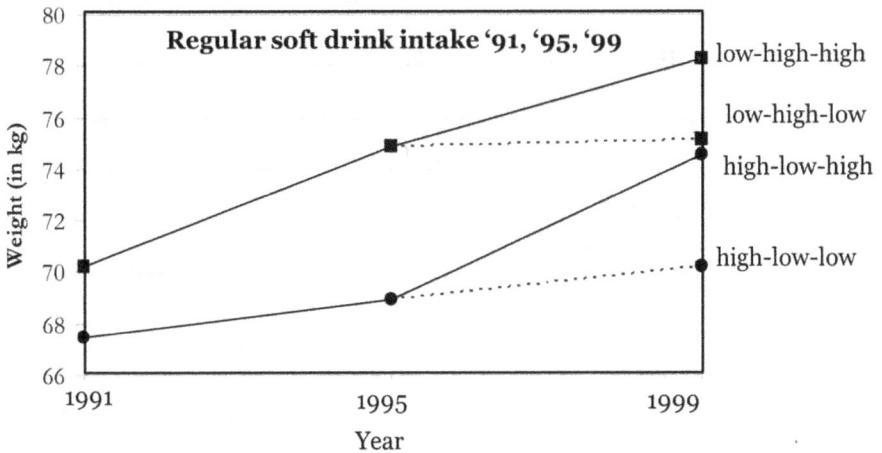

Figure 44 Consumption of SSBs and weight gain

The European EPIC Studies show one can of SSB a day increases weight by 0.5 kg every four years. In the Framingham Offspring Study with an average duration of four years and over 4000 participants, showed those who consumed less than one soft drink per day still had a 37% higher risk of obesity than those who drank infrequently. Since this analysis included both diet and regular soft drinks, it is difficult to disentangle the independent effect of SSBs, as consumers of diet soft drinks may be weight-conscious or trying to lose weight. Hu concluded in 2013 that:

- Prevention of long-term weight gain through dietary changes such as limiting consumption of SSBs is more important than short-term weight loss in reducing the prevalence of obesity in the population. Once an individual becomes obese, it is difficult to lose weight and keep it off.

- We should consider the totality of evidence rather than selective pieces of evidence (e.g. from short-term RCTs only).

231

- We should act now. While recognizing that the evidence of harm on health against SSBs is strong, we should avoid the trap of waiting for absolute proof before allowing public health action to be taken.

Not surprisingly the giant global SSB manufacturers strongly disagree.

Recent meta-studies show that intake of free sugars or SSBs is a determinant of body weight, and Mann from Otago University in New Zealand showed it was the sugar in itself. If people swapped the free sugar with other carbohydrates, they did not have the weight increase.

The pathways from SSBs to disease is shown below. The caramel colouring is important as the advanced glycation end products are implicated in type 2 diabetes. Most research has focused on the high fructose and calorie loading component from SSB consumption, and the inflammatory markers that result from that.

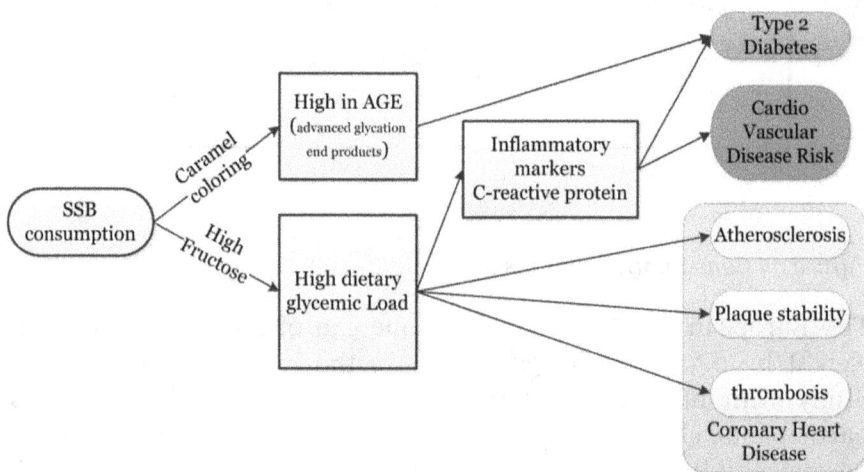

Figure 45 Mechanism of SSB Weight Gain

The mechanism for increased weight is thought to be that sugars in liquid beverages may not suppress further eating. I.e. There is no feedback loop for further eating. Many studies show greater energy intake and weight gain following isocaloric consumption of beverages, as opposed to solid food. The pathway for this feedback is being studied. It is not clear what exactly causes the excess weight, whereas the reasons for some of the other intermediate outcomes are known. Obesity is more of a marker than MetS. SSBs cause a rapid rise in blood glucose and insulin concentrations, which together with the large quantities contribute to a high dietary glycaemic load (GL). High GL diets are thought to stimulate appetite and promote weight gain.

Fructose compared with glucose is preferentially deposited as visceral and ectopic fat, and is worse for lipid metabolism, *de novo* lipogenesis, blood pressure, and insulin sensitivity. Glucose helps adsorption of fructose in the gut. In most SSBs, high fructose corn syrup (HFCS) is the preferred sweetener over sucrose due to lower costs. This mix of glucose and fructose (and not sucrose) might accelerate the problem. Appetite is increased not decreased when you consume fructose. Fructose depresses leptin. With leptin intolerance satiety is further reduced. Therefore appetite is increased.

Even in the 1950's, fructose was demonstrated to induce insulin resistance in rats. We know fructose causes oxidative stress and all the features of Metabolic Syndrome. Most recent studies show confirm this activity. Johnson and colleagues administered a diet of water and glucose to 3 groups of mice. One group acted as a control, and two others lacked enzymes that help the body process fructose. The normal or control mice got sick, and developed a fatty liver and became resistant to insulin. The other groups which could not process the fructose were protected. The body's conversion of glucose to fructose, therefore, seems to help spur metabolic woes. Glucose is isomerized to fructose in the glycolysis cycle in the cytosol of cells. It is just one of the series of steps in the overall decomposition of glucose.

Both Vasanti Malik and Frank Hu, both lead researchers in this area conclude:

Although more research is needed, the weight of the evidence based on previous systematic reviews and meta-analyses of prospective studies shows clear and consistent associations between SSBs and obesity and related cardio-metabolic diseases. This evidence is also supported by findings from mechanistic and experimental studies.
.....Despite attempts from the beverage industry to obfuscate the issue by funding biased analyses and reviews, and by providing misleading information to consumers, many regulatory strategies to reduce intake of SSBs are already in place.

What are SSB Alternatives?

- Water.

233

- Milk, of which one serving provides 85 Calories – half that of an SSB. The fat in the milk reduces appetite and provides protein, calcium, magnesium, zinc, vitamin A, and vitamin D and decreases risk for osteoporosis and bone fractures.

- Diet soda, which has no calories, but the intense, attractive, sweet flavour may stimulate appetite. Diet soda may cause the drinker as an excuse to eat more. Diet SSB drinkers may be diabetic and affect results from the epidemiological studies. Furthermore, coloured soda increases AGE, and that is implicated in type 2 diabetes.

- Tea and coffee.

- Fruit juice, but fruit juice can have more fructose than SSBs. It's best not to drink fruit juice. Eat whole fruit instead. In some countries, processed fruit juice nutritional values are not required to be listed on the food label, and consumers do not realize the high calorie and sugar content of the juice.

Dental Health and Sugars

The focus on SSBs has been on obesity and health, but dental health and caries is also much affected by the consumption of sugar (average of 50 g per person per day globally). There is convincing evidence, collectively from human intervention studies, epidemiological studies, animal studies and experimental studies, for an association between the amount and frequency of free sugars intake and dental caries. Although other fermentable carbohydrates may not be totally blameless, epidemiological studies show that consumption of starchy staple foods and fresh fruit are associated with low levels of dental caries. The introduction of fluoride reduces caries risk but has not eliminated dental caries and many countries do not have adequate exposure to fluoride.

Evidence shows that when free sugars consumption is <15-20 kg/yr (approximately 6-10% energy intake), dental caries is low. As consumption rises past the 10% of daily calories from sugar, so do cavies rates. In addition, the frequency of consumption of foods containing free sugars should be limited to a maximum of 4 times per day.

Conclusion

Sugar sweetened beverages and fruit juices are equally implicated in obesity. As much as possible reduce or eliminate both SSBs and fruit juices. As discussed in the obesity section, hot countries, where alcohol is not consumed, have much higher population rates of diabetics and metabolic syndrome sufferers, and it is almost certainly due to their drinking more SSBs and fruit juices. In my view, SSBs and fruit juices should be labelled with a health warning every bit as severe as trans-fats or tobacco warnings, and taxed as much.

Furthermore, because fructose is part of "added sugar" in foods, elimination or reduction of fructose to less than 12g per day means changing what you eat by eating less food *products* and more whole foods. Regrettably, you have to learn to read food labels due to the ubiquitous use of sweeteners by food companies. Avoid anything that is more than 3% sugar (3 g per 100 g); no more than 2 pieces of fruit per day, no product with "Lite" in its name, no product with a Heart Foundation check mark (as they currently do not account for sugar levels) and many food products that say "healthy."

There are more reasons to remove SSBs from your diet when we look specifically at diabetes and SSBS in a later chapter. There are both health and weight advantages of removing fructose from your diet. Replace fructose with more of your favourite foods without fructose or simple carbohydrates.

The WHO and the USDA are both trying to put lower sugar consumption official recommendations. The WHO has recommended, since 2002, that sugar should be less than 10% of total energy per day, and is now going for a recommendation to reduce to 5% per day. That 5% is still 25 g of sugar or 6 teaspoons per day. The Dietary Guidelines Advisory Committee in the USA is proposing guidelines for 10% of daily calories, or 12 teaspoons. Americans currently consume 22 to 30 teaspoons per day. It's a change that food and sugar industries are aggressively fighting.

Removal of fructose is not a trivial task. Many experience what appear to be additive withdrawal symptoms; food choices become harder when you socialize. One of the tactics you need to do when you remove fructose from your diet is to add in food products you like and do not cause health issues. Add back into your diet your favourite foods whether they are avocado, steak, prawns, fish, vegetables, etc. Best of all, the big winners for your efforts will be your heart, liver, kidneys, stomach, brain, and pancreas!

References

a. Malik V, Popkin B, Bray G, Despres J, Hu F. (2010) Sugar Sweetened Beverages, Obesity, Type 2 Diabetes and Cardiovascular Disease risk. Circulation. 23; 121(11): 1356–1364. doi: 10.1161/CIRCULATIONAHA.109.876185

b. Schulze MB, Manson JE, Ludwig DS, Colditz GA, Stampfer MJ, Willett WC, Hu FB. (2004) Sugar-sweetened beverages, weight gain, and incidence of type 2 diabetes in young and middle-aged women. JAMA 292 (8) p. 927-34

c. Hu FB, Malik VS. (2010) Sugar-sweetened beverages and risk of obesity and type 2 diabetes: epidemiologic evidence. Physiol Behav. 26;100(1):47-54. doi: 10.1016/j.physbeh.2010.01.036JAMA. 2004 Aug 25;292(8):927-34.

d. Malik VS, Willett WC, Hu FB. (2009). Sugar-sweetened beverages and BMI in children and adolescents: reanalyses of a meta-analysis. Am J Clin Nutr 2009;89:438–439

e. Hu FB. (2013) Resolved: there is sufficient scientific evidence that decreasing sugar-sweetened beverage consumption will reduce the prevalence of obesity and obesity-related diseases. Obes Rev. 14(8):606-19. doi: 10.1111/obr.12040.

f. Dhingra R, Sullivan L, Jacques PF, Wang TJ, Fox CS, Meigs JB, D'Agostino RB, Gaziano JM, Vasan RS. (2007) Soft drink consumption and risk of developing cardiometabolic risk factors and the metabolic syndrome in middle-aged adults in the community. Circulation 2007;116:480–488

g. DiMeglio DP, Mattes RD. (2000) Liquid versus solid carbohydrate: effects on food intake and body weight. Int J Obes Relat Metab Disord 24:794–800

h. Ludwig DS. The glycaemic index: physiological mechanisms relating to obesity, diabetes, and cardiovascular disease. Jama 2002;287:2414–2423

i. Stanhope KL, Schwarz JM, Keim NL, Griffen SC, Bremer AA, Graham JL, Hatcher B, Cox CL, Dyachenko A, Zhang W, McGahan JP, Seibert A, Krauss RM, Chiu S, Schaefer EJ, Ai M, Otokozawa S, Nakajima K, Nakano T, Beysen C, Hellerstein MK, Berglund L, Havel PJ. (2009) Consuming fructose-sweetened, not glucose-sweetened, beverages increases visceral adiposity and lipids and decreases insulin sensitivity in overweight/obese humans. J Clin Invest 119:1322--1334

j. Black RM, Leiter LA, Anderson GH. (1993) Consuming aspartame with and without taste: differential effects on appetite and food intake of young adult males. Physiol Behav 1993;53:459–466.

k. Almiron-Roig E, Drewnowski A. (2003) Hunger, thirst, and energy intakes following consumption of caloric beverages. Physiol Behav 2003;79:767–773

l. Lanaspa M, Ishimoto T, Li N, Cicerchi C, Orlicky D, Ruzicky P, Rivard C, Inaba S, Roncal-Jimenez C, Bales E, Diggle C, Asipu A, Petrash M, Kosugi T, Maruyama S, Sanchez-Lozada L, McManaman J, Bonthron D, Sautin Y, Johnson R. (2013) Endogenous fructose production and metabolism in the liver contributes to the development of metabolic syndrome. Nature Communications 4, Article number: 2434 doi:10.1038/ncomms3434

m. Ebbeling CB, Leidig MM, Feldman HA, Lovesky MM, Ludwig DS. (2007) Effects of a low-glycaemic load versus low-fat diet in obese young adults: a randomized trial. JAMA 297, 2092–2102

n. Maxwell J. (1992) Beverage Industry Feb 1992, cited by Nestle http://www.nestle-watersna.com/en/about-nestle-waters/industry-overview/beverage-consumption-sales

o. Johnson R, Segal M, Sautin Y, Nakagawa T, Feig D, Kang D, Gersch M,Benner S, Sánchez-Lozada L. (2007) Potential role of sugar (fructose) in the epidemic of hypertension, obesity and the metabolic syndrome, diabetes, kidney disease, and cardiovascular disease. J Clin Nutr 86 (4) 899-906

p. Johnson, RJ, Nakagawa T, Sanchez-Lozada G, Shafiu M, Sundaram S, Le M, Ishimoto T, Sautin Y, Lanaspa M. (2013) Sugar, Uric Acid, and the Etiology of Diabetes and Obesity. Diabetes. 62(10): 3307–3315. doi: 10.2337/db12-1814

q. Morenga L, Mallard S Mann J. (2013) Dietary sugars and body weight: systematic review and meta-analyses of randomised controlled trials and cohort studies. BMJ 2013; 346 doi: http://dx.doi.org/10.1136/bmj.e7492

r. Moynihan P, Petersen P, (2004) Diet, nutrition and the prevention of dental diseases. Public Health Nutr. 7(1A):201-26. PMID: 14972061

s. Touger-Decker R, van Loveren C. (2003) Sugars and dental caries. Am J Clin Nutr. 2003 Oct;78(4):881S-892S. PMID: 14522753

t. Moynihan PJ, Kelly SAM (2013) Effect on Caries of Restricting Sugars Intake. Systematic Review to Inform WHO Guidelines Journal Dental Research. http://jdr.sagepub.com/content/93/1/8

CHAPTER 37
EDUCATION MAKES NO DIFFERENCE

Get the Facts

➢ Education about becoming overweight and obese does not stop weight gain and obesity.

➢ Parents who are informed about weight gain do not make those changes with their young children.

➢ There are many factors regarding obesity that education does not address.

Understand the Science

Do obese children become obese adults? The short answer is probably, but not always. There is some disagreement among researchers. Many studies published in the last decade demonstrate a link between obesity in childhood and obesity in adulthood, however there is little consensus on the age at which childhood weight becomes an accurate predictor of adult weight status. One of the earliest studies tracking weight status over time found that in children under three years of age, the parents' weight was the best predictor of adult obesity, not the child's.

In children over three years old, the child's and parents' weight were equally important predictors of adult obesity. As the child aged, his or her weight status became the best predictor. Based on these results, the authors cautioned against treating overweight children younger than three years of age. Unless one or both parents are obese, overweight young children are unlikely to become obese.

Viner argued that there was no strong relationship, and obesity limited to childhood has little impact on adult outcomes, but did find persistent obesity in women to be associated with poorer employment and relationship outcomes. In another UK review, Baird et al came to the conclusion that children had an increased risk of becoming obese adults if between the ages of three months and two years they had rapid weight gain, were at the higher end of the distribution for BMI, or were classified as obese. Unlike other researchers, they argued that obesity prevention should begin during, or even before, infancy.

Does education work for adults? The short answer would have to be no. If you are educated you are less likely to be obese – but does education make any difference? Back in 1998, the best that the American National Heart and Lung Institute could come up with was:

> *"When assessing the patient's motivation to enter weight loss therapy, the following factors should be evaluated: reasons and motivation for weight reduction; previous history of successful and unsuccessful weight loss attempts; family, friends, and work-site support; the patient's understanding of the causes of obesity and how obesity contributes to several diseases; attitude toward physical activity; capacity to engage in physical activity; time availability for weight loss intervention; and financial considerations. In addition to considering these issues, the health care practitioner needs to heighten a patient's motivation for weight loss and prepare the patient for treatment. This can be done by enumerating the dangers accompanying persistent obesity and by describing the strategy for clinically assisted weight reduction."*

Conclusion

Previously we mentioned the Canadian longitudinal study of over 5000 patients, 50 years or older, and which followed those people after they received an initial diagnosis of chronic illness (heart disease, cancer, stroke, respiratory disease, and diabetes). The results showed that even after being diagnosed, and after being counselled by a health care professional on lifestyle modifications, most people did not make major lifestyle adjustments. You would think anyone with these conditions would change – but not so. So it is most unlikely that obesity will fare any better – even though the illnesses that follow metabolic syndrome are the very same as above. It is even more unlikely that someone of normal weight will change lifestyle, even if shown they may have some of the Metabolic Syndrome symptoms.

It is back to the three reasons why people *will* change: a gain, a loss, or legislation. In society today, without any of these drivers for change, change is unlikely. It is even more unlikely for those who are normal weight, but have metabolic syndrome: first, they are probably unaware, and second, there may be few associated immediate health concerns.

References

a. Boxall, A. (2009) Obesity prevention in young children: what does the evidence say? http://www.aph.gov.au/About_Parliament/Parliamentary_Dep artments/Parliamentary_Library/pubs/BN/0809/ObesityChildr en

b. Baird J, Fisher D, Lucas P, Kleijnen J, Roberts H, Law C. (2005) Being big or growing fast: systematic review of size or growth in infancy and later obesity, British Medical Journal, vol. 331, no. 7522, pp. 929–935.

c. Viner R, Cole T. (2005) Adult socioeconomic, educational, social, and psychological outcomes of childhood obesity: a national birth cohort study BMJ 330 doi: http://dx.doi.org/10.1136/bmj.38453.422049.E0

d. NHLBI Obesity Education Initiative Expert Panel on the Identification, Evaluation, and Treatment of Obesity in Adults (US). 1998. National Heart, Lung, and Blood Institute http://www.ncbi.nlm.nih.gov/books/NBK2008/

Chapter 38
Giraffe Effect

Get the Facts

➤ When you review articles, make sure you look at the whole picture and understand what the real issues are. The real issue is not obesity. It is Metabolic Disease Syndrome and the risks that lead to chronic illness.

➤ Do not believe everything you read. Research, investigate, experiment!

➤ The Giraffe Effect in science means the scientific and political focus will be primarily on the larger issues such as obesity, yet the real consequences can more drastic on the less visible consequences.

Understand the Science

Giraffes are what Yakuel calls "portions of data," which dominate the rest of the data – and hide important insights. Sometimes portions of data even lead to wrong conclusions. Marketers and analysts are always on the lookout for exciting new insights that can translate into action items and provide strategic advantage, but they often miss them. They can even make the wrong decisions because they fail to account for the "giraffe effect" in their data. This should not occur in science, but it can and does.

The Giraffe, the Fox, the Cat, and the Mouse

Let's say you're out watching animals in a nature preserve. Undoubtedly, when you spot a majestic giraffe in your binoculars, you're going to take a good look at him. He stands out, he's taller than the landscape, and he's impressive!

Meanwhile, many of the other smaller animals will all just seem, well, small. You won't even notice that there are significant differences in height among the smaller animals, especially when compared to the giraffe.

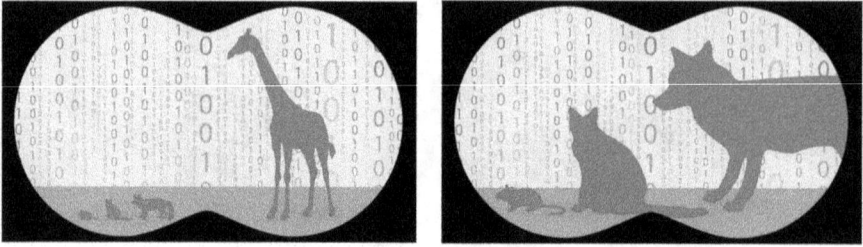

Figure 46 The Giraffe Effect

However, if you can take your eyes off the giraffe for a minute, and you zoom your binoculars into the smaller animals on the plain, an amazing thing happens. You become aware that the differences in size between the animals are actually much larger than you had first realized. This is a very simple example of the giraffe effect. When people look at a set of data which includes some very large and dominant members, important differences, among the rest of the data in the set, often disappear from view.

Conclusion

Everyone is looking at obesity (the giraffe). The real differences are the impacts at the less visible level. The media and press is full of the 65% of the population with obesity, but it is the 38% with metabolic syndrome; the 15% with chronic kidney disease (CKD), or the 4% with life-limiting diabetes. These, or the 20% of normal weight people, with metabolic syndrome and on the path to chronic diseases, are not in the limelight. For example, one in seven hospital admissions in Australia are a result of chronic kidney disease, and 13% of the population is understood to have CKD, compared with 4% with diabetes. It is these lower profile diseases which are churning through the health budgets already. The rise in childhood obesity, and the aging population getting fatter by the day, will present significant challenges to health services.

References

a. Yakuel P. (2013) Beware of the giraffes in your data. Optimove http://gigaom.com/2013/08/24/beware-of-the-giraffes-in-your-data/

CHAPTER 39
POLITICS OF OBESITY – THE FAT WARS

Get the Facts

➤ Obesity has two definitions: scientific, which is defined by BMI, and socio-political.

➤ There is a war going on between those who say obesity is a personal responsibility, and therefore obesity is a personal failure, as opposed to those who say obesity is a result of an unhealthy or obesogenic food environment.

➤ Obesity is big business, even larger than the tobacco industry, and has substantial lobbying power.

➤ A paradox of obesity is that overweight people are considerably disadvantaged, especially women and young girls.

➤ Obesity is now a disability by law in the EU.

Understand the Science

There's no doubt that obesity has received considerable political attention over the past decade as society is losing the battle of the bulge and rising overweight and obese rates of doubling in 20 or 30 years. Policy responses have focused on downstream interventions, such as social marketing campaigns, and funding for school and community programs. While important, these are expensive responses and unlikely to make a dent in obesity levels. There is little political support for any actual policies that target the upstream drivers of the problem and reduce the toxicity of the food environment. Bans on junk-food marketing to children, effective front-of-pack food labelling, and taxing unhealthy products, are "no go zones" for politicians. Political responses to date have been more about creating the appearance of "doing something," rather than actually solving the obesity problem. Why?

Obesity is a political challenge. Politicians are highly averse to insulting or angering anyone who might possibly vote for them. Because a large portion of the population is now over weight, politicians are very sensitive to the topic.

Obesity has also been called the "climate change of public health" and a "brilliant test of political capability." Rightly so. Tackling the upstream causes of obesity challenges the interests of the powerful food, beverage, and advertising industries. It requires interventions across multiple policy sectors (education, health, media, and finance) at local, national, and global levels.

The complexity of the problem means there is a long list of experts and stakeholders who must be consulted in the policy development process and compared with tobacco, which has 30 years of concerted research, advocacy, and regulation behind it, obesity is a relatively young social issue. It has received political attention for only the last decade. Baker tracked words in the Australian parliament records containing each word. Tobacco word rates have fallen, but obesity, overweight, physical activity words have all increased.

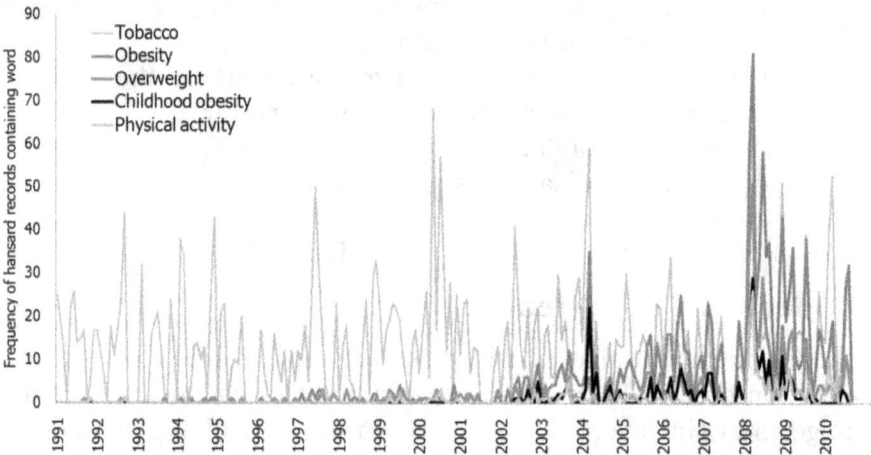

Figure 47 Political attention to obesity (and related issues)

To highlight this politicization of obesity, let's look at a paper from a researcher from The Centre for Disease Control. In early 2013, Katherine Flegan, a senior researcher, undertook a systematic review of 97 studies, over 3m patients, and 270,000 deaths. The study looked at all causes of deaths, and not just overall health risks. Conclusions from that review are:

- People who are overweight with a BMI 25-30 are 6% less likely to die in any given period than people of normal weight of BMI 18.5-25. That's 30% of the USA population.
- Those even moderately obese (BMI 30-35), don't have a higher-than-normal risk of dying.

- Being substantially obese (BMI>35) raises the risk of death by 29%.

This study is the latest, and largest, to document what scientists call the "obesity paradox." Other studies have shown that people with heart disease, diabetes, and other chronic health conditions tend to live longer if they carry excess weight, even though excess weight is associated with heightened risk of heart disease, type 2 diabetes, and several cancers, which in turn raise the risk of premature death.

As you can imagine, the discussion from this study became heated. (I have previously written there is compelling evidence against this sort of result). Early commentators were restrained, but then other researchers started calling this nonsense.

Obesity has a scientific definition and a socio-political definition, and the distinction between the two is increasingly blurred. I also point out that not all obesity winds up causing metabolic syndrome, and that normal weight people also get metabolic syndrome and associated health and mortality consequences. You would have to go back to some of those 97 studies to view the data.

In medical science, obesity has a precise definition: having a BMI of 30 or greater. Overweight means having a BMI of at least 25, but less than 30. These definitions are sometimes accompanied by information regarding waist circumference. The increase in waist circumference has a direct relationship with poorer health.

In policy, media, and lay circles, "obesity" has become shorthand for something quite different from, and much less precise than, the scientific meaning. One meaning is the social stigma with being obese, and the other meaning is the institutionalization of obesity.

You're fat! The problem of people who are above "normal" weight.

Obesity is associated with powerful negatives, stemming from both long-standing prejudice and recent public health framing. These include epidemic threat, devastating impending costs, tragedy (children routinely dying before their parents), as well as character flaws in obese individuals who are frequently said to be lazy, lack willpower, be greedy, or to shirk personal responsibility. This view is used to legitimize the well-documented discrimination experienced by heavier people, especially women, particularly younger women and girls. For people above normal weight, then, public discussion of obesity is complicated. Burgo, an American psychologist, says, "When a person resolves to tackle long-standing weight issues, the inability to follow through can feel like "proof" that one really is a "loser"." He believes the medical profession ignores emotional and psychological issues when confronting a person's weight, "largely because they're unprepared to help the person cope with them."

Recent research shows fat shaming does not help people lose weight; data suggest people experiencing discrimination over their size may even be more likely to put on weight. Researchers from the University College London monitored almost 3000 UK adults over a 4 year period. They found that the 5% who experienced "weight discrimination" gained an average of 1 kg over that time, while those who did not lost an average of 0.7 kg.

The "Institutionalization" of Obesity

Obesity became institutionalized fairly rapidly in universities and governments in the late 20th century. Prior to this, there wasn't any specialization. There are now obesity strategies, government departments responsible for obesity, obesity handbooks, professorial chairs, university research centres, websites, Twitter feeds, and advocacy groups with the word obesity in their titles. Obesity, an amorphous, but potent social and political concept, now raises the stakes in many settings, engendering blame, inducing strong feelings, and providing the focus for many people's professional roles and identities. No wonder it has become such a battleground, nowhere more evident than in the airline industry, under pressure for larger seats and less over-charging for space. It is a battle between the bulge and the buck! Further, in December 2014, the European Court of Justice (ECJ) ruled that morbid obesity could be considered a disability under the Equal Treatment in Employment Directive if the employee is prevented from fully participating in professional life because of his or her weight. Even though obesity is caused by the person themselves, they need to be treated the same as other disabilities. The Court stopped short of saying that obesity needed specific protection under the EU anti-discrimination laws. The full ramifications are yet to be worked out. (The employee had a BMI of 54, and weight of 350 lb, 25 stone, 160 kg). Some of the USA states already have anti-discrimination laws against obesity.

Questioning the relationship between obesity and health has become socially and politically analogous to questioning the relationship between smoking and health. In the case of smoking, the socio-political problem maps fairly neatly onto the scientific problem: the object of concern is people lighting and inhaling from small sticks.

Smoking causes cancer, with little argument now. The arguments are now about the diminishing rights of smokers to smoke in public places. For obesity, however, the socio-political and scientific problems are now hopelessly divergent.

Back to the claim by Flegal and colleagues that overweight is associated with lower all-cause mortality than normal weight was precise, limited, and cautiously interpreted. It was also potentially scientifically important (and not without precedent) and thus worth discussing. However, the socio-political claim that "obesity may not kill you" seems to be regarded by many as potentially treasonous, because the socio-political meaning of obesity is so imprecise and has so much riding on it. Socially and politically, the claim that "obesity may not kill you" may be the equivalent of implying that weight is irrelevant to health (untrue); that we should stop caring about non-communicable diseases (unsupportable); or that urbanization, sedentary work and leisure, car dependence, and radical changes in the food supply are unrelated to health (ridiculous).

The message that "obesity may not kill you" has even starker implications for overweight or obese individuals (who may view it as demonstrating that "the prejudice against me is unfounded and I am vindicated") and for professionals who may view it as implying that "their personal university chair, handbook, advocacy organization, blog, career, or professional identity are deeply misguided or irrelevant." No wonder there was such a passionate exchange. Do I believe the findings from Flegen are "true?" I don't. It is the same issue as often that correlation is not causation.

Conclusion

The inability to manage every factor in trials makes analysis of the data a very tricky business, and it is even trickier when you review dozens of trials in meta-studies. When you combine disparate trials together you lose information, or the process you use can make big differences to the conclusions. Using correlation to prove cause is bad science. Mortality is one thing; quality of life is another, and most of these do not measure these. So being alive, but under medical care / taking drugs / or with dementia is far from optimal. The understanding I have come to is that obesity is a marker of health. If your diet results in increased weight, there is every probability that your health is sub-optimal, and you will suffer a decreased quality of life. If, you are as overweight as the Dane in the EU test case, you undoubtedly will have serious health issues, and the prognosis for a long healthy life are poor. He said "I don't feel my weight is a big problem, but the same as most big people, I'd like to lose some weight."

References

a. Flegal K. (2013) Association of All-Cause Mortality with Overweight and Obesity Using Standard Body Mass Index Categories - A Systematic Review and Meta-analysis. JAMA. 2013;309(1):71-82. doi:10.1001/jama.2012.113905

b. Carter S, Walls HL (2013) JAMA Forum: Separating the Science and Politics of "Obesity" http://newsatjama.jama.com/2013/02/14/jama-forum-separating-the-science-and-politics-of-obesity/

c. Baker P. (2012) Why we're losing the battle of the bulge: the politics of obesity prevention. http://theconversation.com/why-were-losing-the-battle-of-the-bulge-the-politics-of-obesity-prevention-8304

d. Kersh R (2009) The Politics of Obesity: A Current Assessment and Look Ahead. Milbank Q. 2009 March; 87(1): 295–316. doi: 10.1111/j.1468-0009.2009.00556.x

e. Vayle A. (2013) Are you ashamed to lose weight. http://www.smh.com.au/lifestyle/diet-and-fitness/are-you-too-ashamed-to-lose-weight-20130606-2nsku.html

f. European Court of Justice rules obesity can be a disability.(2014) Jurist. http://jurist.org/paperchase/2014/12/european-court-of-justice-rules-obesity-can-be-a-disability.php

CHAPTER 40
NEED FOR VITAMINS – FACT OR FICTION

Get the Facts

➢ We have outsourced responsibility for our health. We don't want to change the way we live despite documentation that lifestyle is one of the most powerful determinants of health.

➢ The question isn't whether people need vitamins. They do. The questions are how much do they need, and do they get enough in foods?

➢ I'm very sceptical of anyone who takes a pill to cure the man-made epidemics of our time (and you should be too).

➢ Nutrition experts argue that people need only the recommended daily allowance – the amount of vitamins found in a routine diet. "Routine" is not often well defined.

➢ Vitamin manufacturers argue that a "regular diet" doesn't contain enough vitamins, and that more is better.

➢ Most people assume that, at the very least, excess vitamins can't do any harm. It turns out, however, that scientists have known for years that large quantities of certain supplemental vitamins can be quite harmful. And most recently, the editors of Annals of Internal Medicine finally said that vitamins are a waste of money and offer no health benefits. That is pretty radical for medicos!

➢ Sales are good. One in three people take supplements. Which confirms my view people don't trust science.

Understand the Science

Vitamins and supplements as a category includes a large range of ingestible products, from vitamins and calcium pills, to protein shakes, diet pills, and energy drinks. Derived from "vita," meaning life in Latin, vitamins are necessary to convert food into energy. When people don't get enough vitamins, they suffer diseases like scurvy and rickets. These diseases are now almost unknown in developed societies.

The vitamin market is also referred to by various names such as nutritional supplements, dietary supplements, and simply, supplements. By whatever the name, this is a lucrative market. The USA Market in 2013 is about $30b, with vitamin sales about $12b, and with 10% annual increases. Over 39% of adults take vitamins and 54% take supplements. Australia's complementary and alternative medical industry is worth at least $4b, and the vitamins and supplement market size is estimated at over $1.8b and likewise growing at 12%.

According to Adams, Professor of Public Health and Director of the Australian Research Centre in Complementary and Integrative Medicine at UTS, the growing use of alternative medicine is part of the development of a "paradigm of wellness" in the community. "People are looking to improve their lot and are thinking more proactively and holistically about health and not just about responding to illness. It's a message the healthcare system in general promotes, whether it's about quitting smoking or having a good diet," he said.

Adams says vitamins and supplements have become firmly entrenched in the way people think about their health, whether or not there is convincing evidence that the products work. "When you look at the data," he said, "one of the most important things you notice is that it's not just a middle-class phenomenon, or people who are wealthy, who are using complementary medicine. It's men and women of all ages and socio-economic groups, right across the country."

From 2002 and onwards, Bjelakovic and others from Copenhagen University reviewed a range of trials in meta-studies. In one review of 815 clinical trials, taking supplements had a detrimental effect on lifespan. You die earlier. Those who took beta-carotene had a 7% increased risk, and vitamins A and E incurred a 16% and a 4% increased risk, respectively. In another study, there was no benefit found of anti-oxidants on colorectal adenoma; a separate study found that older women increased their risk of cardiovascular or cancer death by taking a daily vitamin, especially an iron supplement.

Most recently, Edgar Miller from the Mayo Clinic, one of the Editorial Committee of the Annals of Internal Medicine, commented on three articles in the December 2013 issue and said, "These vitamins should not be used for chronic disease prevention. Enough is enough."

One study analysed 24 previous trials involving 450,000 people and found no beneficial effect on mortality from taking vitamins. A second examined 6000 elderly men and found taking pills had no positive effect on cognitive decline after 12 years, and a third piece of research followed 1700 men and women with heart problems and discovered no benefit in those who had taken supplements.

> The evidence is pretty clear. Multivitamins, β-carotene, antioxidants, Vitamin E, folic acid, B vitamins, and mineral supplements are harmful or ineffective for chronic disease prevention.

It is not worth further trials. Vitamin D supplementation, however, is an open area of investigation, particularly in deficient persons. Clinical trials have been equivocal and sometimes contradictory.

If you want to read dissenting views to Millers editorial, read the comments that were subsequently posted. There are many who say that nutrition is not optimal and vitamins should be taken especially during pregnancy. To my thinking this comes back to, "Eat Food. Not too much. Mostly plants." If your diet is mostly a Western diet with high sugar and processed food products, vitamins might be necessary. Alternatively, just eat whole foods.

Sometimes you see a study and you are left scratching your head. E.g. A study with 14,641 male doctors older than 50 for over 13 years (1997-2011) showed Centrum Silver multivitamins reduced the risk of cancer by about 8% but not site specific cancers such as prostate or colorectal. But what was the doctors' diet? And what was their lifestyle? Why was this study done, without trying to get to some of the interactions between diet and supplements? We just don't know. We are left with that vague feeling that vitamins might prevent some ills, but could also possibly do harm.

Buying vitamins can definitely do some harm to your wallet! Ditch the pills, buy whole food. Try an apple a day. That was as good as statins for mortality reduction.

Omega-3 Supplements

About eight years ago, I started taking fish oil supplements. A family member had said it was beneficial for mild depression, and there appeared to be some relationship with dementia onset from a couple of media articles. However, when I thought we had found a supplement with unquestionable benefit, our hopes of ensuring good health by religiously swallowing the right pill are dashed. There was a recent report that stated that taking fish oil increased prostate cancer risk. We will discuss this more in the next chapter. Health-minded consumers have propelled annual fish oil sales to more than $6b in products and fortified foods.

How did fish oil get on our medical radar and become a $6b industry? It can be very informative to trace the origins of any accepted health practice; especially the whole claim that dietary cholesterol increases heart attacks. Sometimes there is a small experiment or more likely an observation. It may prove to be wrong, but then research can go for years trying to prove there is an advantage. Consumers follow this like lemmings!

In the early 70s, Danish investigators noted a dramatically lower incidence of cardiovascular disease among 130 Greenland Inuit in a study. This is what they said in the abstract.

> *Most types of lipid were decreased, compared with Danish controls and Eskimos living in Denmark. The most remarkable finding was a much lower level of pre-β-lipoprotein and consequently of plasma-triglycerides in Greenlandic Eskimos than in Danish controls. These findings may explain the very low incidence of ischæmic heart-disease and the complete absence of diabetes mellitus in Greenlandic Eskimos.*

I would suggest it might also be due to the lack of a Westernized diet with high sugars and carbohydrates. If these Inuit have high Omega-3 blood levels due to their diet, do they have a high prevalence of prostate cancer? Turns out the Inuit have an extraordinarily low prevalence of prostate cancer. Clearly the prostate-cancer Omega-3 story is more complicated. The Inuit data proved all the more interesting in light of the evolution of their health over the past 50 years. As so often happens, with the westernization/modernization of the Inuit lifestyle, the incidence of cancer has increased dramatically, except for one. Prostate cancer remains incredibly rare amongst the Inuit regardless of dietary fish oil or Omega-3 blood levels. This is not the first time a supplement has been embraced as a therapeutic agent, and subsequently found to have no effect or even a negative one. Vitamins A, C, and E, beta carotene, and selenium supplementation, in the absence of a deficiency, have all proven ineffective or something that increased mortality. It is another example of hype without substance.

There are two overarching reasons as to why this keeps happening.

- The reductive nature of Western science, as explained by Ahn lends itself to a certain kind of thinking. If a population is observed to have a particularly low incidence of a disease, we study them in an attempt to define the one factor that might explain it. We attempt to isolate the therapeutic agent. In this Inuit cash it was Omega-3s.

- The second cause of repeated disappointment in health supplements has to do with our unrealistic expectations. We have outsourced responsibility for our health. We don't want to change the way we live (or eat) despite documentation that lifestyle is one of the most powerful determinants of health. In this regard, we collude with the reductive scientific thinking. We don't want to go and change our lifestyle to that of the primitive Inuits, but if we pop a fish oil pill, that sounds easy!

We want to continue to do the same things and get a different result by swallowing a magic pill.

Commercial interests understand this proclivity very well. They have created a panoply of products (magic pills and potions) that are supposed to make you lose weight, put on muscle, and live longer, disease-free lives without any change in behaviour. In earlier times these products were called snake oil. And sales are good.

We are a tough species. Ten thousand generations of evolution have crafted humans that are remarkably effective at absorbing and using the essential nutrients from food. For better or worse, our body is programmed to work on food, not pills or powders. The "housing" of these nutrients and vitamins in food seems to be an important part of how they are adsorbed and utilised. Evolution has also wired us for lots of movement.

We have inadvertently conducted a global experiment on the consequences of sedentary behaviour and the consumption of huge caloric loads of processed foods. The results are in: an epidemic of obesity, diabetes, hypertension, and cardiovascular disease. As we understand more of our human biome, the bacteria that live in and on us, it seems they are healthier when we eat whole food.

Conclusion

We like simple stories that provide simple solutions and don't ask us to change. Most like a solution of once a day taking a "natural supplement". It seems more "scientific", or so it says on the bottle, than eating whole food. "Proven by clinical trials." Or "As used by a celebrity." If we can appreciate the benefits of whole foods, we should be able to understand the need for thinking about whole people. Many variables determined the Inuit's remarkable health, including lots of physical activity, clean air and water, a close community of supportive social connections, a relatively homogenous population with similar genetics, and yes, their diet too.

Anyone claiming to have a pill to cure the man-made epidemics of our time smells a little fishy to me. If you change to eating whole foods, and especially the complex carbohydrates, some fish, some meat then vitamins and supplements have no role.

References

a. Ahn AC, Tewari M, Poon CS, Phillips RS. (2006) The Limits of Reductionism in Medicine: Could Systems Biology Offer an Alternative? PLoS Med 3(6): e208. doi:10.1371/journal.pmed.0030208

b. Bjelakovic G, Nikolova D, Lotte Gluud L, Simonetti R, Gluud C. (2007) Mortality in Randomized Trials of Antioxidant Supplements for Primary and Secondary Prevention: Systematic Review and Meta-analysis JAMA. 2007;297(8):842-857. doi:10.1001/jama.297.8.842.

c. http://www.nytimes.com/2013/06/09/opinion/sunday/dont-take-your-vitamins.html

d. Bjelakovic G, Nikolova D, Simonetti RG, Gluud C. (2004) Antioxidant supplements for prevention of gastrointestinal cancers: a systematic review and meta-analysis. Lancet. 2-8;364(9441):1219-28. PMID: 15464182

e. http://www.huffingtonpost.com/paul-spector-md/fish-oil-myths_b_3789813.html

f. Bang H, Dyerberg J, Nielsen A. (1971) Plasma Lipid and lipoprotein pattern in Greenlandic West Coast Eskimos The Lancet, Volume 297, Issue 7710, Pages 1143 – 1146 doi:10.1016/S0140-6736(71)91658-8Cite or Link Using DOI

g. Eskimos and Cancer. (2008) Lifestyle Changes Lead to Dramatic Cancer Increase among Inuit People. http://www.cancermonthly.com/iNP/view.asp?ID=228 from Friborg JT, Melbye M. (2008) Cancer patterns in Inuit populations. The Lancet Oncology.Vol 9:892-900

h. Guallar E, Stranges S, Mulrow C, Appel L, Miller E. (2013) Enough Is Enough: Stop Wasting Money on Vitamin and Mineral Supplements. Vol 159 (12) http://annals.org/article.aspx?articleid=1789253

i. Gaziano J.M, Sesso H, Christen W, Bubes V, Smith J, MacFadyen J, Schvartz M, Manson J, Glynn R, Buring J. (2012) Multivitamins in the Prevention of Cancer in Men. The Physicians' Health Study II Randomized Controlled Trial JAMA. 2012;308(18):1871-1880. doi:10.1001/jama.2012.14641.

CHAPTER 41
OMEGA-3 AND PROSTATE DISEASE

Get the Facts

➢ Fish oils seem to provide some benefit in fighting prostate cancer, but a recent study showing adverse effects was published that said taking fish oil supplements increased rates.

➢ How do you decide? You have to look at better designed trials. You have to weigh pros and cons based on other health benefits.

Understand the Science

In general, I come down pretty hard against taking any vitamins or supplements. So it is a bit tricky to admit that I have taken fish oil to help with moisturizing my skin. Since childhood, I have had skin that tends to have eczema and sensitivity to lanolin and other compounds. About ten years ago, someone suggested taking fish oil (Omega-3 supplements) as it appeared to lessen the dry skin condition in low humidity environments.

A male friend takes fish oil as he swears that it helps to minimize depression. I have heard many others also state that fish oil supplements help them with depression. I'm inclined to wonder if the positive effects are more a result of the decision to "do something positive" than to the pill itself.

In mid-2013, a published article received a lot of media attention. The article reported that higher levels of long-chain Omega-3 fats (EPA, DPA, and DHA) in blood were associated with a 43% increased risk of prostate cancer and a 71% increased risk of aggressive prostate cancer. These Omega-3 fats are found in salmon, mackerel, herring, lake trout, sardines, and albacore tuna. Blood levels reflect dietary intake of Omega-3s, something that has been promoted for the prevention of heart disease and cancer. What was the study, and was it good science or did it have design limitations? Like many studies, this is an "epidemiological" study, and not a randomized experiment, and as we know, correlation is not causation as I explain in more detail in the science and studies chapter. The bottom line is that we cannot determine from this study design whether the intake of Omega-3 fatty acids will cause prostate cancer and raise a man's risk for high-grade disease. The media probably sensationalized the risk associated with Omega-3 fatty acid intake, and concerns about the study design were not mentioned at all. The initial study showed that selenium and Omega-3 intake were correlated with reduced prostate cancer. For those who had prostate cancer, it increased a man's risk. We would need better-designed trials that are prospective and randomized to be able to determine the causes beyond reasonable doubt. Until that is done, we will have to weigh the pros and cons of taking Omega-3 fatty acids in terms of its other potential health benefits to decide what to do. Whether or not it causes prostate cancer was not determined by the results of this trial.

The study was a prospective case-control study that involved comparing the blood levels of various fatty acids, including the long-chain Omega-3 fatty acids, in a group of 834 men who developed prostate cancer (156 the high grade, aggressive form), against 1393 who did not. The subjects were all part of the SELECT (Selenium and Vitamin E Cancer Prevention) trial that aimed to evaluate the effects of vitamin E and selenium supplements on prostate cancer. Note that the SELECT trial found that those who took selenium supplements alone experienced a 20% reduction in absolute risk of prostate cancer, while those who took both selenium and vitamin E benefited even more, with a 60% risk reduction. High dose vitamin E (alpha-tocopherol) alone exposed study subjects to a 160% increase in absolute risk.

Prostate cancer expert Prof Anthony D'Amico points out that the authors failed to adjust their calculations for the main risk factors associated with prostate cancer. Key factors such as ethnicity, age, body mass index (BMI), and prostate-specific antigen (PSA) level were not accounted for, despite being listed in the table of baseline patient characteristics and SELECT trial cancer outcomes. D'Amico, who developed a classification method widely used for prostate cancer risk said "The study really cannot make the conclusion that it's trying to. These types of studies are not cause and effect. These studies are simply associations. They didn't account for the known predictors of prostate cancer when they were making the calculation. You're left with a weak association."

In the section on biochemistry of oils, we spoke of the issue that polyunsaturated fats oxidize (technically lipid peroxidation). Of all fatty acids, long-chain Omega-3 fats are the most readily peroxidized. Peroxidation of polyunsaturated fatty acids generates highly toxic compounds, such as aldehydes, which mutate DNA and turn proteins into advanced lipoxidation end products (ALEs). These lipid peroxidation products have been implicated as causal factors in cancer. Further, oxidation products of DHA promote angiogenesis, which is the creation of new blood vessels to feed tumours. These products make cancers grow rapidly. We are left with an uneasy feeling. What don't we know? Does fish oil increase, or decrease, prostate cancer? The evidence is just not conclusive.

Fish Oils and Brain Boosting Power

Omega-3s are often touted as brain boosters, but they don't appear to slow mental decline. Eric Ammann reported from the University of Iowa where they analysed Omega-3 levels in blood samples taken from 2100 women aged 60 to 80 with no dementia. Over six years, the women took tests for fine motor speed, verbal memory, visual memory, spatial ability, verbal knowledge, verbal fluency, and working memory. No difference in cognition was found between women with high and low levels of Omega-3 at the start of the study, nor in how quickly cognitive skills declined in people with consistently low or high omega-3. As I mentioned at the beginning, Omega-3 supplement research is unclear as there is some Omega-3 in most diets – and the supplements just boost the intake. It may be that people who eat lots of fish and nuts are more affluent and health-conscious – like you, the reader. They may have less junk food, lower levels of simple carbohydrates, or they may do more physical or mental exercise. As these were not measured or presented, it's hard to know. Those factors could be the true force behind studies that seem to show Omega-3s' protective effect on cognition. It is a little different if you are a rat and fed on rat chow in a controlled and restricted environment!

Conclusion

In conclusion, what does one do? Moderation perhaps? If you want to take them because you believe they do good, then keep on doing so. They should be encouraged if they help your mental state (that second leg of the dietary stool). If you think taking them will somehow change a prognosis: don't bother. Eat more green leafy vegetables or buy an extra shellfish serving a week depending on your dietary preferences. If you have prostate cancer, stop taking them. If you have a particular condition, such as dry skin or some depression symptoms, test it on your symptom. Use it. Stop using it. Start again. Measure any changes. Keep an open mind that the changes you notice might be a placebo effect. Look for other factors that might be implicated. It seems like this one of the areas of science where we just do not have enough information to be certain of the science.

I've changed. I ditched the fish oil tablets to an additional extra fish meal (salmon) or snack (prawns, oysters, mussels) per week. The nice part is that these high value food of prawns and oysters turned out to be no more expensive than fish oil supplements!

References
a. Brasky TM, Darke A, Song X, Tangen C, Goodman P, Thompson I, Meyskens F, Goodman G, Minasian L , Parnes H, Klein E, Kristal A. (2013) Plasma Phospholipid Fatty Acids and Prostate Cancer Risk in the SELECT trial. J Natl Cancer Inst. 105(15):1132-41. doi: 10.1093/jnci/djt174
b. Brasky TM, Till C, White E, Neuhouser ML, Song X, Goodman P, Thompson IM, King IB, Albanes D, Kristal AR. (2011) Serum phospholipid fatty acids and prostate cancer risk: results from the prostate cancer prevention trial. Am J Epidemiol. Vol 15;173(12):1429-39. http://pmid.us/21518693.
c. Lippman SM, Klein EA, Goodman PJ, et al. (2009) Effect of selenium and vitamin E on risk of prostate cancer and other cancers: the Selenium and Vitamin E Cancer Prevention Trial (SELECT). JAMA. 301:39-51
d. Spector, P (2013) Something Fishy About Omega-3's: Prostate Cancer, Fish Oil and Panaceas http://www.huffingtonpost.com/paul-spector-md/fish-oil-myths_b_3789813.html
e. http://www.anh-europe.org/news/a-tide-of-evidence-washes-away-flawed-fish-oil-prostate-cancer-study
f. Botelho A. (2013) Fish Oil and intelligence? New Scientist 2936 http://www.newscientist.com/article/mg21929363.800-fish-oils-dont-boost-brain-power.html
g. Ammann E, Pottala J, Harris W, Espeland M, Wallace R, Denburg N, Carnahan R, Robinson, J. (2013) Omega-3 fatty acids and domain-specific cognitive aging - Secondary analyses of data from WHISCA. Neurology 10.1212 doi: 10.1212/WNL.0b013e3182a9584c
h. Hulbert AJ, Pamplona R, Buffenstein R, Buttemer WA. (2007) Life and death: metabolic rate, membrane composition, and life

span of animals. Physiological Rev 87(4):1175–213, http://pmid.us/17928583.

i. Hulbert AJ. (2010) Metabolism and longevity: is there a role for membrane fatty acids? Integrative and Comparative Biology Vol 50(5):808–17, http://pmid.us/21558243.

j. Nair, U, Bartsch H, Nair J. (2007) Lipid peroxidation-induced DNA damage in cancer-prone inflammatory diseases: a review of published adduct types and levels in humans. Free Radic Biol Med. Vol 43(8):1109-20. http://pmid.us/17854706.

k. D'Amico AV, Keshaviah A, Manola J, Cote K, Loffredo M, Iskrzytzky O, Renshaw AA. (2002) Clinical utility of the percentage of positive prostate biopsies in predicting prostate cancer-specific and overall survival after radiotherapy for patients with localized prostate cancer.Int J Radiat Oncol Biol Phys. 1;53(3):581-7.

Chapter 42
Antioxidants

Get the Facts

➤ Consumers don't know that taking mega-vitamins can increase their risk of cancer and heart disease and shorten their lives.

➤ Don't take vitamins to get "anti-oxidants." Instead of eating sugar and cheap, simple carbohydrates, eat complex carbohydrates.

➤ Save your money and buy and eat some additional green vegetables.

Understand the Science

Bear with me! I am going to deal with antioxidants in a little more detail than vitamins, as everything these days promotes "healthy antioxidants" as if they are miracle workers.

Antioxidants are not necessarily vitamins, but some vitamins are antioxidants.

Anti-oxidation vs. oxidation has been billed as a contest between good and evil. It takes place in within cells in organelles called mitochondria, where the body converts food to energy — a process that requires oxygen (oxidation). One consequence of oxidation is the generation of atomic scavengers called free radicals (evil). Free radicals can damage DNA, cell membranes, and the lining of arteries. Not surprisingly, they've been linked to aging, cancer, and heart disease.

To neutralize free radicals, the body makes antioxidants (good). Antioxidants can also be found in fruits and vegetables, specifically in selenium, beta carotene, and vitamins A, C, and E. Some studies have shown that people who eat more fruits and vegetables have a lower incidence of cancer and heart disease, and they live longer. The logic is obvious. If fruits and vegetables contain antioxidants, and people who eat fruits and vegetables are healthier, then people who take supplemental antioxidants should also be healthier.

It hasn't worked out that way. It could be that people who eat fruits and vegetables also eat less sugar and simple carbohydrates or any of the other multiple confounding behaviours. Antioxidants have always been questioned about their efficacy and their safety. Back in 1994, 29,000 Finnish men, all smokers, were given daily vitamin E, beta carotene (precursor to Vitamin A), both, or a placebo. The study found that those who took beta carotene for five to eight years were 18% more likely to die from lung cancer or heart disease.

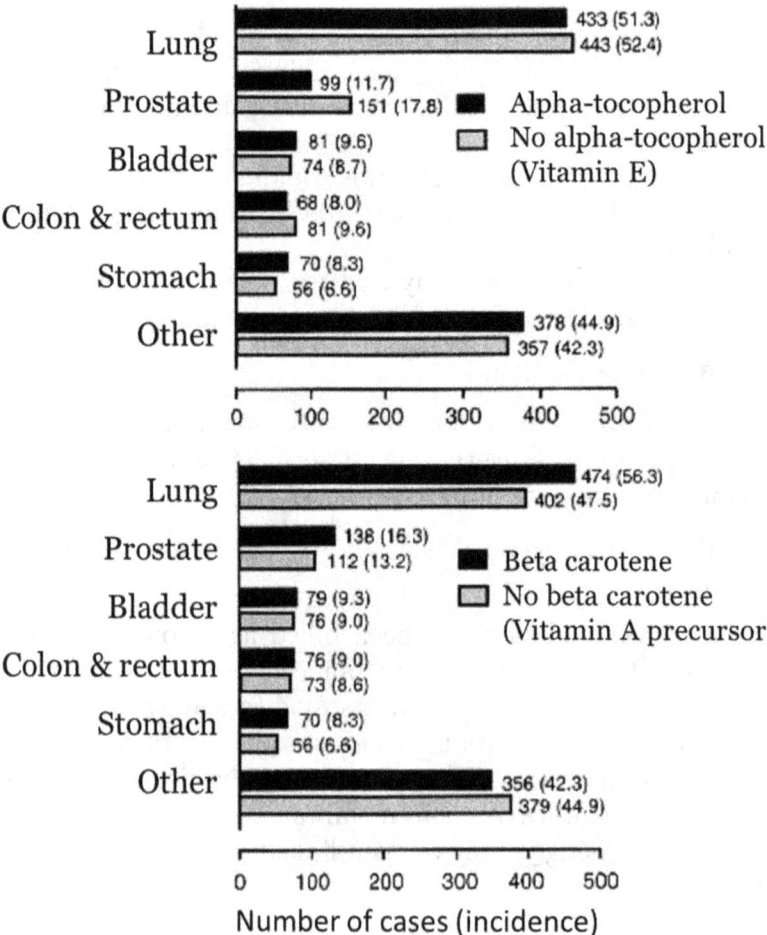

Figure 48 The Antioxidant Cancer Prevention Study

Two years later, the same journal (*NEJM*), published another study on vitamin supplements. In it, 18,000 people who were at an increased risk of lung cancer because of asbestos exposure or smoking, received a combination of vitamin A and beta carotene, or a placebo. Investigators stopped the study when they found that the risk of death from lung cancer for those who took the vitamins was 46% higher. Then, in 2004, a review of 14 randomized trials for the Cochrane Database found that the supplemental vitamins A, C, E and beta carotene, and a mineral (selenium) taken to prevent intestinal cancers, actually increased mortality.

The National Cancer Council (USA) reported on the nine randomized controlled trials of dietary antioxidant supplements for cancer prevention. Overall, these nine randomized controlled clinical trials did not provide evidence that dietary antioxidant supplements are beneficial in primary cancer prevention. They say, though, that the lack of benefit in these trials can be explained by differences in the effects of the tested antioxidants when they are consumed as purified chemicals, as opposed to when they are consumed in foods, which contain complex mixtures of antioxidants, vitamins, and minerals.

The likely explanation is that free radicals aren't as evil as advertised. In fact, people need them to kill bacteria and eliminate new cancer cells. And when people take large doses of antioxidants in the form of supplemental vitamins, the balance between free radical production and destruction might tip too much in one direction, causing an unnatural state where the immune system is less able to kill harmful invaders. Researchers call this the *antioxidant paradox*. Because studies of large doses of supplemental antioxidants haven't clearly supported their use, respected organizations responsible for the public's health do not recommend them for otherwise healthy people. But that is not the case for the commercial interests.

Back in 1972, concerned that people were consuming larger and larger quantities of vitamins, the USA FDA announced a plan to regulate vitamin supplements containing more than 150% of the recommended daily allowance. Vitamin makers had to prove that the "mega vitamins" were safe before selling them. Not surprisingly, the vitamin industry saw this as a threat, and set out to destroy the bill. Speaking in support of the bill, the lawyer for the Consumers Union set eight cantaloupes in front of her, and she said, "You would need to eat eight cantaloupes, a good source of vitamin C, to take in barely 1000 milligrams of vitamin C. But just these two little pills, easy to swallow, contain the same amount." She warned that if the legislation passed, "One tablet would contain as much vitamin C as all of these cantaloupes, or even twice, thrice, or 20 times that amount. And there would be no protective satiety level." But the bill passed and now anyone can sell multivitamins and call them good. The only prohibition is against claiming specific health benefits such as a cure. In looking at the advertisements on TV and the internet using celebrities and sports-people the claims for health benefits are pretty strong, and regulatory authorities seem to turn a blind eye to their claims.

Conclusion

Before researching the research, I thought that antioxidants were a little over-hyped but generally ineffective. We can see now that if you want to run the risk of increased cancer, take anti-oxidants. Eating some fruit and vegetables (note: fruit juice is not fruit) will reduce your weight and improve your health.

It seems like this claim for health from consuming antioxidants has no evidence. This is not a book on household budgeting, but for me any money spent on this sort of stuff is a complete waste of money. I'd rather give the money for clean water projects in Africa, or some other charity. At least it will do some good rather than line the pockets of the antioxidant companies.

References

a. The Alpha-Tocopherol Beta Carotene Cancer Prevention Study Group (1994) The Effect of Vitamin E and Beta Carotene on the Incidence of Lung Cancer and Other Cancers in Male Smokers. N Engl J Med 330:1029-1035 doi: 10.1056/NEJM199404143301501
b. Offit P (June 2013) Don't Take Your Vitamins. http://www.nytimes.com/2013/06/09/opinion/sunday/dont-take-your-vitamins.html?pagewanted=all&_r=2&Revv
c. National Cancer Institute fact sheet: Antioxidant. (2013)
d. http://www.cancer.gov/cancertopics/factsheet/prevention/antioxidants

CHAPTER 43
KIDNEY DISEASE

Get the Facts

➢ Chronic Kidney Disease (CKD) is an epidemic in Australia with 13% having CKD.

➢ One in seven hospital admissions is from CKD.

➢ You can lose 95% of your kidney to disease before symptoms appear.

➢ Sugar is a major contributor to CKD.

Understand the Science

The kidneys are incredibly robust organs. Generally, there are few symptoms unless kidney functions fall to less than 5%, but when they do, the treatment has to be prompt or death occurs. CKD is a major public health problem. On the basis of clinical practice guidelines established by the National Kidney Foundation, 20m adults (about 13%) in the United States have CKD, with 8m of these classified as having moderate or severe kidney disease. In dialysis patients, cardiovascular disease (CVD) mortality rates are 10 to 30 times higher than in the general population. In high-risk patients, defined by the presence of either CVD or cardiovascular risk factors, less severe kidney disease is an independent risk for CVD. The numbers have increased three times since 1991. The Aboriginal community in Australia has the highest rate of CKD globally. It so happens that they also have the highest consumption globally per capita of Coca-Cola, but in fairness to this book, this is correlation and not causation.

The numbers in Australia in 2007 highlight that CKD is one of those huge costs in our increasingly toxic Standard American Diet.

• One in ten deaths were CKD related.

• Three times more were treated for CKD in 2007 than 1991.

• One in two cases are treated with dialysis.

- One in seven hospitalizations were for dialysis.

- Six times more indigenous Australians are treated for CKD than non-indigenous.

- One in three Australians have high blood pressure leading to 30% of CKD cases.

- One in 25 have diagnosed diabetes, causing 35% of CKD cases.

The causes for CKD aren't always known, but anything that damages blood vessels or other structures in the kidneys can lead to kidney disease. The most common cause of chronic kidney disease is diabetes. Diabetes causes about 35% of all chronic kidney disease. The high blood sugar levels caused by diabetes damage blood vessels in the kidneys, and if the blood sugar level remains high, this damage gradually reduces the function of the kidneys.

High blood pressure (hypertension) causes another 30% of all kidney disease. Because blood pressure often rises with chronic kidney disease, high blood pressure may further damage kidney function even when another medical condition initially caused the disease. Other conditions that can damage the kidneys and cause chronic kidney disease include polycystic kidney disease, pyelonephritis, glomerulonephritis, or a kidney problem with which you were born.

A narrowed or blocked renal artery can cause CKD, as the renal artery carries blood to the kidneys. Long-term use of certain medicines can damage blood vessels in the kidneys, including non-steroidal anti-inflammatory drugs (NSAIDs), such as ibuprofen (Advil) and celecoxib (Celebrex), and some antibiotics used by diabetics.

CKD is generally measured by how well the kidneys are dealing with the blood that flows through them. The measure used is a globular filtration rate (GFR), and normal rates are between 60 and 90 ml/min per 1.73 m². If there is chronic kidney disease values will be down from 60. Less than 15 is kidney failure. It is often indirectly measured by serum creatinine which is part of most standard blood tests. It may not always be accurate, but if your creatinine levels should be between 55 and 110 umol/L. If higher you may need to do further tests. When I took my base measurements prior to starting this program, my creatine levels were 115 to 120umol/L which is one reason for my lifestyle change.

So, while there are studies from the Framingham Study group of over 22,000 inclusions that CKD is a risk factor for CVD, the problem with experiments on humans is that ethically you cannot give people a diet that may give them CKD and consign them to a life on dialysis. It's difficult to see where you could recruit volunteers for such service to humanity. That sort of trial has to be done in animals. However, you can take people with existing CKD and see if low or high fructose makes any difference on other markers. That's what Brymora did with 28 patients with existing CKD. They switched from a regular 60g/day fructose to 12 g/day for six weeks and then back again for a further six weeks. In this small trial, they showed that low-fructose diets in patients with CKD reduced inflammation with some potential benefits on blood pressure. It was, however, only a six week trial.

But for trials which introduce fructose you have to look at animal studies. Gersch and the team from University of Florida took three groups of rats with 60% fructose, 60% Glucose, or standard rat chow over a six-week initial period and then continued for a further 11 weeks. All the measures of those on a high fructose diet were worse. Larger kidneys, worse glomerular sclerosis, tubular atrophy, tubular dilatation, and cellular infiltration rates, and increased monocyte chemo attractant protein-1 (MCP-1). The moderation in sugar proponents say these rates of fructose ingestion are out of all normality – just say that to my son when he was 16 and living on a diet of Coca-Cola and white bread. In hindsight, I wonder if his diet was even higher than 60% sugar!

Conclusion

Diet has damaging impacts on chronic kidney disease. The effects are more than just consequential from higher blood pressure and diabetes.

- Firstly, CKD is not dependent on blood pressure and diabetes, so even you don't have these, you can still have CKD.

- Secondly, high levels of fructose causes significant damages within six weeks in animals. What will six years or 60 years of exposure do?

- Thirdly, is there a safe level of consumption? We know damage can be irreversible, and may have an effect for the rest of your life. Given that the only remedy is consistent dialysis, or a scarce transplant, prevention seems the order of the day.

The prudent approach is to take-out fructose rich products from your diet to keep your fructose consumption under 30gm per day. One apple is about 14g of fructose, so 2 apples per day should a maximum.

References

a. Chronic Kidney Disease in Australia (2013). http://www.aihw.gov.au/chronic-kidney-disease/
b. Weiner D, Tighiouart H, Amin M, Stark P, MacLeod B, Griffith J, Salem D, Levey A, Sarnak M. (2005) Chronic Kidney Disease as a Risk Factor for Cardiovascular Disease and All-Cause Mortality: A Pooled Analysis of Community-Based Studies JASN vol. 15 (5) 1307-1315 doi: 10.1097/01.ASN.0000123691.46138.E2
c. Gersch M, Mu W, Cirillo P, Reungjui S, Zhang L, Roncal. C, Sautin YY, Johnson RJ, Nakagawa T. (2007) Fructose but not dextrose accelerates the progression of chronic kidney disease. Am J Physiol Renal Physiol. 293(4):F1256-61 PMID: 17670904
d. Brymora A, Flisiński M, Johnson R, Goszka G, Stefańska A, Manitius J. (2012) Low-fructose Diet Lowers Blood Pressure and Inflammation in Patients with Chronic Kidney Disease. Nephrol Dial Transplant. 2012;27(2):608-612

CHAPTER 44
DIABETES, METABOLIC SYNDROME, AND SSBS

Get the Facts

➢ Sugar consumption has a starring role in the development of hypertension, adverse lipid parameters, inflammation, and coronary vascular disease (CVD).

➢ One in three Australians have MetS (Metabolic Syndrome), the pre-cursor to diabetes and CVD.

➢ One in ten adults have diabetes which is about the same as breast cancer in women or prostate cancer in men.

➢ Over 371m have diabetes globally, with over 1m in Australia.

➢ If you consume one SSB (sugar sweetened beverage) per day, you have an 83% greater risk of diabetes or a 43% chance of MetS.

➢ Do not drink SSBs.

Understand the Science

Metabolic Syndrome (MetS) can still be blamed on eating too much and exercising too little, but it is crucial to understand why some foods are particularly harmful, and why some people gain more weight than others. In particular, part of this is due to high consumption of SSBs. One debate concerns the villainy of the glucose found in starches, and fructose found in fruits, table sugar, and, not surprisingly, high-fructose corn syrup. Diets with a high "glycaemic index" raise glucose levels in the blood and seem to promote metabolic problems.

One type of calorie may be metabolized differently than another. The effect of a particular diet depends on a person's genes and bacteria, and that person's bacteria are determined in part by their diet.

MetS, it seems, hinges on an intricate relationship between food, bacteria, and genetics.

If scientists can understand this relationship, they will illuminate one of the world's most current common ailments. In a previous chapter we discussed the scourge of SSBs, and a major consequence

269

of consuming SSBs is obesity. The other consequence is diabetes. In the meantime, eliminate SSBs and added sugar from the "Western diet" and a large percentage of the diabetes problem will disappear.

Diabetes

Diabetes is a major health issue in itself, with tiredness, increased thirst, frequent urination, and blurred vision. Diabetes goes broader than that as it is a risk factor for other diseases.

- Stroke. The risk is up to 4 times as likely.

- Blindness. Diabetes is the leading cause of blindness.

- Heart Attack. If you have diabetes, you have a 3 times more likely risk and with heart disease, 4 times as likely.

- Kidney Failure. Diabetes is a major cause of kidney failure, and kidney disease is 3 times more likely.

- It is the leading cause of non-traumatic lower limb amputations.

The American Heart Association says prevalence of diabetes for all age groups worldwide was estimated to be 2.8% in 2000 and is projected to be 4.4% in 2030. That's double! The diagnosed rate of diabetes in the USA was 5.1% for adults aged 20 or over back in 1998. The total number of people with diabetes is projected to rise from 171m in 2000 to 366m in 2030. Diabetes consumes about 10% of the UK NHS budget, and is similar in other countries. Diabetes is one of the major costs in health care and even if you don't have it, you are paying for others who do.

There are 3 forms of diabetes.

- Type 1 diabetes (also known as juvenile-onset diabetes) is where there is an absolute requirement for insulin in order to ensure survival. Type 1 is about 5% of cases

- Type 2 diabetes mellitus (T2DM) results from insulin resistance, a condition in which cells fail to use insulin properly, sometimes combined with an absolute insulin deficiency. This form was previously referred to as non-insulin-dependent diabetes mellitus (NIDDM) or "adult-onset diabetes." T2DM is 95% of all cases.

- A third form, gestational diabetes, occurs when pregnant women, without a previous diagnosis of diabetes, develop a high blood glucose level. It may precede development of T2DM and is often corrected after delivery of the baby.

In type 1 diabetes, immune cells are thought to destroy the pancreatic islet beta-cells that normally make insulin, thereby causing the disease, and in T2DM, the pancreatic hormone amylin is thought to adopt an unusual shape that renders it toxic to beta-cells that it probably destroys over a longer period.

As well as producing insulin, cells in the pancreas also produce the hormone amylin. Insulin and amylin normally work together to regulate the body's response to food intake. If they are no longer produced, then levels of sugar in the blood rise resulting in diabetes and causing damage to the heart, kidneys, eyes, and nerves if blood sugar levels aren't properly controlled.

However, some of the amylin that is produced can get deposited around cells in the pancreas as toxic clumps, which then, in turn, destroy those cells that produce insulin and amylin. The consequence of this cell death is diabetes. It was suspected that this was the causative mechanism in T2DM and research suggested type 1 diabetes results from the same mechanism. It was not until 2014 that research by Cooper confirmed both type 1 and T2DM are caused by the formation of toxic clumps of amylin.

Type 1 disease starts at an earlier age and progresses more rapidly compared to T2DM because there is more rapid deposition of toxic amylin clumps in the pancreas. The results, based on 20 years' work in New Zealand, suggest that type 1 and T2DM could both be slowed down and potentially reversed by medicines that stop amylin forming these toxic clumps. Another mechanism to avoid T2DM diabetes is through diet. The prevalence in adults throughout the world ranges from Iceland at 2 per thousand, to 10% in USA and Mexico. The incidence is strongly correlated with obesity. The trend is increasing. Australia has gone from 1.5% to over 4%.

The annual number of people with diabetes in Australia commencing
kidney dialysis or having a kidney transplant (1980-2009)

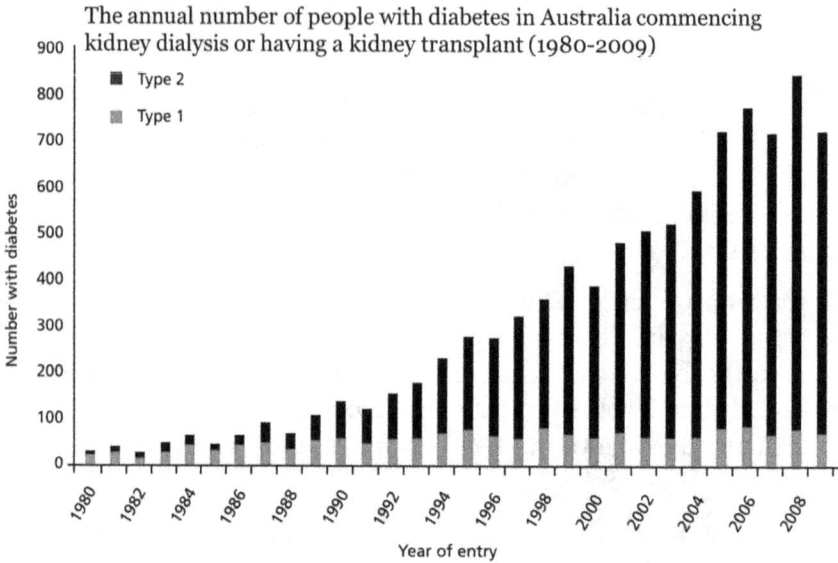

Figure 49 Kidney dialysis or transplants in Australia

Australian data as of June 2013 is similar to that in other obese
nations. The percentage of Type 1 diabetes has remained constant,
and all of the increase is from T2DM.

- About 1m have diabetes. Type 1 is 9%, 70% type 2, 9%
  gestational, and 11% unknown. The cost in Australia was $1.5b,
  or 2.3% of health expenditure.

- In 2011 there were 2,367 Type 1 new registrants, but 73,000 new
  T2DM registrants. Only 196 were aged under 15, and over
  55,000 under 35 years.

- Males make up a greater percentage with 56%, compared to
  females at 44%.

- Approximately 96% of people with diabetes are aged over 35,
  and 43 were aged over 65.

- Indigenous people have 4 times the rate of diabetes or high sugar
  levels than other Australians.

- Over 213,310 (23%) with T2DM require insulin to manage their
  diabetes, and it costs over $1.3b per year with 8.2m scripts.

- The annual healthcare costs of diabetes in Australia per person is between $8,000 and $16,698 depending on complications are micro or macro-vascular complications.

Diabetes incidence increases with age.

Australians diagnosed with diabetes by age group in 2007-2008 (Diabetes Australia)

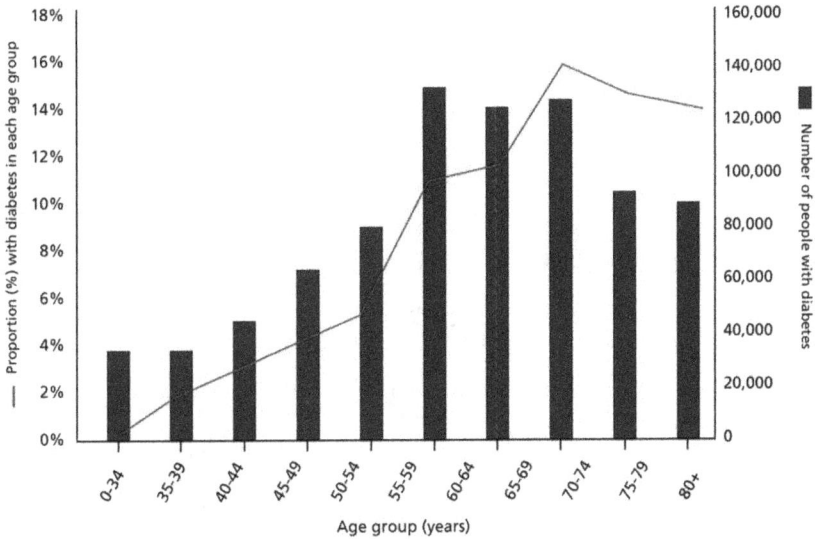

Figure 50 Age distribution of diabetes in Australia.

Very few people under 35 have diabetes and most are Type 1. T2DM seems to take time to get going. The great increase is between 50 and 65 years, and that corresponds with obesity increases. This next figure shows that the diagnosed diabetes is only about a third of those with un-diagnosed diabetes or MetS symptoms of impaired fasting glucose. (NHANES III study, as reported by Harris.)

So what is the relationship between SSBs and the risk of T2DM and MetS? The best indicators have been these same studies with large numbers and long follow-up. They have to be long term so that the disease symptoms (chronic disease etiology) actually appear. Most disease needs time between the cause, the disease initiation, and disease detection. Here are just four studies:

- 50,000 women, over eight years showed a 83% increased risk of T2DM if they drank ≥ 1 SSB per day compared with those consuming <1 SSB per month. BMI accounted for about half of the excess risk.

Prevalence of Diagnosed, and Un-diagnosed Diabetes and Impaired Fasting Glucose

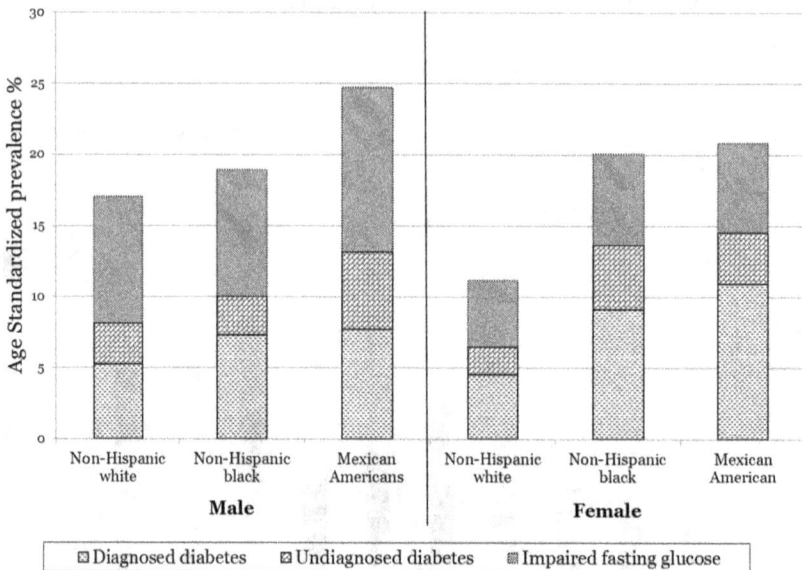

Figure 51 Diabetes and un-diagnosed from NHANES III Study

- 40,000 women over ten years (Black Women's Health) showed a 24% increased risk for those who drank > 1 SSB per day compared to those who consumed < 1 SSB per month. BMI accounted for the majority of effect.

- 70,000 over 18 years showed a 31% greater risk if they drank 2-3 SSBs per day, compared with those <1SSB per month. Because this study adjusted for BMI and total energy intake, both of which are potential mediators of effect, the association between SSB intake and T2DM risk may actually be underestimated.

- With a study of 12,204 men and women over nine years there was no correlation. (Atherosclerosis Risk in Communities Study). In this study participants were older and heavier than in other studies, and the BMI and age probably accounted for the lack of correlation.

- In the Framingham Offspring study with 6000 participants over four years, individuals who consumed ≥1 soft drink per day had a 39% greater risk of developing MetS over the course of four years than non-consumers. This analysis combined diet and regular soft drinks, and it can be assumed that the majority of this effect was due to regular soft drink consumption. Other studies of MetS have found marginal effects of SSBs, but since they adjusted for total energy intake, the results may have been underestimated.

Malik showed in his meta-analysis there is no risk of type 2 diabetes with less than 1 SSB per month. With 1 to 4 per month, the risk is up 6%. At greater than 1 per day, the risk is now up 80%. When Malik computes out the effect of increased BMI, the risk is still 40% higher. So when someone says a can of a sugar beverage a day is ok, the data says otherwise.

Metabolic Syndrome

Metabolic Syndrome (MetS) is the stage before T2DM. MetS is diagnosed when a number of metabolic abnormalities (including insulin resistance and obesity) occur at the same time in an individual. Individuals who have the syndrome are more likely to develop cardiovascular disease and T2DM than those who do not. MetS is defined by the International Diabetes Federation as: Central obesity, indicated by a waist circumference (ethnicity specific) plus any two of the following:

- Increased triglycerides.

- Increased high density cholesterol.

- High blood pressure.

- High fasting plasma glucose.

MetS is an alarmingly common health condition that occurs in some 20–25% of the world's population. In Australia, it is estimated that one in three people over the age of 25 years have Metabolic Syndrome. Individuals diagnosed with Metabolic Syndrome are up to three times more likely to develop cardiovascular health problems, and up to five times more likely to develop T2DM than individuals who do not have Metabolic Syndrome. The studies for MetS and SSB are in line with findings from studies evaluating T2DM.

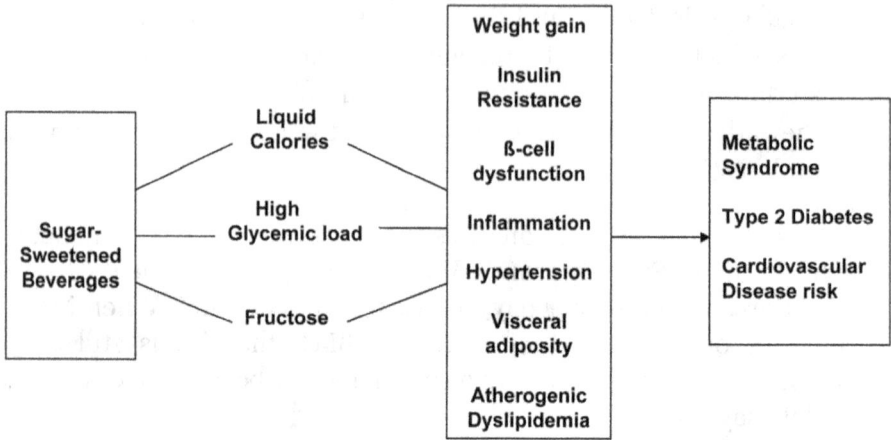

Figure 52 Biological mechanisms underlying the effect of consuming SSBs (Malik)

SSBs have multiple cascading effects and not just increased weight gain. SSBs increases weight. It is the other health risks which are more serious. The linkages between MetS and disease are clear. In Maliks diagram, he missed one of the other factors implicated in damage to health: caramel colouring. This produces advanced glycation end products (AGE) and it seems AGE is responsible for some of the type 2 diabetes seen in SSB drinkers. A single serving of cola provides 16.3 kU of AGEs, and increases insulin resistance and inflammation. The advice to switch from regular sodas to diet sodas looks like it ignores the role of AGE. Lastly, sodas generally have high levels of food acid as well as sugar. Sugar causes cavities, but food acid softens teeth enamel, and a consequence of that softening is more cavities.

Conclusion

Diabetes is a major health issue. Type 2 diabetes is costing billions of dollars annually, and as people age, they can look forward to a life on insulin and the associated high risk of cardiovascular disease and other diseases. There are large numbers of people with un-diagnosed diabetes, or impaired fasting glucose function. Independent of weight gain, SSBs, with their high fructose level and high glycaemic loading, increase the risk of MetS, T2DM, and cardio vascular disease. Furthermore, it does not take long to increase the risk of CVD. In just a few years the risk can be substantially higher and anyone who is overweight and in their early 30's needs to address the health risk then; not wait until their 50's. As the disease progresses from impaired fasting glucose function to type 2 diabetes, it may be too late to reverse the damage and they will spend the rest of their life on insulin.

There is only one conclusion from the research. Don't get type 2 diabetes. Just say "NO!" to caramel sodas – regular or diet. The risk is not minor and it is not about weight gain, but it is all about health.

References

a. Malik, V., Popkin, B., Bray, G., Despres, J., Hu, F. (2010) Sugar Sweetened Beverages, Obesity, Type 2 Diabetes and Cardiovascular Disease risk. Circulation. 23; 121(11): 1356–1364. doi: 10.1161/CIRCULATIONAHA.109.876185

b. Wikipedia Diabetes Mellitus http://en.wikipedia.org/wiki/Diabetes_mellitus

c. WHO. New Data highlight increases in hypertension, diabetes incidence. http://www.who.int/mediacentre/news/releases/2012/world_health_statistics_20120516/en/

d. Harris MI, Flegal KM, Cowie CC, Eberhardt MS, Goldstein DE, Little RR, Wiedmeyer HM, Bryd-Holt DD. (1998) Prevalence of diabetes, impaired fasting glucose, and impaired glucose tolerance in U.S. adults. The third National Health and Nutrition Examination Survey, 1988-1994. Diabetes Care 21(4):518-24.

e. Australian Institute of Health and Welfare (2014) http://www.aihw.gov.au/diabetes/

f. AIHW 2011. Diabetes prevalence in Australia: detailed estimates for 2007-08. Diabetes series no. 17. Cat. no. CVD 56. ISBN 978-1-74249-180-6

g. Diabetes Australia (2013) Diabetes: the Silent Pandemic and its impact on Australia. http://www.diabetesaustralia.com.au/

h. Schulze MB, Manson JE, Ludwig DS, Colditz GA, Stampfer MJ, Willett WC, Hu FB. (2008) Sugar-sweetened beverages weight gain and incidence of type 2 diabetes in young and middle-aged women. Jama 2004;292:927–934 doi: 10.2337/diacare.21.4.518

i. Palmer JR, Boggs DA, Krishnan S, Hu FB, Singer M, Rosenberg L. (2008) Sugar-sweetened beverages and incidence of type 2 diabetes mellitus in African American women. Arch Intern Med 2008;168:1487– 1492.

j. Liu S, Willett WC, Stampfer MJ, Hu FB, Franz M, Sampson L, Hennekens CH, Manson JE. (2000) A prospective study of dietary glycaemic load, carbohydrate intake, and risk of coronary heart disease in US women. Am J Clin Nutr 2000;71:1455–1461

CHAPTER 45
CARDIOVASCULAR DISEASE

Get the Facts

➢ The majority of cardiovascular disease (CVD) is preventable.
➢ CVD is both cardiac heart disease (CHD) and Ischaemic strokes.
➢ Manageable risk factors include high blood pressure, adverse lipid parameters, obesity, tobacco use, diabetes, depression and lack of exercise.
➢ Some risk factors such as age, gender and genetics cannot be changed.
➢ Stop fructose consumption if you want to be healthy and manage your weight.

Understand the Science

An estimated 17m people die of cardio vascular disease (CVD), particularly heart attacks (CHD) and strokes, every year. A substantial number of these deaths can be attributed to tobacco smoking, which increases the risk of dying from coronary heart disease and cerebrovascular disease 3-fold. Over 80% of the world's deaths from heart disease occur in low and middle-income countries. The top five countries with the highest rates of heart disease deaths are Russia, Bulgaria, Romania, Hungary, and Argentina, and the top five countries with the lowest rates are France, Australia, Switzerland, Japan, and Israel. The major risk factors (excluding tobacco) include:

● High blood pressure: 75% of people with chronic heart failure have high blood pressure. And half of adults with hypertension don't have it under control.

● High cholesterol: People with high cholesterol are twice as likely to develop heart disease as people with normal cholesterol levels.

● Diabetes: People with diabetes are 3 to 4 times likely to develop cardio vascular disease as people who don't have it.

- Depression: People with depression are 25% to 40% more likely to die from heart disease than people without depression.

- Obesity: Coronary artery disease is present ten times more often in people who are obese and have a BMI greater than 30.

The WHO put this into a chart. Over 300 risk factors have been associated with CHD and stroke. The major risks meet three criteria: high prevalence; significant independent impact on the risk; and treatment and control reduce the risk.

For coronary heart disease, the two risks are high cholesterol and elevated systolic blood pressure. The highest risk for ischaemic stroke is systolic blood pressure over 115 mmHg.

Note: Systolic blood pressure is the higher of the two blood pressure numbers. Normal is 120/80 mmHg. Pre-hypertension is 120 to 140, and high blood pressure is 140 to 160. Over 180 is emergency room!

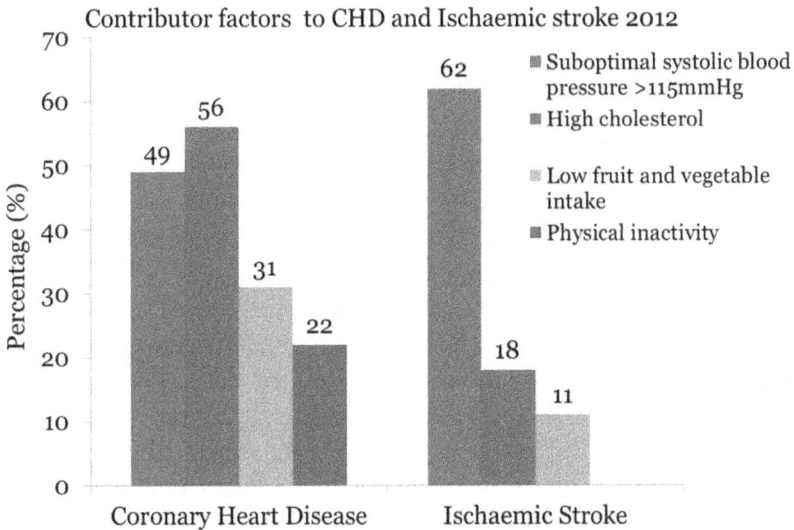

Figure 53 Consequences of Metabolic Syndrome (WHO)

Risk factors

You have to remember that when interpreting this information, the WHO and others have developed risk factors. Risk factors are not necessarily the cause. They are just risks.

- High blood pressure means you have a high risk of CVD. High blood pressure increases the risk of kidney disease and diabetes. High blood pressure is not an illness in itself - it increases risk of other illness. Why do you get high blood pressure? That is the interesting question, and there seems to be a range of reasons.

- Elevated cholesterol is a factor in CVD, but what increases cholesterol levels? In the discussion on cholesterol, there is some controversy about this linkage, and there are a range of complications.

- Weight is a risk factor. Why does obesity increase the risk of CVD?

- Why does exercise reduce the risk of CVD?

Researchers, such as Malik, have followed these studies to understand more fully what increases these risk factors. We know that one of the consequences of having Metabolic Syndrome (MetS) is the progression to either Diabetes or Cardiovascular Heart Disease (CVD). Various studies have looked at the relationship of sugar sweetened beverages (SSBs) to CVD – hypertension, lipids, and cholesterol. Malik showed your relative risk increased by 80% if you have more than 1 can of a SSB per day (adjusted for BMI).

The Framingham Offspring Study looked at SSB intake in the context of MetS components in over 6154 adults who were followed for four years, and found that individuals who consumed ≥ 1 soft drink per day had a 22% higher incidence of hypertension (≥ 135/85 mm hg or on treatment) compared to non-consumers. In the Nurses' Health Studies I and II, women who consumed ≥ 4 SSBs per day had a 44% or 28% higher risk of incidence of hypertension compared to infrequent consumers. The response to SSB for other CVD markers such as lipids follows the same trend with a 22% higher incidence of hypertriglyceridemia in the Framingham Study, and a 28% higher in the MESA Study (4000 people). LDL-cholesterol was worse compared to non-consumers in both studies. In the Nurses' Health Study tracking 88,000 women over 24 years, SSB intake ≥ 2 SSB per day had a 35% greater risk of CHD (nonfatal myocardial infarction or fatal cardiac heart disease). In the NHANES Study, adolescents' blood pressure and SSB intake were tracked in a ten-week intervention study comparing the effects of sucrose and artificially sweetened foods/beverages on markers of inflammation. The researchers found that serum levels of haptoglobin, transferrin, and C-reactive protein (CRP) increased in the sucrose group and decreased in the sweetener group.

The conclusion from these studies shows just one component of diet (a SSB) is strongly correlated with weight, with diabetes, with MetS, hypertension and cholesterol levels. Hypertension and cholesterol are the major risk factors for CVD. Lower them and you reduce the risks. There is an optimum level, so lower blood pressure and cholesterol to an optimum sweet spot of about 70-80mmHg. If the blood pressure is lower than 60 or above 110 the risks go back up.

Conclusion

When reviewing diet and Cardio Vascular Disease, the conclusions are pretty clear:

- Elevated blood pressure increases CVD. You get increased blood pressure from a variety of causes, including obesity.

- Increased SSB consumption is a significant factor, independent of weight gain, and it appears to be the sugar.

- SSB consumption over one per day is risky, creating somewhere between 25% and 45% increased risk of CVD.

- Consider SSB consumption on a par with tobacco. A can of soda might be much cheaper than a packet of cigarettes, but the risk of disease is similar.

Is it worth it? You would have to really crave these SSBs in your high-sacrifice value food groups to consider them. Consuming SSBs isn't as risky as using tobacco, but comes pretty close when you consider they are strongly associated with increased weight, increased diabetes risk, increased MetS and increased CVD. Find alternatives, but not fruit juices because of the fructose. My tactic is to drink water, tea, coffee, or a lower alcohol beer.

References

a. Maier, R. (2014) Heart disease statistics. http://www.healthline.com/health/heart-disease/statistics
b. WHO Cardio Vascular Disease (2014) http://www.who.int/cardiovascular_diseases/en/cvd_atlas_03_risk_factors.pdf
c. Dhingra R, Sullivan L, Jacques PF, Wang TJ, Fox CS, Meigs JB, D'Agostino RB, Gaziano JM, Vasan RS. (2007) Soft drink consumption and risk of developing cardio metabolic risk factors and the metabolic syndrome in middle-aged adults in the community. Circulation. 2007;116:480–488.

d. Winkelmayer WC, Stampfer, MJ, Willett WC, Curhan GC. (2005) Habitual caffeine intake and the risk of hypertension in women.Jama.294:2330–2335.

e. Nguyen S, Choi HK, Lustig RH, Hsu CY. (2009) Sugar-sweetened beverages, serum uric acid, and blood pressure in adolescents.J   Pediatr.2009;154:807–813.[PMC   free article][PubMed]

f. Sorensen LB, Raben A, Stender S, Astrup A. (2005) Effect of sucrose on inflammatory markers in overweight humans.Am J Clin Nutr.2005;82:421–427.[PubMed]

g. Schulze MB, Hoffmann K, Manson JE, Willett WC, Meigs JB, Weikert C, Heidemann C, Colditz GA, Hu FB. (2005) Dietary pattern, inflammation, and incidence of type 2 diabetes in women.Am J Clin Nutr.2005;82:675–684.quiz 714-675.

h. Liu S, Manson JE, Buring JE, Stampfer MJ, Willett WC, Ridker PM. (2002) Relation between a diet with a high glycaemic load and plasma concentrations of high-sensitivity C-reactive protein in middle-aged women.Am J Clin Nutr.2002;75:492–498.[PubMed]

i. Fung TT, Malik V, Rexrode KM, Manson JE, Willett WC, Hu FB. (2009) Sweetened beverage consumption and risk of coronary heart disease in women.Am J Clin Nutr.2009;89:1037–1042.

j. Malik V, Popkin B, Bray G, Després JP, Hu F. (2010) Sugar Sweetened Beverages, Obesity, Type 2 Diabetes and Cardiovascular Disease risk Circulation. 121(11): 1356–1364. doi: 10.1161/CIRCULATIONAHA.109.876185

CHAPTER 46
THYROID AND WEIGHT LOSS

Get the Facts

➤ Many overweight individuals have the majority of the symptoms that are associated with a hypothyroid-like condition.

➤ The symptoms are more common for those with a history of yo-yo dieting or who have difficulty losing weight by cutting back on calories and trying to exercise more.

➤ Inactive thyroids (or "sluggish thyroid") are more likely to be the result of being over-weight. Not the cause.

Understand the Science

Thyroid and weight loss is an active area of research; for many women, the term "sluggish thyroid" is used as an attribution for poor weight loss success, lack of energy, and general ill health. As we will discover, this is probably the result of weight and diet. Rather than try to address the issues with medication, diet and weight loss may be the remedy. Celebrities such as Oprah have publicized sluggish thyroid conditions, and there are plenty of potions and pills on the internet to "get your thyroid working again."

Most thyroid complications are associated with autoimmune disorders. Autoimmune disorders can affect nearly every organ and system of the body and there are over 80 ranging from mild to debilitating diseases. Some autoimmune disorders include:

• Diabetes (Type I) affects the pancreas.

• Thyroid diseases including Graves' disease, Hashimoto's disease and other thyroid complaints. Symptoms vary but can include weight loss without dieting, elevated heart rate, anxiety and diarrhoea.

- Inflammatory bowel disease which includes ulcerative colitis and possibly, Crohn's disease. Symptoms include diarrhoea and abdominal pain.

- Multiple sclerosis affects the nervous system. Depending on which part of the nervous system is affected, symptoms can include numbness, paralysis and vision impairment.

- Psoriasis affects the skin. Features include the development of thick, reddened skin scales.

- Rheumatoid arthritis affects the joints. Symptoms include swollen and deformed joints. The eyes, lungs and heart may also be targeted.

- Scleroderma affects the skin and other structures, causing the formation of scar tissue. Features include thickening of the skin, skin ulcers and stiff joints.

- Systemic lupus erythematosus affects connective tissue and can strike any organ system of the body. Symptoms include joint inflammation, fever, weight loss and a characteristic facial rash.

The thyroid gland is situated at the front of the throat, below the larynx (Adam's apple), and comprises two lobes that lie on either side of the windpipe and looks like a butterfly. The thyroid gland secretes hormones to regulate many metabolic processes, including growth and energy expenditure. The thyroid gland itself is controlled by the pituitary which is turn is controlled by the hypothalamus in the brain.

If the thyroid gland is overactive or sluggish, metabolism appears to be affected, leading to a variety of symptoms that are easily misdiagnosed. Around one in 20 people will experience some form of thyroid dysfunction in their lifetime. Women are more susceptible than men. Common problems include over-activity (hyperthyroidism) and under-activity (hypothyroidism) of the thyroid gland. Common causes of thyroid disorders are Hashimoto's Disease and Grave's Disease, and enlargement of the thyroid gland is a "goitre". The thyroid gland produces two primary hormones – thyroxin (referred to as T4), and tri-iodothyronine (referred to as T3). The numbers 3 and 4 refer to the number of atoms of iodine in the hormones. Iodine is essential for the production of thyroid hormones and humans need about 150 ug (millionths of a gram) each day. Iodine is found in most foods, iodized salt, and especially seafood.

Of the two hormones produced, T3 is more active than T4, but is produced in much smaller quantities. T4 has a lesser effect, but most is converted to T3 by enzymes that remove one iodine atom. The greater the amount of T3 and T4 circulating in the blood, the faster the metabolism. Lower amounts of T3 and T4 result in a reduced metabolism.

The control process is:

- The hypothalamus prompts the pituitary gland to make a chemical called thyroid-stimulating hormone (TSH).

- The pituitary gland checks the amount of T4 and T3 in the blood and releases TSH if the T4 and T3 levels need to be topped up.

- It is thought that the thyroid gland secretes T4 and T3 depending on the "order" it receives from the pituitary gland but generally speaking, the more TSH the thyroid receives, the more T4 and T3 it secretes.

Hashimoto's Disease, also known as Hashimoto's thyroiditis, chronic lymphocytic thyroiditis, or autoimmune thyroiditis, is a common cause of hypothyroidism (underactive thyroid), but is the result of an autoimmune condition. Immune system cells attack the thyroid gland, causing inflammation. This inflammation reduces the thyroid's ability to make hormones.

A great deal of confusion has existed among patients and the medical community regarding the precise role that thyroid hormones play in obesity. This is partly because thyroid lab tests often don't correlate with the patient's hypothyroid symptoms. I.e. The patient is complaining, yet the lab tests seem okay or not too far off. And it is partly because many people who are normal weight or underweight also have hypothyroid-like symptoms or clear cut hypothyroidism by lab test. Researchers now believe that even small elevations in TSH (thyroid stimulating hormone), rather than indicating a looming thyroid problem, can actually predict an emerging leptin and insulin problem associated with weight gain. It was found that when weight was lost, TSH scores returned to normal. Another study showed very clearly that leptin-driven weight gain actually inflames the thyroid gland and induces thyroid auto-antibodies to form. Thyroid auto-antibodies levels returned to normal when weight was lost.

The picture is murky when you look at Hashimoto's Disease, which traditionally was thought to be a result of autoimmune disease. Radetti and a team from Italy, looked at 137 obese or overweight children and compared them with normal weight children. They got both. Some children showed alterations of thyroid structure and function but no autoimmune involvement, while others did show changes of thyroid function and structure, suggestive of Hashimoto's Thyroiditis, but no thyroid autoimmunity. There must be other things going on. There are anecdotal accounts that some of this confusion is due to diet. Some have found that eliminating sugar from their diet fixes the thyroid condition, even with Hashimoto's Disease.

Visini and others systematically reviewed over 329 articles regarding clinical, experimental, and pathophysiological data on the relationship between obesity, adipokines – namely leptin, adiponectin, resistin, visfatin – and various immune-mediated conditions, including rheumatoid arthritis (RA), systemic lupus erythematosus (SLE), inflammatory bowel disease (IBD), multiple sclerosis (MS), type 1 diabetes (T1D), psoriasis and psoriatic arthritis (PsA), and thyroid autoimmunity (TAI), especially Hashimoto Thyroiditis (HT).

Obesity is a conclusive risk for rheumatoid arthritis, MS, psoriasis and PsA, and implicated strongly for Irritable Bowel, Type 1 diabetes, and thyroid autoimmunity. In other words, obesity may not be the whole cause, but part of the cause of these diseases. Moreover, obesity worsens the course of RA, SLE, IBD, psoriasis and PsA, and impairs the treatment response of RA, IBD, psoriasis and PsA. All the extensive clinical data and experimental models show adipokines are involved in these autoimmune diseases.

Conclusion

What is the overriding conclusion from current research? Obesity appears to be a major environmental factor contributing to the onset and progression of autoimmune diseases. Within those 329 studies there will be a range of complications, but if there is one take home from the science it is to reduce weight. Gut bacteria are also very much involved in autoimmune diseases, and treatment of autoimmune diseases has been successful using techniques such as faecal implants to modify populations of gut bacteria an effective treatment especially for irritable bowel syndrome.

It appears convenient to blame a sluggish thyroid for inability to reduce weight when dieting. It is more probable a sluggish thyroid is the result of excess weight, and not the cause. Our biology is exceedingly complex so it is simplistic to blame one thing, such as the thyroid, for failure of weight management and obesity.

References

a. Versini M, Jeandel JP, Rosenthal E, Shoenfel Y. (2014) Obesity in autoimmune diseases: Not a passive bystander. Autoimmunity Reviews. DOI: 10.1016/j.autrev.2014.07.001
b. Richards B. (2013) Leptin, Thyroid, and Weight Loss http://www.wellnessresources.com/weight_tips/articles/leptin _thyroid_and_weight_loss
c. Radetti G, Kleon W, Buzi F, Crivellaro C, Pappalardo L, di Iorgi N, Maghnie M. (2008)Thyroid Function and Structure Are Affected in Childhood Obesity Volume 93(12) doi: http://dx.doi.org/10.1210/jc.2008-0823

CHAPTER 47
CANCER AND DIET

Get the Facts

➤ Some forms of cancer are preventable through diet and lifestyle.

➤ Most forms of cancer are "bad luck" and risk factors such as age, gender and genetics cannot be changed.

➤ More than 42% of cancers could be prevented by changes in lifestyle.

➤ The take-out diet addresses the known risks for cancer.

Understand the Science

Cancer is a generic term for a large group of diseases that can affect any part of the body. Other terms used are malignant tumours and neoplasms. One defining feature of cancer is the rapid creation of abnormal cells that grow beyond their usual boundaries, and which can then invade adjoining parts of the body and spread to other organs, the latter process is referred to as metastasizing. Metastases are the major cause of death from cancer. Cancer is a leading cause of death worldwide, accounting for 8.2 million deaths in 2012 The most common causes of cancer death are cancers of:

- lung (1.59 million deaths)

- liver (745 000 deaths)

- stomach (723 000 deaths)

- colorectal (694 000 deaths)

- breast (521 000 deaths)

- oesophageal cancer (400 000 deaths)

In comparison with other causes of death, here are the figures from 1900 to 1990 in the USA.

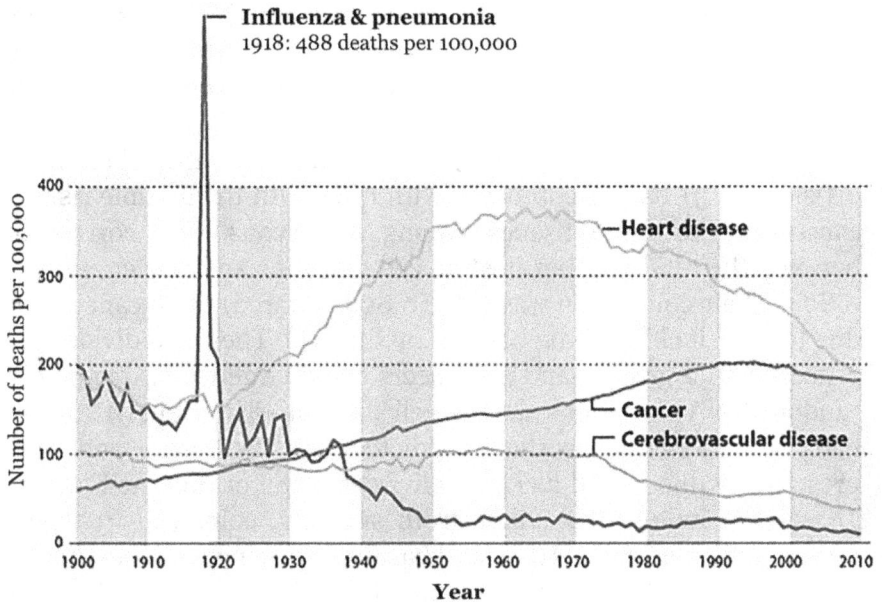

Figure 54 USA Mortality rates 1900 to 2009

The data comes from Jones, and the infographic from R Toro. In 1900, the leading cause of death was influenza and pneumonia, but the introduction of antibiotics and vaccines saw that drop and since 1950 it is a minor cause. Death from cancer has increased up to 2000, but has since decreased. This may because there is earlier diagnosis and better treatments. Heart disease has fallen possibly because of better treatment. These figures have to be viewed with some discretion, as we just don't know whether the cause of death was correctly diagnosed correctly in 1900.

What causes cancer?

Cancer arises from one single cell. The transformation from a normal cell into a tumour cell is a multistage process, typically a progression from a pre-cancerous lesion to malignant tumours. Cancer arises when tissue-specific stem cells make random mistakes, or mutations, when one chemical letter in DNA is incorrectly swapped for another during the replication process in cell division. The more these mutations accumulate, the higher the risk that cells will grow unchecked, a hallmark of cancer. These changes are the result of the interaction between a person's genetic factors and three categories of external agents, including physical, chemical and biological carcinogens.

289

In early 2015, Tomasetti and Vogelstein from the Johns Hopkins Kimmel Cancer Center created a statistical model that measures the proportion of cancer incidence, across many tissue types, caused mainly by random mutations that occur when stem cells divide. They analysed data from other research on the number of stem cell divisions in 31 tissues compared with rates with the lifetime risks of cancer in the same tissues among Americans. The correlation between the total number of stem cell divisions and cancer risk was 0.804. Their conclusion was 65% (0.804 squared) of all cancers are due to "bad luck" and the balance by lifestyle. They also divided the cancers into 2 groups, and 22 cancers could largely be explained by random DNA mutations during cell division. The other 9 cancers had incidences higher than predicted by "bad luck" and were presumably due to bad luck and environmental or inherited factors. These 9 included lung cancer from smokers, colorectal (3 types), thyroid follicular, HPV, HCV, and basal cell carcinoma. Note this is a correlation analysis but it does confirm that generally most researchers previously proposed the link between cancer and diet is no more than 30 to 40%. This may be so in the research world, but are there other factors?

The question remains: does diet and health change what happens after a random mutation occurs? In an overweight, sedentary person, is that mutation more likely turn into a cancer than if you are not overweight, fit and have a good diet? Even more broadly, what is the mechanism for dealing with a mutation and remaining cancer free?

Diet and Cancer

Specific links between diet and cancer are tenuous for most cancers. In the 1990's it became popular from the epidemiological studies to implicate diet with increased cancer rates, but we now know there are few such links. Lung cancer for smokers or colorectal cancers are exceptions. The World Cancer Research Fund and the American Institute for Cancer Research carry out ongoing reviews for colorectal cancers with over 1000 papers cited and their most recent findings are:

- Physical activity protects.
- Consumption of red meat, processed meat increases rates of cancer.
- Alcohol increases rates.

- Body fatness and abdominal fatness increase rates.

- Consumption of garlic, milk and calcium probably protect.

- Limited evidence that non-starchy vegetables and fruits protect.

- Limited evidence foods containing sugar and fructose increases rates.

- Supplements / vitamins / "super-foods" have little or no effect.

Colorectal cancer is one of the easiest cancers to diagnose, and easy to treat if diagnosed early. Some countries, including Australia, have taken steps to implement national screening programs. There is less evidence for most other cancers. Alcohol and tobacco do cause cancers. Those who are overweight or obese seem to be at higher risk, but the reasons are not clear. Is obesity the cause? Is it the type of food overweight people eat? Do overweight people do more sitting and less physical exercise? Most Cancer Councils say a correct lifestyle would prevent 40% of all cancer cases. UK data says cancer could be prevented by not smoking (19% of new cases per year), healthy weight (5%), eating fruit and vegetables (5%), less alcohol (4.6%), be sun smart (3%), eat less processed red meat (3%), or being active (1%). Some cancers such as prostate don't appear preventable, whereas lung cancer from smoking is more than 89% preventable, and melanoma 86%. Occupational exposure prevention was 4.9%. The lifestyle therefore is not smoking, keeping a healthy body weight, cutting back on alcohol, keeping active, a healthy diet, staying safe in the sun, and avoiding infections such as HPV.

Less than 3% of people know that being overweight increases cancer risks. The direct relationship between diet and cancer is at most 30%.

Conclusion

The direct relationship between diet and cancer is at most 30% except for a couple of specific cancers and cancer agents such as alcohol. We get mutations in our genes. Some give rise to cancers. Others don't. No-one yet has found why stem cells turn cancerous, or how our body deals with them normally. Nor do we know conclusively what can be done to prevent this happening. Some propose inflammation sets off cancer, but how and how much is unclear. If 35% of cancer is environmental, and not "bad luck" what is needed to minimize that risk. For me, I won't reduce red meat consumption. I have taken-out simple carbohydrates, taken-out added sugar and reduced alcohol consumption. I eat more complex carbohydrates and more whole food. I don't bother to take supplements or super-foods. Intermittent fasting may have some value. I try to do some additional exercise. Lastly I make sure I get regular screening for bowel cancer, prostate cancer, skin cancer and an annual general check-up.

References

a. WHO (2014) Fact Sheet No 297 http://www.who.int/mediacentre/factsheets/fs297/en/
b. UK Cancer Council (2014) Statistics on preventable cancers. http://www.cancerresearchuk.org/cancer-info/cancerstats/causes/preventable/
c. Parkin DM, Boyd L, Walker LC. (2011). The fraction of cancer attributable to lifestyle and environmental factors in the UK in 2010. Summary and conclusions. Br J Cancer 2011;105 (S2):S77-S81. doi:10.1038/bjc.2011.489
d. Tomasetti, C, Vogelstein, B. (2015) Variation in cancer risk among tissues can be explained by the number of stem cell divisions. Science 347 (6217) p.78-81 DOI: 10.1126/science.1260825
e. Jones, D, Podolsky, S, Greene, JA. (2012) The Burden of Disease and the Changing Task of Medicine. Engl J Med 2012; 366:2333-2338 DOI: 10.1056/NEJMp1113569
f. Nilsson LM, Winkvist, A, Johansson I, Lindahl, B, Hallmans G, Lenner P, Van Guelpen B. (2013)Low-carbohydrate, high-protein diet score and risk of incident cancer; a prospective cohort study. Nutr J. 7;12:58. doi: 10.1186/1475-2891-12-58.
g. WCRF/AICR. Colorectal Cancer 2011 Report. http://www.dietandcancerreport.org/cancer_resource_centre/downloads/cu/Colorectal-Cancer-2011-Report.pdf
h. Donaldson M. (2004) Nutrition and cancer: A review of the evidence for an anti-cancer diet. Nutrition J 3:19 doi:10.1186/1475-2891-3-19 http://www.nutritionj.com/content/3/1/19

CHAPTER 48
STATINS AND CHOLESTEROL

Get the Facts

➤ Coronary Vascular Disease (CVD) is the leading cause of death.

➤ Nearly 40 years ago, research showed the risk of CVD and levels of cholesterol were correlated.

➤ Latest research has shown this association to be bad science and false. There is no correlation.

➤ Diets were implicated, as well as smoking and lifestyle, but taking a pill is an easy solution. Doctors and drug companies thought so, too.

➤ The drug class of statins was developed to reduce cholesterol levels, which they do.

➤ There is evidence that statins are most effective for CVD as a secondary prevention strategy. They have questionable benefits (i.e. don't work) in those with elevated cholesterol levels but without previous CVD.

➤ The protective mechanism may not be the lowering of cholesterol per se, but reduction in other enzymes.

➤ Drug companies have pushed statins even to those with moderate cholesterol over the past ten years. Ten years ago, they were 88% over-prescribed, and use has now gone up six times.

➤ Many argue the focus on cholesterol reduction with statins has been misguided, very expensive, ineffective, and the real culprit is the increased diet of simple carbohydrates; and in particular fructose consumption.

➤ The cheapest way to reduce CVD? Take-Out fructose and reduce take-out simple carbohydrates!

➤ Another cheap way to reduce CVD is to eat an apple every day.

Understand the Science

This whole area of cholesterol, heart disease, drug use (statins), and dietary advice is complicated and divisive. Like me, you may be left confused about what the reality is, and what the best health strategies are. Is there a right and wrong? Coronary Vascular Disease (CVD) is also called Coronary Artery Disease (CAD), Atherosclerotic Heart Disease, Coronary Heart Disease (CHD) or Coro or ischemic heart disease (IHD).

CVD is the most common type of heart disease, the cause of heart attacks, and is the biggest cause of death in the world. Symptoms include angina and heart attacks.

The disease is caused by plaque building up along the inner walls of the arteries of the heart, which narrows the arteries and reduces blood flow to the heart. Causes include genetics, smoking (54% of cases), hypertension, diabetes, and obesity (20% of cases). Treatment is with angioplasty (stents), bypass surgery, or medication. Conventional prevention is drugs (statins), lifestyle, diet, and exercise.

The statin class of drugs lowers cholesterol levels by inhibiting the enzyme HMG-CoA reductase, which plays a central role in the production of cholesterol in the liver. Statins lower the level of LDL cholesterol (bad) and increase HDL cholesterol (good), and cut the number of plaques that form in the arteries. Statin drugs include simvastatin, atorvastatin, fluvastatin, lovastatin, pitavastatin, pravastatin, and rosuvastatin. Like all drugs, they have side effects. Simvastatin and pravastatin appear to have fewer and less severe side effects. The best-selling statin is atorvastatin, which in 2003 became the best-selling pharmaceutical in history, with Pfizer reporting sales of $12.4b in 2008.

Statins are promoted as being effective in decreasing mortality in people with pre-existing CVD. They are also currently advocated for use in patients at high risk of developing heart disease. On average, statins can lower LDL cholesterol by 1.8 mmol/l (70 mg/dl), which translates into an estimated 60% decrease in the number of cardiac events (heart attack, sudden cardiac death) and a 17% reduced risk of stroke after long-term treatment. The causes of this have been unclear, but recent studies say this effect is not from reducing cholesterol, but through other processes.

Ten years ago in Canada, a study concluded that practices for prescribing statins need to be realigned with more recent research evidence. This study showed that 88% of patients should not have been prescribed statins. Women and the elderly should not have been prescribed the drugs. Drug use should be directed towards men with CVD. Ten years later, little has changed. The ABC Australia (Oct. 2013) ran two Catalyst documentaries questioning the worth of statin prescriptions. Women suffer 300% less heart disease than men, in spite of having higher average cholesterol levels. As far back as 1992, Jacobs showed there was absolutely no relationship between total cholesterol levels and mortality from CVD as analysed over 11 major studies with over 125,000 women in those studies. And none since.

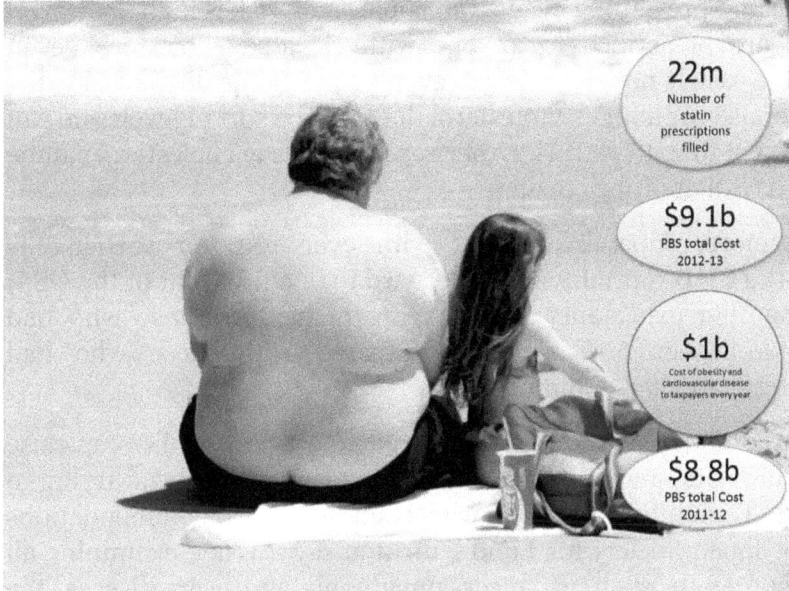

Figure 55 Statin Use and Health Costs in Australia

In Australia, obesity and cardiovascular disease cost taxpayers nearly $1b a year in medication alone. The two most-prescribed statin drugs on the Australian Pharmaceutical Benefit Scheme were atorvastatin ($0.46b with a government contribution of $0.4b), and rosuvastatin ($0.7b with a government contribution of $0.6b). Another statin, simvastatin, appeared 12th on the list and cost taxpayers $0.1b. In 1995, 5% of people over 45 were prescribed statins and by 2013 it was 30% which is a staggering 22 million scripts! The PBS scheme in total runs to $9.1b, so nearly 10% of the health budget is poured into this drug.

University of NSW Professor of Clinical Pharmacology, Prof Day, said the figures were symptomatic of a sedentary culture, rising obesity, and poor nutritional choices. *"They get a pill to fix it up easy, while not making any changes to their lives. There was no doubt that many Australians had been prescribed statins needlessly, as their total risk of heart disease was not high. Statins are even over-prescribed for young people. If the only risk factor for Cardiovascular Disease is higher cholesterol, you could argue statins are not the answer."*

On the prescription side, it is true that cardiovascular disease is the most prevalent disease in our community, and takes the lives of about half the people who die. Statins have been shown to be very effective in reducing recurrent events in people with known vascular disease, and preventing events in people when risk is high. However, statins are prescribed to anyone with elevated cholesterol, even when the case is not clear. What level is safe? Some doctors, say diet and exercise cannot get cholesterol down to the sort of levels you can get it down to with statins. Other researchers say cholesterol can be reduced with appropriate diet.

Furthermore, Japanese studies with over 160,000 participants found the CHD mortality rate one third to one fifth that of the USA, and that life expectancy was 5 years higher for those who had cholesterol over 6.18 mmol/l compared with those who had cholesterol about 3.18 mmol/l.

This is yet another example where epidemiological studies can raise intriguing data, and leaves scientists scratching their head trying to explain. Tomohito Hamazaki who compiled the recommendations for The Japan Society for Lipid Nutrition says "When examining all causes of death, such as cancer, pneumonia and heart disease, the number of deaths attributable to LDL cholesterol levels exceeding 3.62mmol/l is less than people with lower LDL cholesterol levels."

I don't think the issue is clear cut. There are complications to this cholesterol/statin story. White in 2013, reported on the longest and largest study of CVD (Australian research) and followed over 9000 patients who had a medical history presenting angina or heart attack (myocardial infarction or ischemic events). As they say in their study, one of the causes of CVD is plaques. Plaques come in hard and soft forms, and stick to the inside of the artery. When they break off and float away, they cause heart attacks, or worse, strokes. Elevated levels of the enzyme Lipoprotein associated phospholipase A2 (Lp-PLA$_2$) levels, are associated with CVD risk in both healthy individuals and in patients who have had angina or heart attacks. Products of Lp-PLA$_2$ are found in plaques and are pro-inflammatory and pro-apoptotic (rapid cell death). Lp-PLA$_2$ is also a marker of vulnerable plaques. Cholesterol levels were between 4.0 to 7.0 mmol/L so they weren't particularly high. After one year, 6500 patients were event free (i.e. no CVD). The researchers followed 7863 patients over the next six years, and the results suggest it is not the cholesterol lowering reduction from the statins that reduced further CVD, but it is the reduction of the Lp-PLA$_2$. Lower Lp-PLA$_2$ accounted for over 60% of lower CVD, and statin effect on cholesterol reduction was less than 10%. So it comes back to this inflammation reduction story. Stop taking statins unless you are at risk of CVD.

The continuing message from the medical fraternity is "take a pill." It is not "drop the fork," or more importantly, change what you eat. Animal study data shows diet is very effective in reducing inflammation. There are many kinds of inflammation, so a sweeping generalization that fructose and polyunsaturated oils cause inflammation has to be viewed carefully, and the pathways have to be understood. Current research is showing the very things that the medical profession say you should eat more of, such as "balanced carbohydrates," and polyunsaturated oils, are possibly the absolute opposite of what is needed. The warning signs are there. The Australian Heart Foundations currently focuses on fat as cause of heart disease, whereas there is ample evidence that sugar is the major contributor.

Patients on intermittent fasting (including the 5:2 Diet) show reductions of one to two whole points of cholesterol. The levels ofLp-PLA$_2$ do not appear to have been studied with this diet, but it seems like a good research project.

How do Statins Work?

Cholesterol is produced by cells as part of our normal processes. Statins inhibit an enzyme in this process, reducing the level of mevalonate, and reducing cholesterol. But this process is pretty important, and other processes that rely on mevalonate are also blocked.

Side Effects

There are side effects with statins, as complications are part of drug use. Drugs are registered/approved if they are safe (i.e. cause no major side effects), and benefits outweigh complications. Chemotherapy drugs, for example, cause severe side effects, but cancer is slowed. When statins were first introduced, it was believed high cholesterol caused cardiovascular disease, and as statins reduced cholesterol, the benefits outweighed any side effects. Side effects include myositis, or inflammation of the muscles; elevated levels of CPK or creatine kinase which causes mild inflammation and muscle weakness; and rarely, rhabdomyolysis or extreme muscle inflammation and damage.

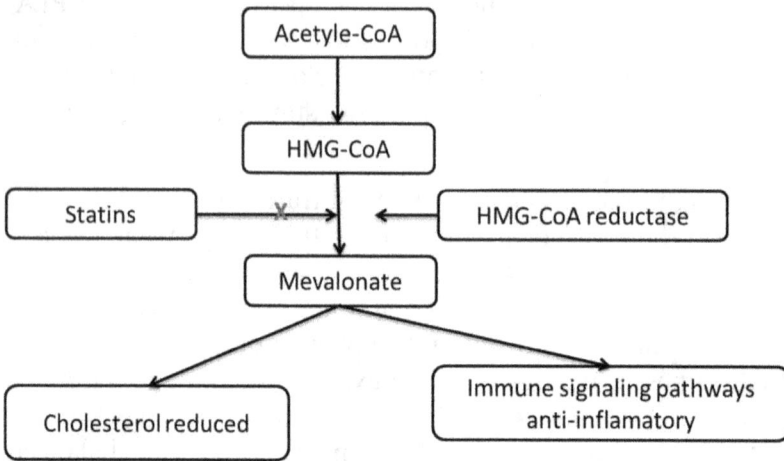

Figure 56 Statin Actions

Are Current Risk Factors Correct?

In December 2013, Silverman, looking at the Multi-Ethnic Study of Atherosclerosis (the MESA study), suggested millions of patients put on the medications were being "over treated," exposing them to potential side effects, while other patients were more likely to suffer a heart attack were not targeted. Most patients are put on statins because they have high cholesterol, high blood pressure, or other conditions such as diabetes. But the study of almost 6700 adults found that the risk factors were not an accurate way of predicting the likelihood of a heart attack or a stroke. The Corona artery calcium score (CAC) provides a direct measure of calcium deposits in heart arteries and is easily obtained on a computed tomography (CT) scan. These scans were far better at identifying patients who would suffer a cardiac event. Thirty-five percent of those who were assessed as "very high risk" using conventional screening tools actually had an extremely low chance of having a heart attack. Meanwhile, 15% of those who were told they had a very low chance of such an event, in fact, were at far higher risk, which was indicated by high levels of calcium in the arteries.

According to Nasir, the senior author, the results may encourage a major paradigm shift in how physicians estimate heart disease risk for their patients. "Our study shows that coronary artery calcium testing holds promise as a frontline assessment for people before they develop heart disease symptoms. In the meantime, we believe that doctors should consider offering a coronary artery calcium scan to their patients to markedly improve risk prediction if they are unsure whether they should be on lifelong statin and aspirin therapy."

Statins are Cost Effective

There is reasonable justification for some use of statins. In the West of Scotland Coronary Prevention Study (WOSCOPS) 6500 patients were followed. Some of the men, without a history of myocardial infarction, took statins for 5 years. The researchers tracked the impact on healthcare resource utilization, costs, and quality of life over 15 years. They estimated the 5 years of treatment with pravastatin (40 mg/day) saved the NHS £710,000 per 1000 people, including the cost of pravastatin and lipid and safety monitoring, and gained 136 quality-adjusted life-years (QALYs) over the 15-year period. Benefits per 1000 subjects, attributable to prevention of cardiovascular events, included 163 fewer admissions and a saving of 1836 days in hospital, with 31% fewer admissions for myocardial infarction, stroke, heart failure, and coronary revascularization. There was no excess in non-cardiovascular admissions or costs (or in admissions associated with diabetes or its complications), and no evidence of heterogeneity of effect over sub-groups defined by baseline cardiovascular risk.

Their conclusion was that five years' primary prevention treatment of middle-aged men with a statin significantly reduced healthcare resource utilization, was cost saving, and increased QALYs. They went on to say treatment of even younger, lower risk individuals is likely to be cost-effective, but there is no data to support this supposition. This study has to be viewed like all studies: did the study itself cause an outcome? Intervention through a trial with double blind controls can affect the outcomes. Maybe this was simply the outcome of effective primary health care?

Is the Target for Reduction of LDL Cholesterol Correct?

The widely held view is that LDL is the evil cholesterol, and that HDL is good. This has recently been found to be half true, or half false. It's too detailed in this book to go to the absolute science, but let's follow this a little more.

Cholesterol does not exist in the blood as cholesterol. It is an oil, which is not soluble in water (i.e. the blood) so it has to get around with a lipoprotein surface coating – in the same way "dish washing detergent cuts through grease." It emulsifies it. In the biological world, think of the lipoprotein as the ship, and the cholesterol the cargo. Big ships (HDL) and small ships (LDL). It also turns out the size of the cargo is also important. Think of a bucket of tennis balls, or the same size bucket, but now full of golf balls. The bucket is the same size, and the current cholesterol test measures the bucket. What is important is the size of the balls. The smaller balls are actually the cholesterol that do the damage and inflame the arterial cell walls. Big lipoproteins (HDL) do not damage blood cell walls. With the LDL, it is the particle number, or the smaller ones (the golf balls) that are the real issue. Specific research tests can measure the particle number.

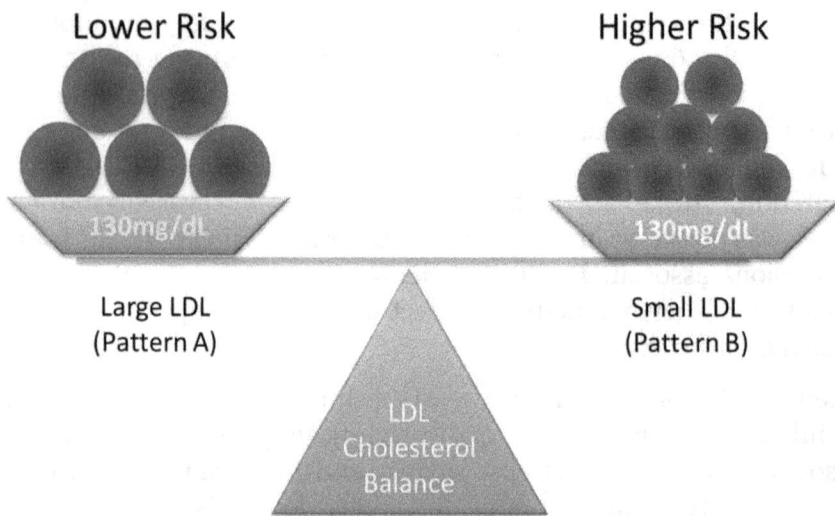

Lower Risk   **Higher Risk**

130mg/dL   130mg/dL

Large LDL (Pattern A)   Small LDL (Pattern B)

LDL Cholesterol Balance

Figure 57 LDL Particle Size

All commercially available tests only measure indirectly the HDL and LDL ones. They do not measure particle number. Some researchers say the current tests you undergo are meaningless and are poor predictors of disease. In the next figure, you might have the same amount of LDL, but the smaller the particle size, the higher the risk.

It may take some time to work this whole process out. As for information about cholesterol, keep in mind that a regular cholesterol test at your doctor won't tell you anything about your small LDL level. The standard tests measure your total cholesterol, LDL and HDL. But they don't distinguish between the dangerous small LDL and benign or protective large LDL. The fastest and cheapest, albeit most indirect, route is to test your blood sugar both before, and then 60 minutes after a meal. (It is called a post-prandial glucose test). The reason a post-prandial blood glucose test can be a rough indicator for small LDL is because the same foods that trigger a rise in blood sugar also increase small LDL. Namely, carbohydrates. In the meantime, consider changing your diet.

Apples are Even More Cost Effective

The original 1866 proverb states "eat an apple on going to bed, and you'll keep the doctor from earning his bread". In late 2013, Briggs from Oxford University looked at previous studies which demonstrated the benefits of fruit consumption for cardiovascular health and decreased mortality. They then compared that to similar mortality figures for statin users. Around 5.2m people are currently eligible for statins in the UK. If everyone over the age of 50 was prescribed statins it would mean an extra 17.6m people would take the drug, and 9400 more deaths would be prevented each year.

The researchers assumed there would only be a 70% compliance rate if apples were prescribed. But they said that even at that level, it would prevent 8500 deaths a year. If there was a 100% take-up, it could prevent more than 12,000 deaths a year. Biggs said, "Prescribing either an apple a day or a statin a day to everyone over 50 years old is likely to have a similar effect on population vascular mortality. Choosing apples rather than statins avoids the side effects of statins, which would be more than a 1,000 excess cases of myopathy (skeletal muscle weakness) and more than 12,000 excess diabetes diagnoses."

As far as diet goes, understand dietary cholesterol has a negligible effect on total blood LDL cholesterol levels. Worse, replacing saturated fats with carbohydrates increases the risk of heart disease by reducing HDL, and it increases small, dense LDL. So ignore the advice from various Heart groups. The typical standard medical advice is still stuck on this bad science. Go ahead and eat eggs every day as you will reduce small, dense LDL, which in turn reduces the risk of heart disease.

Conclusion

Statins are over prescribed by orders of magnitude. Statins were introduced at a time the relationship between dietary fat, serum cholesterol, and CVD were not proven, but the thought was if it does no harm, then it is good insurance against CVD. The drug companies have been spectacularly successful in selling the medication, and the medical profession is "negligent" in continuing to over prescribe. I am glad that I was reluctant to start taking statins, although five years ago I did seriously consider taking a "poly pill" of statin, aspirin, and a blood pressure to further reduce risk from CVD. My cholesterol is on the higher side of "normal," but genetically our family has elevated levels.

The reduction in weight and waist measure, elimination of simple carbohydrates including sugar, and no tobacco use, makes any such cholesterol measures unhelpful, but worse the side effects are too often discounted. To take preventative poisonous, disruptive drugs where there is no risk and questionable benefits (at best) seems the height of stupidity and ignorance. The best way to lower small, dense LDL and protect yourself from heart disease is to eat fewer simple carbohydrates, reduce your weight, and do some exercise. And eat an apple a day!

Regrettably, as per the 3 legged stool model, drug companies and the social environment would suggest the entrenched conventional view of statin prescription will continue for many years.

References

a. Coronary artery disease. http://en.wikipedia.org/wiki/Coronary_artery_disease
b. http://www.smh.com.au/national/health/statins-offer-quick-fix-for-heart-for-a-price-20130921-2u6na.html
c. Statin. http://en.wikipedia.org/wiki/Statin
d. Taylor F, Ward K, Moore TH, Burke M, Davey Smith G, Casas JP, Ebrahim S. (2011). Statins for the primary prevention of cardiovascular disease. In Taylor Fiona. Cochrane Database Syst Rev (1): CD004816. doi:10.1002/14651858.CD004816.pub4. PMID 21249663.
e. Savoiea I, Kazanjian A. (2002) Utilization of lipid-lowering drugs in men and women: a reflection of the research evidence? Vol 55 (1) January 2002, Pages 95–101 doi:10.1016/S0895-4356(01)00436-X
f. Mark D. (2013) Heart Foundation "shocked" at ABC decision to run Catalyst program on cholesterol drugs statins http://www.abc.net.au/news/2013-11-02/heart-foundation-shocked-at-abc-decision-to-run-catalyst-report/5065298
g. White H, Simes J, Stewart R, Blankenberg S, Barnes E, Marschner I, Thompson P, West M, Zeller T, Colquhoun D, Nestel P, Keech A, Sullivan D, Hunt D, Tonkin A, The LIPID Study Investigators. (2013). Changes in Lipoprotein-Associated Phospholipase A2 Activity Predict Coronary Events and Partly

Account for the Treatment Effect of Pravastatin: Results from the Long-term Intervention with Pravastatin in Ischemic Disease Study. J Am Heart Assoc. Vol 2:e000360. doi: 10.1161/JAHA.113.000360

h.   McConnachie A, Walker A, Robertson M, Marchbank L, Peacock J, Packard C, Cobbe S. and Ford S. (2013) Long-term impact on healthcare resource utilization of statin treatment and its cost effectiveness in the primary prevention of cardiovascular disease: a record linkage study. Eur Heart J(2013) doi:10.1093/eurheartj/eht232

i.   Briggs A, Mizdra A. (2013) A statin a day keeps the doctor away: comparative proverb assessment modelling study BMJ 2013; 347 doi: http://dx.doi.org/10.1136/bmj.f7267

j.   Silverman G, Blaha M, Krumholz H, Budoff M, Blankstein R, Sibley CT, Agatston A, Blumenthal R, Nasir. K. (2013) Impact of Coronary Artery Calcium on Coronary Heart Disease Events in Individuals at the Extremes of Traditional Risk Factor Burden: The Multi-Ethnic Study of Atherosclerosis. Eur. Heart J. 2013 PMID: 24366919

k.   Lafeber M, Spiering W, van der Graaf Y, Nathoe H, Bots ML, Grobbee DE, Visseren FL (2013) The combined use of aspirin, a statin, and blood pressure-lowering agents (polypill components) and the risk of vascular morbidity and mortality in patients with coronary artery disease. Am Heart J. 166(2):282-289.e1. doi: 10.1016/j.ahj.2013.04.011

l.   Jacobs D, Blackburn H, Higgins M, Reed D, Iso H, McMillan G, Neaton J, Nelson J, Potter J, Rifkind B, et al. (1992) Report of the Conference on Low Blood Cholesterol: Mortality Associations. Circulation Sep;86(3):1046-60.

m.   Okayama A, Ueshima H, Marmot M, Nakamura M, Kita Y, Yamakawa M (1993) Changes in Total Serum Cholesterol and Other Risk Factors for Cardiovascular Disease in Japan, 1980–1989 Int. J. Epidemiol. (1993) 22 (6): 1038-1047.doi: 10.1093/ije/22.6.1038

n.   Iso H. (2008) Heart Disease in Asia, Changes in Coronary Heart Disease Risk Among Japanese. Circulation. 118: 2725-2729 doi: 10.1161/CIRCULATIONAHA.107.750117

o.   Tonegawa M. (2010) High levels of cholesterol said better for longevity. Physorg. http://phys.org/news203844242.html

CHAPTER 49
FATTY LIVER DISEASE

Get the Facts

➢ Fatty Liver Disease was once a disease of excess alcohol consumption.

➢ In the last 20 years, the incidence has skyrocketed, and now an estimated one in three has fatty liver disease.

➢ The prevalence is 80% to 90% in obese adults.

➢ It may start as a mild condition, but leads to serious health issues such as cirrhosis, and cancer of the liver.

➢ Animal studies show fructose is a cause, even in the absence of weight gain.

➢ Minimize fructose consumption. Keep consumption as low as you can, and fruit to maybe two pieces per day.

➢ Consider fructose to be as damaging to health as alcohol.

Understand the Science

Fatty liver, also known as Fatty Liver Disease (FLD), is a reversible condition where large vacuoles of triglyceride fat accumulate in liver cells via the process of steatosis (i.e. abnormal retention of lipids within a cell). Vacuoles are spaces or vesicles within a cell, with a membrane, and filled with fluid. Fatty liver can be considered a single disease that occurs worldwide in those who drink too much alcohol, too often, and in those who are obese (with or without effects of insulin resistance). Alcoholic FLD or non-alcoholic FLD (NAFLD) are hard to distinguish and both show micro-vascular and macro-vascular fatty changes at different stages. By definition, alcohol consumption of over 20g/day (about 25 ml/day) makes it alcoholic FLD, not non-alcoholic FLD. The extreme form of NAFLD is NASH (Non-alcoholic steatohepatitis), and is regarded as a major cause of cirrhosis of the liver of unknown cause. The progression of severity goes from Fatty Liver Disease, then hepatitis, and then cirrhosis of the liver. Fatty liver disease is reversible, hepatitis is variable, while cirrhosis is not reversible.

Alcoholic FLD is a universal illness of heavy alcohol drinkers, and up to 40% of those with modest alcohol intake ($\leq$ 10g/day) also exhibit fatty changes. In an autopsy study, a threshold daily alcohol intake of 40g is necessary to produce pathologic changes of alcoholic hepatitis in men. Consumption of more than 80g per day is associated with an increase in the severity of alcoholic hepatitis. It comes down to a clear dose-dependent relation between alcohol intake and the incidence of alcoholic cirrhosis. A daily intake of more than 60g of alcohol in men and 20g in women significantly increases the risk of cirrhosis. Steady daily drinking, as compared with binge drinking, appears to be more harmful. The more you consume alcohol, the worse the level of alcoholic fatty liver disease.

Non-alcoholic Fatty Liver Disease (NAFLD) is rapidly becoming the most common liver disease worldwide. The prevalence of NAFLD in the general population of Western countries is 20-30%.

About 2-3% of the general population is estimated to have non-alcoholic steatohepatitis (NASH), which may progress to liver cirrhosis and hepatocarcinoma. Estimates range from 9% to 36.9% of the population of Japan and China. The USA is at approximately 20%, but increasing, and is higher in Hispanics. Experts blame high rates of obesity and type 2 diabetes for the higher rates. Non-alcoholic Fatty Liver Disease is also more common among men than women in all age groups until age 60 and is due to the protective nature of oestrogen. The prevalence of NAFLD is 80-90% in obese adults, 30-50% in patients with diabetes, and up to 90% in patients with hyperlipidaemia. The prevalence of NAFLD among children is 3-10%, rising up to 40-70% among obese children. Moreover, paediatric NAFLD increased from about 3% a decade ago to 5% today, with a male-to-female ratio of 2:1. Sobering increases!

Detection of Fatty Liver Disease is done through routine blood tests, with treatment being weight loss or (surprise!) drugs. The role of dietary fructose in the development of obesity and fatty liver diseases remains controversial, with previous studies indicating that the problems resulted from fructose plus a diet too high in calories. Soft drinks have been linked to NAFLD through the presence of high fructose corn syrup, which may cause increased deposits of fat in the abdomen, and the consumption of sucrose shows a similar effect, likely due to its breakdown into fructose.

Genetics play a role, with Indian men having a higher prevalence of NAFLD than non-Indian. Two genetic mutations for this susceptibility have been identified, and these mutations provide clues to the mechanism of NASH and related diseases.

Most patients with NAFLD have few or no symptoms. Patients may complain of fatigue, malaise, and dull, right-upper-quadrant abdominal discomfort. Mild jaundice may be noticed, although this is rare. More commonly, NAFLD is diagnosed following abnormal liver function tests during routine blood tests. NAFLD is associated with insulin resistance and metabolic syndrome (obesity, combined hyperlipidaemia, diabetes mellitus (type II) and high blood pressure).

Recent studies with monkeys demonstrated fructose rapidly caused liver damage even without weight gain. Wake Forest Baptist Medical Center researchers led by Kylie Kavanagh found that over the six-week study period, liver damage more than doubled in the animals that were fed a high-fructose diet as compared to those in the control group. They allowed one group to eat as much as they wanted of low-fat food with added fructose for six weeks, and compared these ad-lib eaters to a control group fed a low-fructose, low-fat diet for the same time period. Not surprisingly, the animals allowed to eat as much as they wanted of the high-fructose diet gained 50% more weight than the control group. They developed diabetes at three times the rate of the control group and also developed hepatic steatosis, or Non-alcoholic Fatty Liver Disease.

The big question for the researchers, was what caused the liver damage? Was it because the animals got fat from eating too much, or was it something else? To answer that question, a study was designed to prevent weight gain.

Ten middle-aged, normal weight monkeys that had never eaten fructose were divided into two groups based on comparable body shapes and waist circumference. Over six weeks, one group was fed a calorie-controlled diet consisting of 24% fructose, while the control group was fed a calorie-controlled diet with only a negligible amount of fructose, approximately 0.5%. Both diets had the same amount of fat, carbohydrate, and protein, but the sources were different. The high fructose group's diet was made from flour, butter, pork fat, eggs, and fructose (the main ingredient in corn syrup). This is similar to what many people eat. The control group's diet was made from healthy complex carbohydrates and soy protein. Every week the research team weighed both groups and measured their waist circumference, then adjusted the amount of food provided to prevent weight gain. At the end of the study, the researchers measured bio-markers of liver damage through blood samples and examined what type of bacteria was in the intestine through faecal samples and intestinal biopsies.

"What surprised us the most was how quickly the liver was affected and how extensive the damage was, especially without weight gain as a factor," Kavanagh said. "Six weeks in monkeys is roughly equivalent to three months in humans." In the high fructose group, the researchers found that the type of intestinal bacteria hadn't changed, but that they were migrating to the liver more rapidly and causing damage there. "It appears that something about the high fructose levels was causing the intestines to be less protective than normal, and consequently allowing the bacteria to leak out at a 30 percent higher rate," Kavanagh said. "We studied fructose because it is the most commonly added sugar in the American diet, but based on our study findings, we can't say conclusively that fructose, rather than glucose, caused the liver damage. What we can say is that high added sugars caused bacteria to exit the intestines, go into the blood stream, and damage the liver. The liver damage began even in the absence of weight gain. This could have clinical implications because most doctors and scientists have thought that it was the fat in and around tissues in the body that caused the health problems."

Fructose: A Cause of Fatty Liver Disease

Basaranoglu et al provide two diagrams which show why fructose is now seen as the major cause of NAFLD and NASH. In this first diagram, increased fructose disturbs production of adipokines such as leptin and insulin. Oxidants and antioxidant levels change. We discussed Antioxidants in a previous chapter and their role.

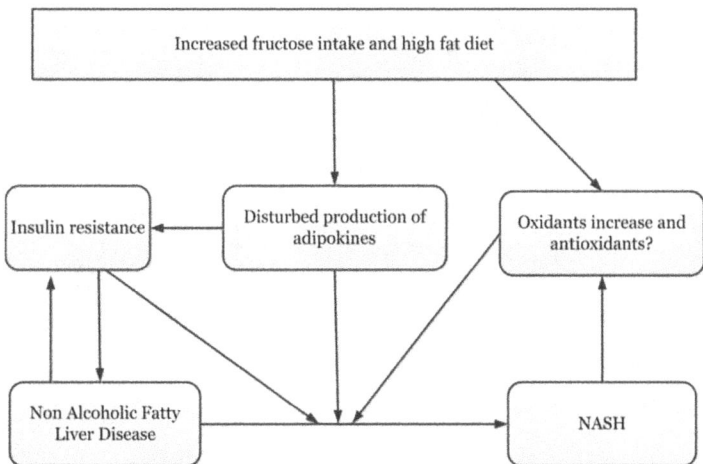

Figure 58 Fatty Liver Disease

Researchers have looked at high fat diets that produce obesity, insulin resistance, and some hepatic steatosis with minimal inflammation with no fibrosis. But when researchers look at a fast food diet, there are other changes. Changes in gene expression lead to liver cell death.

The complicated pathway is shown below.

- Decreased antioxidants.

- Changes the intermediate proteins

- Start to get these Mallory hyaline (or Mallory body) which are damaged filaments within the liver cells, and indicative of liver cell disease.

- Ultimately get cell death (liver fibrosis, inflammation, and lipo-apoptosis.)

This highlights that sometimes medical advice can be really wrong and really slow to change. The anatomic position of the liver places it in a strategic buffering position for absorbed carbohydrates and amino acids. Fructose was previously accepted as a beneficial dietary component because it does not stimulate insulin secretion and was recommended by groups such as diabetic associations. Now people know insulin signalling plays an important role in central mechanisms of NAFLD, yet the recommendation to avoid fructose is still very muted.

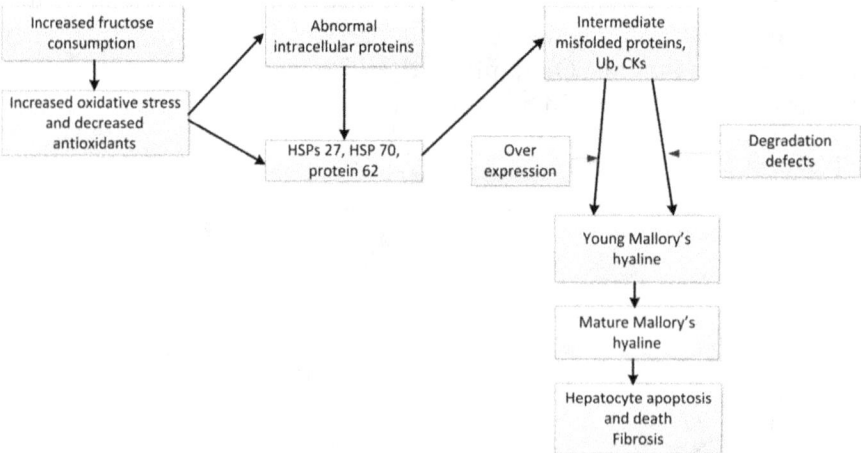

Figure 58 Liver Disease Pathways

Conclusion

Our livers are very forgiving, and can generally recover from both AFLD and NAFLD. There is a very high incidence of NAFLD in the Western world and it is a huge concern for current and future medical costs. There is some death from fatty liver disease, but patients with NAFLD generally have more serious illnesses such as cardio vascular disease and diabetes. Fatty liver disease is not a high contributor to mortality, as you are more likely to die from CVD. Without a liver though, you die. Transplants are expensive and limited by the number of donors.

It is clear that high levels of dietary fructose cause FLD. High fat does not create NAFLD. The fructose does. What is very puzzling is why do the nutritionists and public authorities not come out and say "avoid fructose?" Why are the diabetic societies not more vocal? You do not need to cut out all fructose, and 2 of pieces of whole fruit a day is probably ok. The quest of some to go on a liver cleansing diet, or a juicing diet and over consume fruit will do more damage than good.

For me, it has come down to a simple 80/20 rule. Have a glass of wine, or have a fruit juice. Both do your liver the same damage. Choose the least of the poisons. Not only take-out of your diet empty calories from the added sugar but also avoid serious health complications from fatty liver disease. If you are going to kill yourself, make sure you get as much pleasure as can doing so!

References

a. Non Alcoholic fatty Liver Disease http://en.wikipedia.org/wiki/Non-alcoholic_fatty_liver_disease
b. Kavanagh K, Wylie A, Tucker K, Hamp T,Gharaibeh R, Fodor A, Cullenet J. (2013). Dietary fructose induces endotoxemia and hepatic injury in calorically controlled primates (2013). Am J Clin Nutr ajcn.057331 doi: 10.3945/ajcn.112.057331 (see popular article http://www.sciencecodex.com/dietary_fructose_causes_liver_damage_in_animal_model_study_finds-114381
c. Bellentani S, Scaglioni F, Marino M, Bedogni G. (2010) Epidemiology of non-alcoholic fatty liver disease Dig Dis. 2010;28(1):155-61. doi: 10.1159/000282080
d. Basaranoglu M, Basaranoglu G, Sabuncu T, Sentürk H. (2013) Fructose as a key player in the development of fatty liver disease.

World J Gastroenterol. 19(8):1166-72. doi: 10.3748/wjg.v19.i8.1166.

e. Fairbanks K. (2014) Alcoholic Liver Disease. The Cleveland Clinic Foundation. www.clevelandclinicmeded.com/medicalpubs/diseasemanagem ent/hepatology/alcoholic-liver-disease/

f. Carlquist JF, Muhlestein JB, Anderson JL. (2007) Lipoprotein-associated phospholipase A2: a new biomarker for cardiovascular risk assessment and potential therapeutic target. Expert Rev Mol Diagn. 2007 Sep;7(5):511-7.

CHAPTER 50
GOUT

Get the Facts

➤ Gout is on the increase.

➤ The most likely cause is due to added sugars in the diet. Fructose directly increases uric acid.

➤ The kidney is unable to excrete the additional uric acid, and uric acid accumulates in joints..

Understand the Science

Gout is a type of inflammatory arthritis caused by elevated levels of uric acid in the blood, forming crystal deposits in the joints, tendons, and surrounding tissue. Gout typically affects the feet in general and big toe joint specifically, and causes severe pain and swelling.

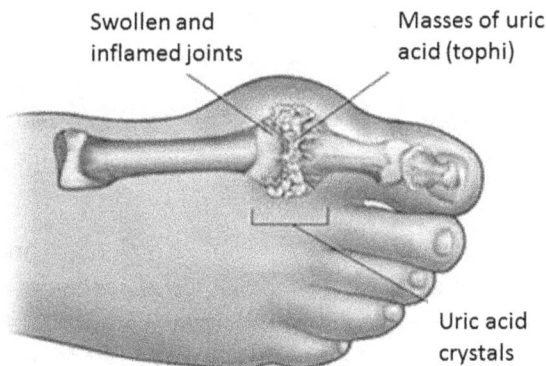

Figure 59 Gout

In the past, gout was referred to as a "rich man's disease," as it typically affected the upper class and royalty who could afford "rich" foods like meat, sugar, and alcohol. It might have also been due to the lead content in their food and drinking vessels! Numerous risk factors for the development of gout have been established, including hyperuricemia, genetic factors, dietary factors, alcohol consumption, metabolic syndrome, hypertension, obesity, diuretic use, and chronic renal disease. If you have osteoarthritis, you are predisposed to local crystal deposition.

Uric acid is a by-product of the metabolism of purines, one of two types of nitrogenous bases that form the basic structure of DNA and RNA. While purines are present in all foods, they are typically higher in red meat, turkey, organ meats, and certain types of fish and seafood. Even cauliflower has high levels of purines. Patients with gout are often advised to reduce or eliminate these purine-rich foods with the goal of preventing excess uric acid production. Roddy reported that with over 600 gout patients, those who had high purine intakes had a 5 fold increase of acute gout attacks, suggesting that those diagnosed with gout would benefit from a reduction in purine-rich foods. High risk factors are total meat intake, seafood, SSBs, diet soft drinks, and total amount of alcohol consumed (beer and spirits). Foods including dairy products, low fat dairy, coffee, tea, are all low risk. Fructose is a slightly higher risk than alcohol. When we understand the process of uric acid production, it becomes clear why.

While some uric acid in the blood is normal, providing a level of antioxidant protection, excess uric acid is a pro-oxidant, and this is the major causative factor for getting gout. Some researchers even suggest that this excess uric acid in the blood is a major factor in the development of insulin resistance and metabolic diseases. So if you're avoiding excess fructose consumption from high fructose corn syrup and excess sucrose (table sugar), you'll be at a lower risk for gout than someone who's washing their burger down with a can of soda.

While high purine intake is associated with gout attacks in those who already have hyperuricemia, or have high levels of uric acid in the blood, purine intake alone is not enough to trigger these attacks. In fact, uric acid levels are frequently decreased during gout attacks, sometimes to within the normal range. Another factor associated with gout flares is an increase in C-reactive protein (CRP) and interleukin-6 (IL-6), cytokines produced during numerous inflammatory conditions. These inflammatory cytokines are increased in the joint fluid and serum of patients with acute gouty arthritis. Therefore, systemic inflammation is likely a key factor affecting the likelihood of developing gout flares, and as we know, diet plays a significant role in inflammation. While foods like grass-fed beef, sardines, and mackerel are high in purines, they are also higher in Omega-3 fatty acids and low in Omega-6 fatty acids. Since the Omega-3 to Omega-6 balance in your diet modulates the inflammatory response, a diet with sufficient long-chain Omega-3 fats like EPA and DHA will reduce systemic inflammation and may reduce the risk of forming the uric acid crystals that cause joint pain.

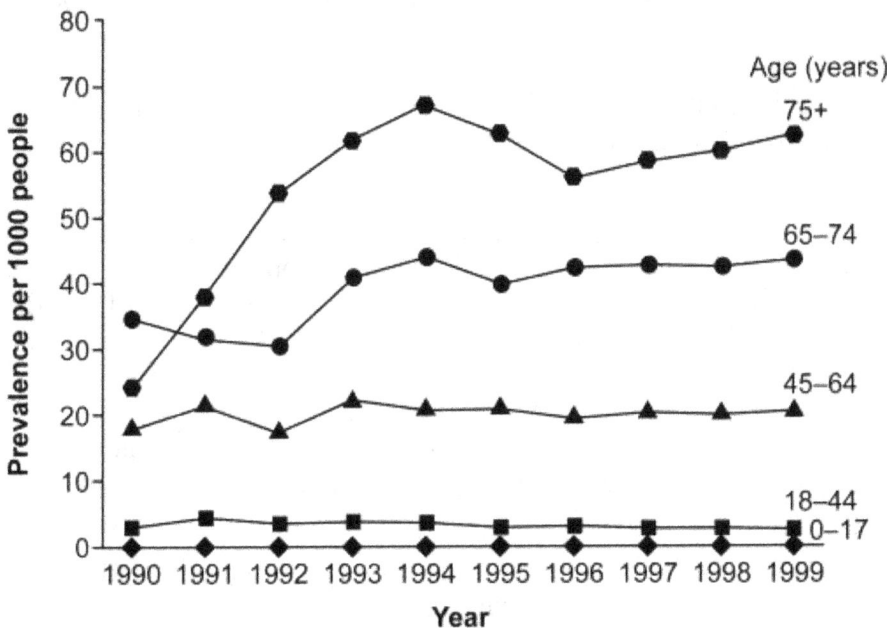

Figure 60 Prevalence of gout in USA men, 1990–99

Incidence of Gout

In New Zealand, gout from 1958 to 1992 increased from 3 per 1000 among Europeans and 27 per 1000 in Maori, up to 30 per 1000 and 70 per 1000 respectfully. Data from a large managed care database in the USA indicated that the unadjusted prevalence of gout increased from 2.9/1000 people in 1990 to 5.2/1000 people in 1999. There were 3.9% or 8.3m sufferers in 2009. Men were 5.9% and women 2%. Numbers have likely doubled since then. Age is important but we have seen that obesity is higher in this group as well.

Does Fructose Cause Gout?

Fructose increases blood uric acid concentrations. The Western diet is a risk factor and may mask the effects. While fructose in naturally occurring amounts is relatively benign (similar to alcohol if taken as small quantities of red wine), research shows higher intakes of fructose involved in many of the abnormalities seen in Metabolic Syndrome, including elevated triglycerides, due to increases in uric

313

acid production. Fructose elevates uric acid, both by producing excess uric acid and reducing its excretion in the urine. We know gout is associated with insulin resistance and Metabolic Syndrome. Why? Molley and her collaborators say uric acid could be the cause of Metabolic Syndrome; not the outcome. Uric acid is a normal waste product removed from the body by the kidneys and intestines and released in urine and the faeces. It has been unclear whether uric acid itself is causing damage or is simply a by-product of other processes that lead to dysfunctional metabolism.

Molley says their work in mice showed that the gut is an important clearance mechanism for uric acid. A protein called GLUT9 is an important transporter of uric acid. GLUT9 stops working in the gut, essentially blocking the body's ability to remove uric acid from the intestine. In their study, the kidney's ability to remove uric acid remained normal. Other work shows fructose increases the production of uric acid in the kidney, so it is a double whammy. There is more uric acid production, and less uric acid removal. The consequence is more gout. Fructose also increases Metabolic Syndrome.

A major reason that many conventional physicians and health professionals see red meat consumption as a significant risk factor for gout is that red meat is typically a component of an overall "Western diet pattern," a pattern that is also high in sugar, vegetable oils, sweetened beverages, refined grains, and processed meats, while being low in fruits and vegetables. It is nearly impossible for epidemiologists to separate meat consumption from this general pattern of eating when studying modern cultures. After all, most "health conscious" eaters in our generation believe that meat is unhealthy and typically eat less of it.

While most epidemiological studies attempt to isolate through statistics these confounding factors, the truth is that most high consumers of meat are generally prone to other unhealthy habits such as smoking and drinking, and are typically more overweight than low meat consumers. And like all epidemiological studies, they cannot prove causation, only correlations.

Conclusion

Gout is pretty painful arthritic disease. If it were just an outcome of eating rich purine foods, and what you needed to do was eat less of them – that could be acceptable, even though that means avoiding alcohol and sugar sweetened beverages. We now know that fructose is a particularly insidious dietary additive – not just a cause for gout, but more importantly increased Metabolic Syndrome. If you have gout, you are also likely to have Metabolic Syndrome. When you reduce your consumption of sugar, you will also reduce your Metabolic Syndrome risk and reduce gout incidence.

References

a. Kresser C (2013) Will eating a paleo diet cause gout? http://chriskresser.com/will-eating-a-paleo-diet-cause-gout

b. Angelopoulos TJ (2009) The effect of high-fructose corn syrup consumption on triglycerides and uric acid. J Nutr. 2009 Jun;139(6):1242S-1245S. doi: 10.3945/jn.108.098194. Epub 2009 Apr 29.

c. Takahiko (2006) A causal role for uric acid in fructose-induced metabolic syndrome. American Journal of Physiology - Renal Physiology Vol. 290 no. F625-F631DOI: 10.1152/ajprenal.00140.2005 (http://ajprenal.physiology.org/content/290/3/F625.full)

d. Roddy E, Doherty M. (2010) Gout. Epidemiology of gout. Arthritis Res Ther. 12(6): 223. PMCID: PMC3046529 doi: 10.1186/ar3199.

e. Angelopoulos T, Lowndes J, Zukley L, Melanson KJ, Nguyen V, Huffman A, Rippe JM. (2009). The effect of high-fructose corn syrup consumption on triglycerides and uric acid J Nutr. 139(6):1242S-1245S. doi: 10.3945/jn.108.098194

f. Cordain L, Eaton SB, Sebastian A, Mann N, Lindeberg S, Watkins B, O'Keefe J,Brand-Miller J. (2005) Origins and evolution of the Western diet: health implications for the 21st century Am J Clin Nutr February vol 81(2)341-354

g. Choi HK, Curhan G. (2008) Soft drinks, fructose consumption, and the risk ofgout in men: prospective cohort study.BMJ.336:309–312.Rheumatology (2009) 48 (suppl 2): ii2-ii8.

h. Doherty M (2012) New insights into the epidemiology of gout. Rheumatology. doi: 10.1093/rheumatology/kep086 http://rheumatology.oxfordjournals.org/content/48/suppl_2/ii 2.full

i. Wallace KL, Riedel AA, Joseph-Ridge N, Wortmann R. (2004) Increasing prevalence of gout and hyperuricemia over 10 years among older adults in a managed care population. J Rheumatol 31:1582-7.

j. Johnson RJ, Segal MS, Sautin Y, Nakagawa T, Feig DI, Kang DH, Gersch MS, Benner S, SanchezLozada LG. (2007) Potential role of sugar (fructose) in the epidemic of hypertension, obesity and the metabolic syndrome, diabetes, kidney disease, and cardiovascular disease. Am J Clin Nutr 2007;86:899–906.

k. Nakagawa T, Tuttle KR, Short RA, Johnson RJ. (2005) Hypothesis: fructose-induced hyperuricemia as a causal mechanism for the epidemic of the metabolic syndrome. Nat Clin Pract Nephrol 2005;1:80–86.

l. DeBosch B, Kluth O, Fujiwara H, Schurmann A, Moley K. (2014) Early-onset metabolic syndrome in mice lacking the intestinal uric acid transporter SLC2A9 Nature Communications 5(4642) doi:10.1038/ncomms5642ons.

m. Zhu Y, Pandya BJ, Choi HK. (2011) Prevalence of Gout and Hyperuricemia in the US General Population.(2011) Arthritis & Rheumatism; DOI: 10.1002/art.30520

CHAPTER 51
DEMENTIA

Get the Facts

➤   Dementia reduces Quality of Life in the latter years.

➤   Science does not fully understand why it occurs, risk factors associated with onset, how to reduce the severity or the treatment of dementia.

➤   There are likely preventative strategies.

➤   Exercise appears to reduce incidence, onset, and severity.

➤   Weights exercise improves cognitive therapy.

➤   Diets with high simple carbohydrates such as the Standard American Diet appear to increase dementia onset and severity.

➤   Learning new language appears to reduce the risk of dementia.

Understand the Science

Dementia is a syndrome, usually of a chronic or progressive nature, caused by a variety of brain illnesses that affect memory, thinking, behaviour and ability to perform everyday activities. There are many types of dementia including Alzheimer's disease (70% of cases), vascular dementia, fronto temporal dementia and dementia with Lewy Bodies. Most dementia has the formation of plaques and tangles in the brain, but these might be the result, not the cause of the disease. Dementia can happen to anybody, but it is more common after the age of 65, and affects about 10% of those over 65 years old. The number of people living with dementia worldwide is currently estimated at 35.6 million. This number will double by 2030, and triple by 2050. Australia has over 340,000 Alzheimer sufferers. Dementia is not part of normal ageing, and the economic impact is estimated at $604 billion. About 10% of sufferers are younger than 65 years and it is called Younger Onset Dementia. Dementia is the single greatest cause of disability in older people, and the 3rd leading cause of disability burden overall.

My mother had dementia from the age of 85 until she died at 89, and was the major reason I started to look at diet, lifestyle, and health. Throughout this book, I have noted where these affect dementia risk. Most advice is general and there is little definitive advice. Here are just some of the preventative strategies.

- Exercise. Exercise seems to delay onset, but it is unclear how much and how often we should exercise.

- Weights Exercise. Lifting weights appears to improve cognitive skills. Sydney researcher Singh took 100 adults over 60 years old with mild cognitive impairment, and 1/3rd did weight training, 1/3rd did computer based brain training and others did both for 6 months. The weight trainers did better on Alzheimer's scores, there was no benefit from the brain training, and the benefits from weights persisted 12 months after the supervised training stopped. Another Canadian study which compared aerobic exercise with resistance exercise over 6 months found the resistance training improved cognitive skills and brain plasticity.

- Fasting. As discussed in the 5:2 diet chapter, various researchers are adamant that intermittent fasting reduces cognitive loss in both animal and human studies, and more interestingly fasting appeared to reverse some of the effects.

- Brain Exercises. Learning a new language appears to reduce cognitive loss. Doing things repetitively does not seem to offer advantages. So if you do crossword puzzles, it may not be the type of brain exercise that reduces dementia.

- Alcohol. Moderate consumption which is less than 2 drinks per day may be beneficial, but large quantities of alcohol increases the risk of dementia.

- Social Interaction. Maintaining strong social connections and keeping mentally active as we age might lower the risk of cognitive decline and Alzheimer's. Experts are not certain about the reason for this association. It may be due to direct mechanisms through which social and mental stimulation strengthen connections between nerve cells in the brain.

- Diets. Several conditions that increase cardiovascular disease such as high blood pressure, diabetes and high cholesterol also are associated with the risk of developing Alzheimer's. Some autopsy studies show that as many as 80% of individuals with Alzheimer's also have cardiovascular disease. Diets such as the Mediterranean Diet or the DASH Diet (Dietary Approaches to stop Hypertension) that are focused on reduction of hypertension also appear positive for dementia.

- Drugs. There is some indication that pain killers such as aspirin or paracetamol (or NSAIDs) reduce the risk of dementia. In some studies, statins reduced dementia, but the causes are not clear.

Many groups promote a mix of tactics and lifestyles to reduce dementia risk. For example, the vegan activist non-profit group, the Physicians Committee for Responsible Medicine, have 7 strategies to reduce dementia risk. These strategies include 120 minutes of exercise per week, cutting back on trans-fats, choosing vitamins without iron or copper, chosing aluminium free products, taking 2.4mg of vitamin B12, eating plant based foods, and consuming 15mg of Vitamin E each day. Given what is discussed in various other chapters such as vitamins and minerals, and the general lack of definitive results in dementia research, these recommendations have little science to back up their conclusions.

Conclusions

I did not find anything in the information that gave me confidence science has any real answers about dementia. Neither did Williams in a 770 page report in 2010 in a review of 25 systematic reviews and 250 primary research articles. The disease occurs at the end of life. No-one knows what lifestyle choices 10, 20, or 50 years prior to onset may be important. It might be too late to take preventative actions if you are 60 years old or more. Furthermore, by the time dementia is actually diagnosed it is generally 3 years after the first early signs are present and it is often is too late for some of the treatments to make much difference. The only positive news is that a diet good for the heart is also good for the brain.

References

a. Alzheimers Australia. (2015). http://yourbrainmatters.org.au/
b. Prince M, Bryce R, Albanese E, Wimo A, Ribeiro W, Ferri CP. (2013) The global prevalence of dementia: a systematic review and metaanalysis. Alzheimers Dement. 9(1):63-75.e2. doi: 10.1016/j.jalz.2012.11.007.
c. WHO (2012) 10 facts on Dementia. http://www.who.int/features/factfiles/dementia/en/

d. Alzheimer's Disease International (2013) Policy Brief for Heads of Government: The Global Impact of Dementia 2013 - 2050 http://www.alz.co.uk/research/G8-policy-brief

e. Singh M, Gates N, Saigal N, Wilson G, Meiklejohn J, Brodaty H, Wen W, Singh M, Baune B, Suo C, Baker M, Foroughi N, Wang Y, Sachdev P, Valenzuela M. (2014) The Study of Mental and Resistance Training (SMART) Study—Resistance Training and/or Cognitive Training in Mild Cognitive Impairment: A Randomized, Double-Blind, Double-Sham Controlled Trial. 15 (12)   P   873–880   DOI: http://dx.doi.org/10.1016/j.jamda.2014.09.010

f. Williams JW, Plassman B, Burke J, Holsinger T, Benjamin S (2010) Preventing Alzheimer's Disease and Cognitive Decline: Evidence Report/Technology Assessment Number 193. (Prepared by the Duke Evidence-based Practice Center under Contract No. HHSA 290-2007-10066-I.) AHRQ Publication No. 10-E005. Rockville, MD: Agency for Healthcare Research and Quality.

g. Jick H, Zornberg GL, Jick SS, Seshadri S, Drachman DA. (2000) Statins and the risk of Dementia. Lancet 2000; 356: 1627–31

h. Jordan F, McGuinness B, Murphy K, Passmore P, Kelly JP, Devane D. (2015) Aspirin and anti-inflammatory drugs for the prevention of dementia. Cochrane Library. DOI: 10.1002/14651858.CD011459

i. Nagamatsu L, Handy T, Liang Hsu C, Voss M, Liu-Ambrose T. (2012) Resistance Training Promotes Cognitive and Functional Brain Plasticity in Seniors With Probable Mild Cognitive Impairment   Arch Intern Med. 172(8):666-668. doi:10.1001/archinternmed.2012.379.

CHAPTER 52
ALCOHOL

Get the Facts

➤ Alcohol is a toxin and linked to 60 different medical conditions including cancer.

➤ Alcohol in moderation is OK. No more than 3 to 5 standard drinks per week.

➤ The alcohol related costs to society is estimated to be $14b in Australia, and $223b in USA or about $1.90 per drink.

➤ Alcohol has high calories and can sabotage weight loss.

➤ Teetotallers and heavy drinkers live 5 years less than occasional drinkers.

Understand the Science

I didn't have a chapter on alcohol in the first drafts of this book, as I thought I personally did not need to deal with alcohol. The first time I presented the book to a group, a question was asked from the audience of "Do you need to take-out alcohol?" It made me add this short chapter. I'm what medical people call a "social drinker". Previously, on survey forms I ticked the box that said I consumed alcohol 2 or 3 times per week. Looking back on the records in food diary app gave lie to that as it was more like 6 to 7 drinks per week. Denial of consumption is one reason to record everything eaten or drunk to get a true baseline of your diet and lifestyle. There is no point to start any health or diet program without a baseline, and mine showed I need to manage alcohol consumption. I am not alone. Alcohol is an issue for one of these factors.

● It is a toxin. It causes physiological damage, including liver, cancer and brain damage and is linked to at least 60 different medical conditions.

● Alcoholism doubles the chances of death in women compared with men.

● Alcohol is addictive, with huge individual and society cost. Over 60% of all police attendances are linked to alcohol.

- It is high in calories, close to that of fat, and may cause a "mini-binge" just from a calorific perspective.

- Alcohol lowers inhibition and reduces will power, so it often undoes a weight loss program. You may get "What the Hell" moments. Ever had 1 glass, or two, and then somehow you find you have had the rest of the bottle along with a large pizza. You realize your self-control got lost in the glass.

- It makes you hungrier. Just like fructose and simple carbohydrates, the alcohol disrupts your normal feedback mechanisms. Some drinks are always consumed with sugar-sweetened beverages, e.g. rum and Coke, so the strategy is to avoid those type of drinks.

- The effects of drinking last more than a few hours. You will probably eat more the following day by making you hungrier.

There is some evidence that a little alcohol may extend life compared with those who are tee total or those who drink to excess, but the mechanism is unclear. (hormesis response). Alcohol causes or increases cancers of mouth, pharyngeal, oesophageal, laryngeal, breast, bowel and liver cancer in a number of ways and theories include:

- The production of the by-product acetaldehyde which damages DNA and stops our cells repairing the damage.

- By increasing hormones such as oestrogen.

- By damaging cells such as cirrhosis.

- By making it easier to absorb other carcinogens such as tobacco smoke.

- By producing Reactive Oxygen Species (ROS) which may damage DNA.

Conclusion

Alcohol is part of society and comes with serious health complications and costs. I try to deal with alcohol by not making it forbidden. Some need or choose to not consume at all, but for me that is a change too far. I've learnt to moderate consumption, and now have a sparkling water as a substitute for the alcohol on many occasions. Adopting a 5:2 diet means I have 2 alcohol free days per week. If I drink I choose a glass of dry red or dry white wine or a beer to minimise fructose. I now consciously make choices to have a drink or have additional food. I may have consumed larger quantities of alcohol at times in my life, but now I know some of the consequences of alcohol. Moderation is essential since I started this researching the research!

References

a. Anon. (2014) How to Drink Without Gaining Weight Health.com.
   http://www.health.com/health/article/0,,20670897,00.html
b. Excessive Drinking Costs U.S. $223.5 Billion. 2014
   http://www.cdc.gov/features/alcoholconsumption/
c. Curtin University (2014) National Drug Research Institute.
   http://ndri.curtin.edu.au/research/naip.cfm
d. Drug Info. (2014) Facts and Resources about alcohol and drugs.
   http://www.druginfo.adf.org.au/topics/statistics
e. Cancer Research UK. How Alcohol causes cancer.
   http://www.cancerresearchuk.org/

CHAPTER 53
SCIENCE AND STUDIES

Get the Facts

➤ Good scientific processes separate good information from "data free" observation.

➤ There are 5 steps to rigorous science experimentation.

➤ Regrettably much dietary and health advice is only based on the first 2 steps.

➤ The Reductionism approach to science is most typical, but a systems orientated approach may led to better understanding and improved medical treatments.

Understand (and Question) the Science

We know the story of Newton sitting under an apple tree, seeing an apple fall and making the association about gravity. What we don't see is the years of study that Newton had spent working with mathematics, understanding the cosmos, and trying to fit theory with measurement.

The Scientific Approach

The scientific approach is based around 5 steps.

• Make observations and gather data.

• Form a testable hypothesis.

• Conduct experiments to test this hypothesis.

• Collect valid data from experiments.

• Reach a conclusion based on repeatable data.

Furthermore, experiments are studies, but not all studies are experiments. In medicine, many types of studies are observational studies and only a few are clinical studies. Steps 1 and 2 are the two steps in observational studies, but they are not experiments. Only clinical studies which go from steps 3 to 5 are experiments.

Observational studies have no intervention – they simply observe people and gather data. Researchers look for data that are associated, correlated, or linked (all similar meanings). The huge problem is that scientists may not identify confounding factors and the explanation may be eventually proven incomplete, confused or just plain wrong by doing an experiment.

This science approach applies to most science disciplines. Scientists develop a hypothesis, and then go and devise an experiment to prove or disprove that hypothesis. In Physics, the Large Hadron Collider at CERN is just that sort of venture. It all begins with a collection of theories known as the "standard model." The standard model answers two important and fundamental questions: What is matter made of? And why does it behave the way it does? This was back in the 1960s.

In the search for a Unified Field Theory of matter, mathematicians and physicists including Peter Higgs said the Higgs Boson was the "missing bit". It took 50 years to actually measure this particle, and needed advances in all types of engineering technology – cryogenics, computers, particle detectors, billions of Euros and the brains of 5000 physicists and engineers. Now, they think they have evidence, but it has also raised new theories and new questions.

Lord Rutherford gave us 3 breakthroughs, winning the Nobel Prize in Chemistry in 1908 for his work on transmutation of one chemical element to another in radioactive material. He gave us the nuclear model of the atom with the tiny nucleus surround by orbiting electrons, and his third achievement was to be the first to split the atom. Some call him the world's first successful alchemist. Somewhat biased, he said "All science is either physics or stamp collecting." "Stamp collecting" as described by him was collecting information, and summarizing that information. Experimentation was needed to confirm hypotheses, and he was an avid experimentalist physicist. Our botany and biology systems are often like that stamp collecting. David Brown, sent to Australia in 1801, collected over 4000 new plants. Brown is best remembered for his scientific excellence. He brought a new dimension to the use of the microscope and pioneered new techniques in looking at plants and their various parts. His dedication lifted botany from what had previously been really only a hobby for amateurs and gentlemen into a dedicated, professional branch of the sciences. Most importantly, he was able to present scientific evidence in spectacular style.

Chemistry moved from stamp collecting, mostly due to the discovery of the Periodic Table. Dmitri Mendeleev (1869) is generally credited for the first widely recognized Periodic Table. He developed his table to illustrate periodic trends in the properties of the then-known elements. Mendeleev also predicted some properties of then-unknown elements that would be expected to fill gaps in this table. Most of his predictions were proved correct when the elements in question were subsequently discovered. Until then, chemistry was mostly about measuring reactions. With the introduction of the Periodic Table, chemistry moved from observation to hypothesis, then experimentation as per the Scientific Approach.

Biological systems move slower. Computing and technology brings new understanding every month. Our information about how DNA works is continually changing. First, we thought the important part of DNA was the genes, only a fraction of the DNA. New research showed the "junk" DNA, which was in between the genes, was also just as important. More recently, the environment has been shown to turn genes on or off (epigenicity), which further complicates our understanding. We don't understand our brain with its 80 trillion synapse pathways, yet the brain greatly contributes to our health and well-being.

The Plural of Anecdote is Not Data

People's experiences and stories are valid although the explanation and the cause, or the application to the broader community, may not be. Raymond Wolfinger, from Berkeley, in the 1969-70 academic year, rejoined a student's dismissal of a simple factual statement – by another student or him – as a mere anecdote with the quote that "the plural of anecdote is data." However, it was misheard, and most use it the other way around and say "the plural of anecdote is *not* data". A lot of anecdotes do not make for science data as they are not based on statistical rigour. An example might be "my father smoked two packets of cigarettes all his life, and he lived to be ninety." That is anecdotal (one person's knowledge); is valid data (he did, and was a real person), and it is true some proportion of the population will not die young. But smoking kills. When you get all the anecdotes about who lived long, who died young, smoking reduces life expectancy by 15 years. (That is valid data.) When we looked at the issue of vitamins, many will argue that they take vitamins and they feel better. That's anecdotal. If you have 1000 people take vitamins and they all feel better, that is still anecdotal. If you did a randomized, double blind experiment, and the data was analysed properly, that becomes data. If you wish to find out more, then view the lecture from Tom Naughton's called "Science For Smart People" and it is without a doubt the best (and funniest) crash course in epidemiology that you will see. If you watch this you will know more about health and nutrition science than 99% of people out there.

Double Blind Experiments

The gold standard for science is randomized double blind placebo based trials. For example, in a drug trial on humans, you take a population and split it into three groups. A simple case is to take a sample of 1000 men and women, aged between 50 and 55 (to eliminate age related complications). Patients are randomly allocated into a treatment block. One-third would receive an active pill, one-third receive no pill, and one-third receive a placebo, a pill that looks like the drug but has no drug in it. Then measure what the effect that pill has. Neither the patient nor the researchers know which treatment block the patient is in. The measurements are done not knowing what the treatment was. That is the double blind type of study. Neither the subject nor the researcher knows. Maybe in this case, you can probably figure out the gender! So you might split the trial further into male and female and have 6 groups. It is impossible to do this type of study with food because people know what treatment they have. The trials cannot be double blind. Changing the food that someone eats will change the energy of the food, and the quantities. The patient certainly will know if on their diet they have two drinks of natural fruit juice a day and 50% of their diet as carbohydrate, and another group has the same calories but 5% carbohydrates. They are going to have to eat more fat or protein. Most can tell if they are eating pasta or steak! Their brains AND digestive system will let them know! Furthermore, patients may exercise free will. They might eat more or less, and cheat (unless the research is in a confined space).

Reductionist Approach To Science

As Ahn says, since Descartes and the Renaissance, science, including medicine, has taken a distinct path in its analytical evaluation of the natural world. This approach can be described as one of "divide and conquer," and it is rooted in the assumption that complex problems are solvable by dividing them into smaller, simpler, and thus more tractable units. Because the processes are "reduced" into more basic units, this approach has been termed "reductionism" and has been the predominant paradigm of science over the past two centuries. Reductionism pervades the medical sciences and affects the way we diagnose, treat, and prevent diseases. While it has been responsible for tremendous successes in modern medicine, there are limits to reductionism, and an alternative explanation must be sought to complement it.

Characteristic	Reductionism	Systems-Orientated Approach
Principle	Behaviour of a biological system can be explained by the properties of its constituent parts.	Biological systems possess emergent properties that are only possessed by the system as a whole and not by any isolated part of the system.
Metaphor	Machine, magic bullet.	Network.
Approach	One factor singled out for attention and is given explanatory weight on its own.	Many factors are simultaneously evaluated to assess the dynamic of the system.
Critical factors	Predictors / associated factors.	Time, space, context.
Model Characteristics	Linear, predictable, frequently deterministic.	Non-linear, sensitive to initial conditions, stochastic, chaotic.
Medical concepts	Health is normal. Health is risk reduction. Health is homeostasis.	Health is robustness. Health is adaption and plasticity. Health is homodynamic.
Disease types	Acute Simple.	Chronic Complex diseases.
Examples	Urinary Tract infection. Appendicitis. Aortic aneurysm.	Diabetes. Coronary artery disease. Asthma.

The alternative is a systems orientated approach. The systems perspective is rooted in the assumption that the forest cannot be explained by studying the trees individually. Recent work on the 2 kg of human biome is part of this approach. Our bacteria are now seen to be keeping us healthy, whereas previously bacteria were bad and we should kill them. But bacteria operate on a systems approach, not a reductionist approach. If a patient goes into hospital with a coronary heart condition and diabetes, each is treated separately, rather than as a whole.

Conclusion

My conclusion from reading hundreds of papers is that much of the work in nutrition science is simply stamp collecting! Much of the nutritional information is derived from observational or epidemiological studies. Authors make statements about cause when only correlation is appropriate.

The nutrition world is mostly reductionist, and a systems orientated approach is more suitable for these more complex health issues. As we see throughout this book, a healthy diet is one where you have to look at a unified wholeness. When we look at the failure to fix the obesity pandemic, we see a reductionist approach stated as "eat less, move more," or all food in moderation. This approach has failed, and a systems approach is needed.

References

a. Ahn AC, Tewari M, Poon C-S, Phillips RS (2006) The Limits of Reductionism in Medicine: Could Systems Biology Offer an Alternative? PLoS Med 3(6): e208. doi:10.1371/journal.pmed.0030208
b. Ahn AC, Tewari M, Poon C-S, Phillips RS (2006) The Clinical Applications of a Systems Approach. PLoS Med 3(7): e209. doi:10.1371/journal.pmed.0030209
c. Tom Naughton Science for Smart People. YouTube http://youtu.be/y1RXvBvehto

CHAPTER 54
CHERRY PICKING SCIENCE

Get the Facts

➤ Science evolves rapidly in some ways, but is slow to change in others. Attitudes are slow to change, and scientists generally do not like making statements that are not "proven."

➤ The majority of researchers cherry pick the scientific literature they use to support their cause.

➤ In a scientific experiment, you need to control all the variables, and vary only one or two factors.

➤ In a great number of the experiments over the past 20 years, this basic tenet of controlling all the variables appears to have been overlooked. It is understandable in epidemiological trials, especially where patients self-report. Some scientists do not even appear to understand the science process.

➤ Not all science is published. Nil results are seldom published, and non-conclusive results even more rarely published, if ever. So the ones that are published tend to support only one side of an argument or another.

➤ Don't be concerned about cherry picking. Everyone does it. I've done it. I made hypotheses, reviewed other research, and reported the results. One tries to find a new angle, a new piece of understanding. It may not always be wilful, but occasionally it is.

Understand the Science

How does one select the right information? How can one know what is accurate when it comes to health, diet, and nutrition? In a field rife with interests, prejudices, axes to grind, and products to sell, it is hard to discern the truth. The following are just three peer reviewed publications in the Journal of Nutrition. The first, by White in 2009, says High-Fructose Corn Syrup (HCFS) is maligned. The second says it may be / may not be bad for children. The third says there is enough evidence to show it causes poorer health.

White, in 2009 states:

> *"Misconceptions about high-fructose corn syrup abound in the scientific literature, the advice of health professionals to their patients, media reporting, product advertising, and the irrational behaviour of consumers. Foremost among these is the misconception that HFCS has a unique and substantive responsibility for the current obesity crisis. Inaccurate information from ostensibly reliable sources and selective presentation of research data gathered under extreme experimental conditions, representing neither the human diet nor HFCS, have misled the uninformed and created an atmosphere of distrust and avoidance for what, by all rights, should be considered a safe and innocuous sweetener. In the first part of this article, common misconceptions about the composition, functionality, metabolism, and use of HFCS and its purported link to obesity are identified and corrected. In the second part, an emerging misconception that HFCS in carbonated soft drinks contributes materially to physiological levels of reactive dicarbonyl compounds and advanced glycation end products is addressed in detail, and evidence is presented that HFCS does not pose a unique dietary risk in healthy individuals or diabetics."*

Morgan, in 2013, looked at the issue of HFCS beverages' effects on childhood obesity and "concludes" inconclusive evidence.

> *"The consumption of high-fructose corn syrup (HFCS) beverages has increased since the 1970s. At the same time, childhood obesity is on the rise, causing children to be at risk of heart disease, diabetes and other diseases. Healthcare providers have attributed childhood obesity to the consumption of HFCS in the form of beverages. This article will look at the available research and determine if there is scientific evidence underlying the idea that sweetened soft drinks, especially those containing HFCS, could cause or contribute to childhood obesity. A thorough literature search was performed using the ISI Web of Sciences, PubMed and Scopus databases within the years 2006-2012. The search generated 19 results. The articles were screened, and six were deemed eligible: four systematic reviews and two meta-analyses. Two systematic reviews found that there is no relationship between consumption of HFCS beverages and obesity in children.*

The other two systematic reviews found possible links between HFCS and childhood obesity. The meta-analysis articles found that consumption of HFCS beverages can contribute to childhood obesity, and limitation of sweetened beverages may help decrease obesity in children. Available research studies demonstrate inconclusive scientific evidence definitively linking HFCS to obesity in children."

Ferder et al (2010) says that HFCS produces Metabolic Syndrome, a clear marker of health risk.

"Obesity and related diseases are an important and growing health concern in the United States and around the world. Soft drinks and other sugar-sweetened beverages are now the primary sources of added sugars in Americans' diets. The metabolic syndrome is a cluster of common pathologies, including abdominal obesity linked to an excess of visceral fat, fatty liver, insulin resistance, hyperinsulinemia, dyslipidaemia, and hypertension. Trends in all of these alterations are related to the consumption of dietary fructose and the introduction of high-fructose corn syrup (HFCS) as a sweetener in soft drinks and other foods. Experimental and clinical evidence suggests a progressive association between HFCS consumption, obesity, and the other injury processes. However, experimental HFCS consumption seems to produce some of the changes associated with metabolic syndrome even without increasing the body weight. Metabolic damage associated with HFCS probably is not limited to obesity-pathway mechanisms."

So which do you believe? If the scientists can come up with mixed messages, how can laymen possibly get to the bottom of the science? And it is not just cherry picking in SSBs.

Cherry picking goes on in the diet-heart research area. The hypothesis states saturated fat, and in some versions cholesterol, raises blood cholesterol, and contributes to the risk of having a heart attack. To test this hypothesis, scientists have been studying the relationship between saturated fat consumption and heart attack risk for more than half a century. What have these studies found? The large majority of observational studies have found no connection between habitual saturated fat consumption and heart attack risk. The scientific literature contains dozens of these studies, and Stephen Guyenet on his blog narrowed the field to prospective studies only, because they are considered the most reliable. In these designs, investigators find a group of initially healthy people, record information about them (in this case what they eat), and watch who gets sick over the years.

The results depends which set of publications you follow! Of more than 25 high quality papers, only 4 supported the diet-heart hypothesis. Is that part of the reason the Swedish Government, on advice from the medical experts who reviewed 10,000 papers, say saturated fat is ok. In contrast, the Australian Heart Foundation supports the diet-heart hypothesis, but in response has said it will do its own review sometime soon. One guesses they will come up with another conclusion. Cherry picking at its worst.

Conclusion

All authors select other articles that support their hypothesis, and this makes reviewing science difficult. When I look at the data, my conclusion is clear. I think that Ferder and others are correct and fructose is bad for health. I also think that the Swedish review that concluded dietary fat is not linked to heart disease. It would be good if scientists got their processes of research right, and stopped confusing the policy makers and the public.

References

a. White JS. (2009) Misconceptions about high-fructose corn syrup: is it uniquely responsible for obesity, reactive dicarbonyl compounds, and advanced glycation endproducts? J Nutr. 2009 Jun;139(6):1219S-1227S. doi: 10.3945/jn.108.097998..
b. Morgan RE. (2013) Does consumption of high-fructose corn syrup beverages cause obesity in children? Pediatr Obes. 2013 Aug;8(4):249-54. doi: 10.1111/j.2047-6310.2013.00173.x. Epub 2013 Apr 29.
c. Ferder L. (2010) The role of high-fructose corn syrup in metabolic syndrome and hypertension. Curr Hypertens Rep. 2010 Apr;12(2):105-12. doi: 10.1007/s11906-010-0097-3.
d. Gary Taubes. http://garytaubes.com/2010/12/calories-fat-or-carbohydrates/
e. Guyenet, S. (2009) The Dirty Little Secret of the Diet-Heart Hypothesis. http://wholehealthsource.blogspot.com.au/2009/12/dirty-little-secret-of-diet-heart.html

CHAPTER 55
EPIDEMIOLOGICAL STUDIES

Get the Facts

➤ Beware of epidemiological studies. They are great at identifying trends and getting "overall effects."

➤ Epidemiological studies cannot prove cause. They only show correlations.

➤ They rely heavily on statistics and the populations studied. They always have a range of factors they say they account for, but seldom do. They are always "correlation" and not "causation."

Understand the Science

Epidemiology is the study (or the science of the study) of the patterns, causes, and effects of health and disease conditions in defined populations. It is the cornerstone of public health, and informs policy decisions and evidence-based medicine by identifying risk factors for disease and targets for preventive medicine. Epidemiologists help with study design, collection and statistical analysis of data, and interpretation and dissemination of results (including peer review and occasional systematic review). Epidemiology has helped develop methodology used in clinical research, public health studies and, to a lesser extent, basic research in the biological sciences.

Here is one example of a large epidemiological study done in Europe and a report that soft drink consumption increases diabetes. In a previous

Chapter we discussed the health burden of diabetes in Australia. Romaguera, from Imperial College London, reported the results in *Diabetologia*. They used data on consumption of juices and nectars, sugar-sweetened soft drinks, and artificially sweetened soft drinks collected across eight European cohorts participating in the European Prospective Investigation into Cancer and Nutrition (EPIC study; UK, Germany, Denmark, Italy, Spain, Sweden, France,

Netherlands), covering some 350,000 participants. The EPIC study was designed to investigate the relationships between diet, nutritional status, lifestyle, and environmental factors, and the incidence of cancer and other chronic diseases. We don't know what other factors influenced the results. Researchers try to cover every aspect with questionnaires and physical assessments, but the study relies on subjects' memory and a host of other complications with diets and lifestyle.

- Consumption of every 12-oz can of sugar sweetened soft drink, per day, increased risk of diabetes by 22%.

- Two cans increased the risk by 44%.

- People who drank more artificially sweetened soft drinks were also more likely to get type 2 diabetes, but this association appeared to be because participants with a higher BMI tend to drink more artificially sweetened drinks, and they are also more likely to develop diabetes.

- Drinking pure fruit juice or nectar (diluted juices, sometimes with additives) was not associated with diabetes risk.

A meta-analysis of previous studies, mainly done in North America, found a 25% increased risk of type 2 diabetes for each daily sugar-sweetened drink consumed.

The upshot of this is we are left with many correlations, but no definitive causation. Researchers have concluded that SSBs increase diabetes, to one degree or another. But is this because drinking SSBs increases BMI? And if subjects are overweight or obese it is likely they drink artificially sweetened SSBs? Doing experiments on people is going to be impossible. As we discussed in the chapter on Science, these large, expensive epidemiological studies are "stamp collecting" as Rutherford said. We cannot confirm that SSBs cause diabetes, we can only assume. The evidence is strong, but it is not experimentation.

An example of epidemiology which clearly is wrong is the one by Ancel Keys, an American scientist, who studied the influence of diet on health. Keys was responsible for two famous diets: K-rations formulated as balanced meals for combat soldiers in World War II, and later on the Mediterranean Diet. In particular, he hypothesized that different kinds of dietary fat had different effects on health. He examined the epidemiology of cardiovascular disease in 1950. In 1980, he published his Seven-countries Studies and the study appeared to show that serum cholesterol was strongly related to coronary heart disease mortality both at the population and at the individual level. The only problem is he presented a subset of data. With seven countries, the correlation was linear. More cholesterol, more coronary heart disease. As disclosed later, using all 14 countries, there is no correlation. But this study became the basis of the diet-heart hypothesis.

Conclusion

Why is epidemiology the main methodology in this field of diet and health?

- Firstly, as detailed in the Science and Studies chapter, it is very hard to do experiments on people. While occasional despots and societies have condoned it (think Nazi or Pol Pot regimes), it is not possible from an ethical perspective to undertake experiments that are known or likely to have ill-effects on the subjects.

- Secondly, effects may not show up for decades, and most researchers do not have the budget.

- Thirdly, animal studies may not translate to human behaviour.

In the absence of experiments, the researchers can only measure and try to explain patterns observed. Be particularly concerned when science publication makes it to the media. The media leave out some much of the detail, and in most cases, the reporter will state causation, where there is often clearly none, and we are often left with results that can be contradictory, or worse, wrong.

References

a. Definition of epidemiology. http://en.wikipedia.org/wiki/Epidemiology
b. The latest statistics on diabetes in Australia. (2013) http://www.aihw.gov.au/diabetes/
c. The InterAct Consortium "Consumption of sweet beverages and type 2 diabetes incidence in European adults: results from EPIC-InterAct". Diabetologia 2013. DOI 10.1007/s00125-013-2899-8
d. Ancel Keys (1950). The Biology of Human Starvation. Minneapolis, MN: University of Minnesota Press. p. 262.
e. Keys, A (1980). Seven Countries: A Multivariate Analysis of Death and Coronary Heart Disease. Harvard University Press. ISBN 0-674-80237-3.

f. Kromhout D (1999) Serum cholesterol in cross-cultural perspective. The Seven-Countries Study. Acta Cardiol 1999;54:155–158

g. Katan MB, Beynen AC. (1981) Linoleic acid consumption and coronary heart disease in USA and UK Lancet. 1981 Aug 15;2(8242):371

CHAPTER 56
MAKING SENSE OF STATISTICS

Get the Facts

➢ Statistics help in data interpretation.
➢ Mathematics for biological sciences are an integral part of science analysis.
➢ Statistical analyses cannot show causation. I can show correlation. Experimental design and the experimental techniques must be right if the research is to explore the causes. Statistics cannot make a silk purse out of a sow's ear.

Understand the Science

Biological systems are diverse. Statistics are used in various ways; and the words of Benjamin Disraeli or Mark Twain both who were credited with the quote of "lies, damn lies, and statistics." Statistics can make sense of numbers though. Statistical analysis can be done in many different ways – the choice of methodology can lead to different results and different conclusions.

Most also misunderstand randomness. E.g. in the simplest case, if we take a physical action, such as tossing a coin, we understand that statistics give us confidence about the randomness of this activity. We would expect that in 50% of the tosses we would get heads, and 50% of the time we would get tails. However, if we toss it four times, we are not likely to get the same number of heads and tails (two of each). We may have to toss the coin hundreds of times to get close to an equal number of heads and tails.

Statistics are often used to help researchers to understand if relationships are significant. They never can tell us if there is a causation. Here is an example from the previous section: a study claims drinking soft drinks results in higher diabetes. What the statistical analysis will show is that the more consumers who drink SSBs, the more people have diabetes. But do SSBs actually cause diabetes? The only science method is to do a double blind randomized trial.

Epidemiological studies are great for correlation and good guesses. But researchers generally have to go back to animal studies to find out why. This study is not the same as taking these 1000 people, getting 250 to consume no soft drinks, 250 to drink one can, 250 to drink two cans, and 250 to drink three cans over ten years. Ethically you can't do this; not when you are pretty sure those who consume a lot of soft drinks will develop diabetes. Cost is also an issue – this would not be cheap, and lastly, people cheat when it comes to diet: self-reporting is notoriously poor. Other impediments are because people move, change lifestyle, age, and create other variables in their lives. That's why you must go to an animal lab and do the studies with rats. Hence the reason that researchers like epidemiological studies. They go out with clipboards, ask a few questions, do some statistics, and publish a paper. Quick and dirty, and often flawed.

Use of Statistics in Biology

If one graded strictly on a curve, a class of 100 students may produce the result in the table below. The top two students in the class would be awarded A, the next 14 B, and so forth. This is based on the normal distribution, also called Gaussian Distribution by statisticians. When this normal distribution is plotted on a graph, it produces the famous "bell curve" frequently shortened to "curve."

Statistical assumptions behind the normal distribution include randomness and an entire universe (very large numbers) to choose from. However, in biology, the normal distribution curve is generally not symmetrical, nor do we have an entire universe. We select the least number of test subjects for optimal results. Most populations do not fit the normal population or "Bell Curve." For example, if we look at the average adult weight, there are very few people less than 132 lb (60 kg) and very few larger than 220 lb (100 kg), so the distribution is not "normal". So more sophisticated mathematics are needed to try to factor out these issues, and decide what is "same as others" or "definitely less than others" (presented as 5% confidence or 1% confidence).

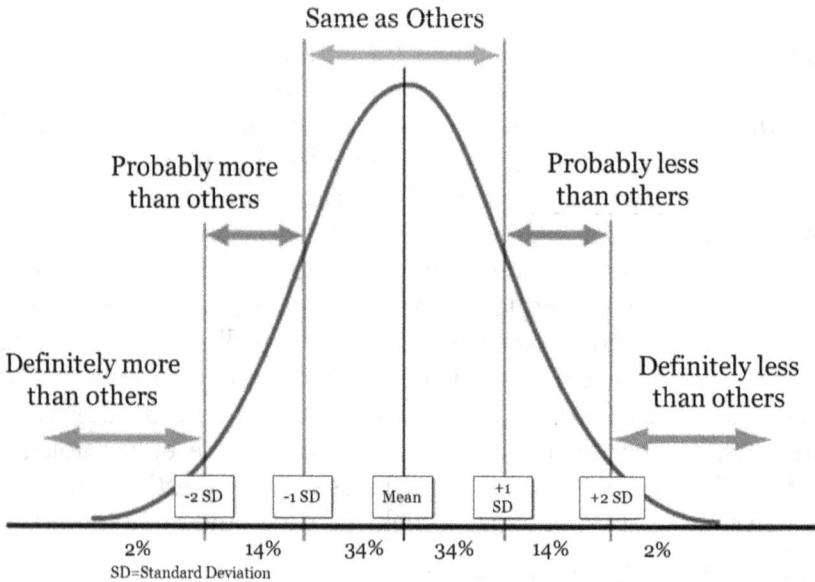

Figure 61 Bell Curve

In addition to the complication from small samples misrepresenting the whole population, there is another reason that strict adherence to the curve suggested by normal distribution is not valid for most research, both clinical or in epidemiological studies. For example, in the Nurses Health studies who were a group of 35,000 nurses from the USA and extensively studied. The nurses are unlikely to be completely representative of society. They are likely to be better educated, mostly female, have some understanding of health, and may not be representative of the broader society based on random selection. Family, education, motivation are all biases in their selection. Therefore, the data from this group, based on a random model, is not entirely applicable or equitable. However, statistical treatment will try to isolate out these biases.

Generally what statistics try to show is that one population (from one treatment) is different from or similar to another and put confidence limits around this. Here are some examples.

Problem 1. Is the population on the left different from the one on the right by a meaningful amount? What is the average, the mean, the population distribution? These are samples, not the whole population.

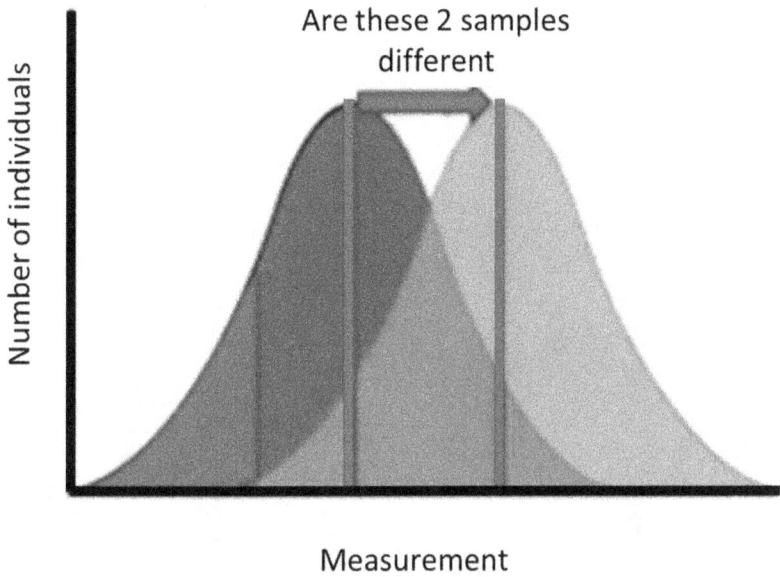

Are these 2 samples different

Number of individuals

Measurement

Figure 62 Statistics - differences in Populations

Problem 2. Based on USA population by age and sex in 2000 and 2010 in the figure above, the "average person" is not that average. The population has a distribution that is not "bell shaped," neither for male or female, nor by age. The average changes over time as you can from this shifting baby boom bulge. As people age, medical issues become more severe and important. This lack of normal distribution in the population requires more sophisticated statistical algorithms and these can be used incorrectly. Populations change over time. Figure 65 shows the projected impact on age as baby boomers age.

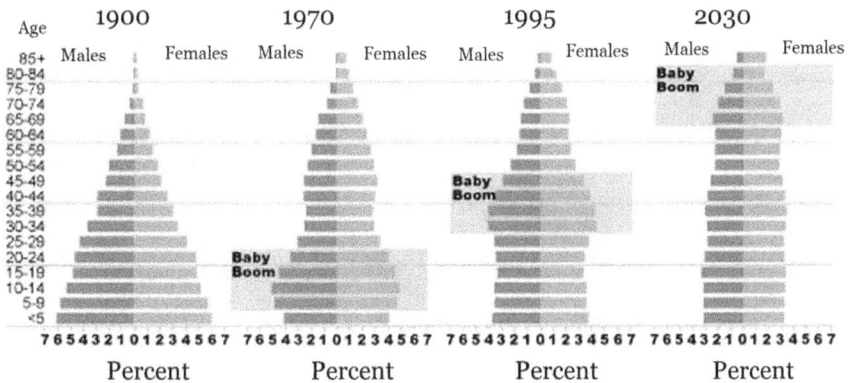

Figure 63 Populations Change over time

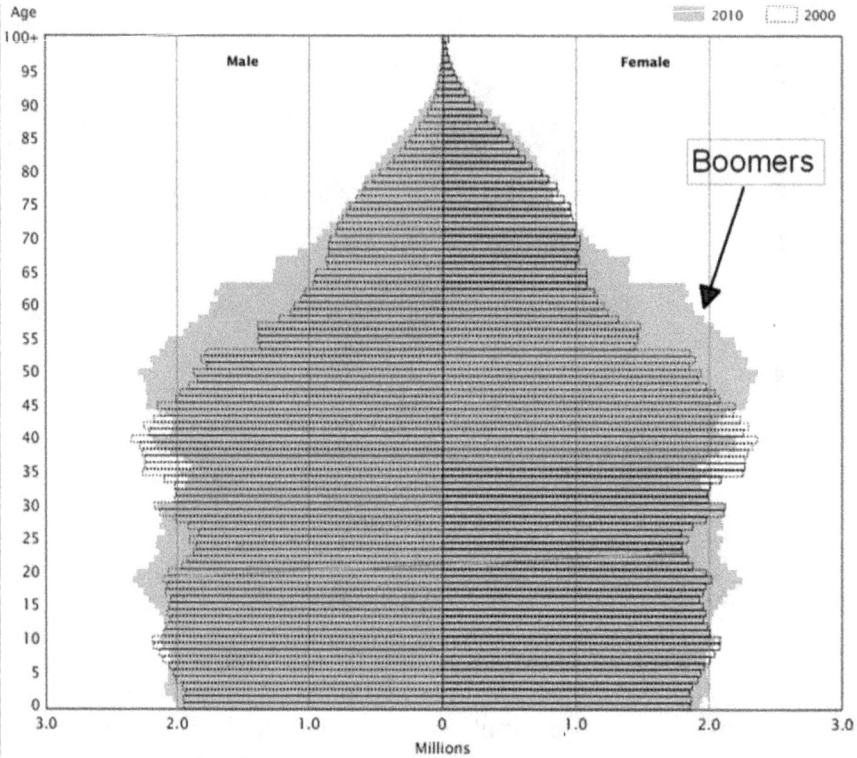

Figure 64 The USA Population is not Equal

Conclusion

Statistics are tools. Used properly they help us to isolate patterns, they remove some biases, and give us confidence that differences measured are actual differences. Used incorrectly they compound the lies. It's been said that given the right statistics, one can prove anything.

References

a. US Census (2010) Age and Sex Composition 2010 https://www.census.gov/prod/cen2010/briefs/c2010br-03.pdf

CHAPTER 57
GLOBALISATION OF FOOD

Get the Facts

➤   Food products are dominated by 20 companies globally.

Understand the Science

As part of the 3rd leg of food and diet, we have to at least understand who creates the food products that many people now eat. This table from Oxfam shows the global ranking of the top 10 food companies and employees.

Company	Revenue (US billion)	Employees
Nestle S.A.	103.5	333,000
Coca-Cola	46.9	136,000
PepsiCo	66.4	274,000
Unilever Group	68.5	174,000
Mondelez International, Inc (ex Kraft)	35.3	107,000
Groupe Danone	29.3	104,000
Associated British Foods PLC	21.1	112,000
General Mills, Inc	17.9	43,000
Kellogg Co.	14.8	30,277
Mars, Inc	33.0	60,000

Others in the top 20 companies include Campbell Soup Company; ConAgra Foods, Inc.; Dunkin' Brands Group, Inc.; Grupo Bimbo; Hillshire Brands Company; H.J. Heinz Company; Hormel Foods Corporation; Krispy Kreme Doughnuts Corp.; Nissin Foods Holdings Co., Ltd.; The Hershey Company; The J.M. Smucker Company and Toyo Suisan Kaisha, Ltd.

As we saw in the Fats chapters, palm oil has taken over as the fat of choice for the "Snack Food 20." Palm oil now makes up 50% of any food you eat out of a bag, a box or package of any kind. Palm oil and its derivatives are used in a remarkable array of products, such as ice cream, cookies, crackers, chocolate, cereals, breakfast bars, cake mixes, doughnuts, potato chips, instant noodles, frozen sweets and meals, baby formula, margarine, and dry and canned soups. Palm oil is also found in detergents, soaps, personal care products, and increasingly as a feedstock for biofuels. How did this happen so quickly? It is due to the changing face of the food industry. The food industry is now dominated by a few corporations. This control by a few select corporations is now the norm across all sectors of the food industry.

- The top 10 seed companies control nearly 50% of the $21b global commercial seed market.

- The top 10 pesticide companies control 84% of the $30b annual pesticide market.

- The top 10 retailers control 24% of the $3.5trillion global food market.

- These top 10 food and beverage companies control 24% of the estimatcd $1.25 trilllion global market for packaged goods.

Conclusion

If you eat food products, the probability is you will be consuming a product from one of these 20 food companies. It makes a diet and a lifestyle very much in the hands of the company, and I do not have the confidence they have my best interests at heart. It makes that 3rd leg of the stool very hard to change. The food companies are immensely powerful and politically connected. Even if you move to eating whole food, you are relying on those top 10 seed and pesticide companies!

References

a. OXFAM (2014) Behind the Brands. http://www.behindthebrands.org/
b. Clapp J, Fuchs D. (2009) Corporate Power in Global Agrifood Governance. MIT Books. Pp 328 ISBN: 9780262012751

CHAPTER 58
THE TAKE-OUT DIET

Get the Facts

➤ Diets should be about health, and a healthy lifestyle. They fail if they only focus on weight.

➤ Science is clear that weight is a marker of health. Fat or thin, anyone can have an unhealthy body and diet.

➤ The change from an unhealthy to a healthy lifestyle, is critical for enjoyment of a full and high quality life.

➤ The 80/20 rule says taking out one or two foods and food products from the diet is more effective than trying to put more in.

➤ Taking out poor food means you eat more good food, most of which you already eat.

➤ Changing your lifestyle requires three factors for success: Biochemistry and hormones, your mind, and interaction with society.

The Take-Out Diet?

How can you use this book to help a 65-year-old friend? How will this book, and the scientific knowledge reviewed, provide direction to her?

She's been on various diets and lifestyles for 35 years, ever since giving birth to her first child. She is overweight by 33 lb (15 kg), with a BMI of 27, elevated blood pressure, and on statins for elevated cholesterol. She has arthritis in a knee, and she's waiting for a hip replacement. My guess is that she has Metabolic Syndrome, some fatty liver disease, and impaired kidney function, which is typical of many her age. She is sick of hearing about diets such as 5:2, Atkins, low carbohydrate, high carbohydrate, and vegetarian. Worse, she is fed up with listening to my opinions. She is not alone in her frustration. By the time the book was published, she had achieved her goal of losing much of that weight, her blood pressure was back to normal, her cholesterol levels had dropped, the operation sucessful, and she has encouraged many of her friends to take up the

Take-Out Diet. She has said she has found it so easy just to focus on a few simple strategies and recognizes this is a lifestyle change that people often talk about, but cannot define. She enjoys this new lifestyle, and is looking to maintain it not for 1 year, but the rest of her life.

Science is not contradictory. The quote at the start of my book was "Half of what we know is wrong, the purpose of science is to determine which half." Science has delivered, and there are good clear practical strategies for her, and for millions of others. Policymakers may not have caught up with science, nor have entrenched stakeholders such as food company oligopolies, drug companies, or "snake oil peddlers." The Science is unambiguous for her, for me, and for you.

- Improvement in diet will led to improvement in health. A good diet will reduce risk factors for cardiovascular disease, cancer, and arthritis. It can eliminate Metabolic Syndrome and a host of autoimmune diseases.

- Some chronic illness risks can be reduced by 5 times within 12 weeks and reduced by more than 100 times for some illnesses within a year.

- Changes in diet will lead to weight reduction, and a low carbohydrate diet is better than most others.

- A weight reduction of 15% of body mass is achievable and sustainable for the rest of your life.

- Associated weight reduction markedly improves recovery from joint operations or any other surgical procedures.

- A good diet gives practical risk mitigation for dementia by orders of magnitude with an increased quality of life, not only for the next few years, but right through your "twilight" years.

Sound fanciful? Science says it is both achievable and conservative. Change Management on the other hand says that planned processes are required. Appropriate Change Management can lead to "lifestyle changes." I believe with specific changes for the first 20 days and then practicing those skills for a further nine weeks will achieve the outcome you want. These life changing first 20 days require only six steps and are in the context of my three-legged stool. These 6 steps address the biochemistry and hormones issues (reduce fructose and

346

low simple carbohydrate consumption), help the brain and mind (calorie count, food sacrifice), and help internal and external social and behaviours (5:2 diet).

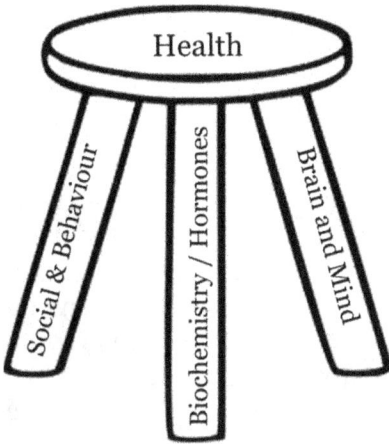

Figure 65 The Three-Legged Stool of the Take-Out Diet

Science is unambiguous when it tells us that a "single" approach to a diet fails. However science provides evidence of what solutions work, and for long term success you probably have to do all of the following six steps. Not one or two or three – all six. If you feel you cannot make the changes, do not start this process or any diet. Clear goals and outcomes are critical for Change Management and while the most important goal is good health, weight and self-worth are essential parts of these steps.

Throughout the book the phrase "*take-out diet*" is used because bad foods, and food products, have increasingly entered Western diets, and these demonstrably damage our health and disrupt our appetite. It's time to take them out!

Removing them is much simpler than trying to add more food products or developing new drugs. "Take-out" may have connotations of loss and deprivation, and maybe a better phrase is "replace and upsize" foods that you already eat. The take-out phrase is to emphasise that these are pro-active changes first and foremost. You won't have to find new foods – you will already have foods that are perfectly fine and enjoyable.

If you like chicken and chicken skin, but previously you took the skin off because you thought the skin was fattening, then eat the chicken skin. But don't eat the bun. If you cut the fat off the steak – don't. If you like eggs, eat more. If you eat beans and legumes, please stop gassing your friends. (It may be good for your microbiome!) If, however, you mistook "Take-Out" to mean the drive-thru window at your favourite fast food emporium, you were mistaken. The drive-thru window is where good health goes to die.

These are the six steps for anyone who is contemplating a change and it is for an initial 20 day period.

1. Take-out fructose from your diet.

Fructose is part of added sugar so that will mean changing what you eat by eating more whole food. You do need to read the nutrition labels of food products because sweeteners are used in nearly every manufactured/package food. Avoid anything that is more than 3% sugar (3 g per 100 g); no more than two pieces of fruit per day, no fruit drinks, no SSBs, no product with "Lite" in its name, no product with a Heart Foundation Tick, and many food products that say "healthy." The upside when you remove fructose, you can eat more of your other favourite foods. These ones will have neither fructose nor simple carbohydrates in them. (NB. The Tick is current policy and could change for the better, sometime, I hope.). Generally, you will have to eat and cook whole food, not food products.

2. Take-out simple carbohydrates.

To manage your glucose levels and avoid insulin spikes, move to a low simple carbohydrate diet. Complex carbohydrates are fine. That means avoiding any food product that is made with flour or rice, potato, and yams. Imagine an Atkins, South Beach, or Paleo type diet without some of the rigidity of those diets.

3. Take-out a calorie counter.

To help take-out your low sacrifice foods and to get some baseline measures of your diet use a calorie counter. For at least two weeks record everything you eat and drink using a calorie counter app. Everything! Be obsessive! Buy, and then use a set of small kitchen scales. These tools help understand portion size, and help you avoid increasing consumption of high density calorie nuts and fat products. These high density foods can undo any calorie reduction and you need weight loss for a win as part of the Change Management process. Adjust your portion size to your appetite. You do not need to continue to count calories, providing that you have re-adjusted your lifestyle. As part of this process of understanding what you eat, and for long-term change, take-out "*low sacrifice high calorie*" foods. Prepare your personal food sacrifice list to ensure that you do not try to eliminate your "*high value sacrifice foods*" and develop some new tactics to ensure you do not have "*Last supper*,"

"*What the Hell*," or "*Deprivation*" moments. By avoiding the mini-binges that follow from these moments, you avoid the failure to meet weight reduction targets. Work out a tactic to "have your cake and eat it."

4. Take-out some food for two days a week.

For 12 weeks, do a 5:2 diet (consume only 25% of daily calories for only two days a week). Do eat as much as you feel you have to on the days you eat normally and do not try to manage the hunger over the first four weeks with calorie restriction on normal days. It is essential you don't feel hungry and so eat more of your favourite healthy foods. If you continue to eat simple carbohydrates you will fell hungrier, which is why a low carbohydrate diet works well with a 5:2 diet. Low carbohydrate diets dampen your appetite with the higher levels of protein and fat. Do not have the two days of calorie restriction on consecutive days (for example Saturday and Sunday). This limited amount of fasting does three things:

- It provides for a decent calorie reduction over a week. It helps avoid the guilt of failure (because you will undoubtedly experience success), and helps offset any mini-binges that will occur as you learn new tactics.

- It retrains the mind and body that hunger is okay. You are not starving. The behaviour of snacking or eating five meals a day changes to eating one to three instead.

- It re-educates you as to what are good food choices. If you want to continue this after 12 weeks – fine. It is a smart tactic for long-term health and provides flexibility to manage our modern social behaviour with its eating out lifestyle. There are other tactics which may work, but retraining the brain improvement is a compelling change gain.

5. Take-Out Sitting Down.

Don't try to exercise more; just try to do less sitting. Sit for no more than 20 minutes at a time and then stand up and walk to another room and back. Minor exercise is still better than sitting. Increasing exercise for health is important long-term, but don't try to increase exercise in these first 12 weeks.

6. Take-out polyunsaturated oils.

Seed oils contain high levels of poly unsaturated fatty acids and these oils increase your health risks. No canola, no safflower, sunflower, rice bran, or sesame oils. None. Swap these polyunsaturated fats with fats from animals and plants, such as butter, olive oil, or coconut oil.

Keep Changes Minimal.

Many other tactics make little or no difference, and will distract you from the changes you are making. So don't exercise any more than you currently do; stop taking any vitamins and supplements, don't get hung up on Omega-3, and you don't switch to organic, Paleo, Weight Watchers or any other strategy. Don't change any prescription medication. Leave that for after this 12 week period and only in consultation with a knowledgeable medical professional. Go as hard and fast as you can on this weight reduction – the faster you lose weight, the more likely this will continue. The rewards are to do with your beauty, self-worth and motivation factors rather than just the health benefits. The more reasons to change, the more changes becomes cemented into behaviour. Success builds upon success.

Take-Out For Success

At 20 days, review and assess which of these changes need more practice. Why 20 days?

- Fructose and simple refined carbohydrates appear to be addictive.

- Sugar cravings will have passed.

- With three weeks of 5:2 and keeping food intake on the normal days to TDE, you will have lost about 7 lb (3 kg) and that should measurable, satisfying, and rewarding. If mini-binges have crept in, the weight loss might be lower, but equally, your weight loss may be more if you are male, do a lot of exercise, or have truly restricted calories.

The key issue is to assess how these changes suit your lifestyle. If you like the lifestyle, continue for the balance of the 12 weeks. Remove the words "guilt", "bad" foods, and replace them with "smart choices." You will feel smart eating an apple instead of drinking apple juice. As with quitting smoking, if the program becomes too hard or too much of a change, stop. Take the skills learned, and then try again when your mind is in the right space. It is up to you to "manage" the Change Management process and everyone comes from a different space. The 3rd leg of the stool, the social environment you live in. It may present the most difficulties. Everyone will use different smart tactics to get around those challenges. You can't change the whole world, but you can change one or two things around you.

At the end of 12 weeks, a weight loss of 20 to 35 lb (8 to 15 kg) is likely. More importantly, many of the internal, unseen health benefits will have already happened, and the liver, kidney, heart, pancreas, thyroid, and microbiome will be forever grateful. Good luck. The next phase is practicing these new found lifestyle skills, so in 6 months, 2 years, 5 years you are still in that lifestyle and have better health outcomes.

It has been a rewarding effort for me to research this book. I could have spent many more years in researching information about health and wellbeing, but would I have met my criteria of the 80/20 principles? How much knowledge do I really need to make a change?

I am now 30 lb (14 kg) lighter, and my waist is now less than half my height. I am clearer on the science and am able to protect myself for the next 60 years. All the metabolic data is looking good for me. This effort has been priceless. I've managed 2 years, and know that this lifestyle is sustainable for life through everyday living, parties, family events, and travel. My hope is that it is for you as well.

EPILOGUE

At the start of my journey in 2013, I believed science had answers, if only I could find them among the confusion. In the process of researching the researchers, I found a mix of excellent science, good science, incompetent science, and deceit and you can see why the answers about health and diet are so muddled. The medical profession and the nutrition science discipline has a great deal to answer for. Changes for the better are glacially slow. It is left to us to do our own analysis. We can better equip ourselves to improve our chances for a better quality of life. Without some knowledge, we will read the headlines and, more often than not, make wrong lifestyle choices.

When I started two years ago, I thought I might need to lose 2 kg (5 lbs), at most, to be at optimum weight for health. I could enjoy most foods in moderation, and there were no "bad" foods, except those high fat products. That surely has changed! I now look at lifestyle in the context of the 3-legged stool. I now understand some clear principles and I need to follow them this next week, the next year and the next 50 years if I want the best chance for good health. I should not put off changes until next week! Using skills and experience from business practice, I simply cannot "fail to plan" or I will be "planning to fail." I won't now leave it to chance. I made a decision to change, made the plans to support that change and taken the least number of defined steps. I have implemented key performance "lead" measures. The "lag" measure will be my funeral!

Those changes have led to a 14 kg (32 lb) weight loss and a 12 cm (6 in) waist reduction. While there were no changes in serum total cholesterol, there is a 30% reduction in triglycerides and 20% improvement in LDL/HDL ratios, but these are irrelevant if the latest science theories are correct, even though it keeps my doctor happy. It has led to a 30% improvement in kidney function markers. And the best estimate for dietary changes is that my risk of cardiovascular disease and cancers is much lower. How much is less certain, but it could be as high as 100 times. Some strategies for delay of dementia are also part of this new lifestyle.

I am fortunate that I was not severely overweight or obese or my journey may have been more difficult. It astounds me that I am back to the same weight, 45 years from my teenage years. If I knew what I know now, that journey to 100 kg and back could have been avoided, and the cost of clothing halved. The most important understanding is that science does have the answers now. But it has the same problems it always has of being too narrow in its viewpoint, too entrenched in dogma, and too close to commercial interests such as food companies.

Health needs to be holistic. The lifestyle to maintain good health cannot be just biochemistry, hormones and DNA. Our mind and our society are just as important in changing from unhealthy to healthy. Using our 3-legged stool model, the 3 legs have to work in unison. You cannot make a lifestyle change without considering all 3 aspects and I trust I have shown you need changes to every part. You have to change the food you eat. You have to recognize your behaviour and work within those parameters. And you have to do all this in the context of continuing to live in the society we live in, our social interactions and the food that big business puts in front of us. The best practices from business say we have to make those changes as small as possible, be committed, take positive steps and so increase the chance of success.

- Use best business practice tactics such as planning, the 80/20 principle, Performance Measures, and Change Management processes.

- Using the 3-legged stool model, accept that change is needed across all three aspects of this lifestyle.

- Adopt the Take-Out Diet process. Six Steps, 3 weeks pilot program, and 12 weeks in total.

- Maintain the Take-Out Diet Lifestyle for ever.

- Enjoy and live a full, long, and healthy life!

TABLE OF FIGURES

www.ingramcontent.com/pod-product-compliance
Lightning Source LLC
Chambersburg PA
CBHW050451270326
41927CB00009B/1690